The Digest Diet Cookbook

150 All-New Fat Releasing Recipes to Lose up to 26 Pounds in 21 Days!

BY LIZ VACCARIELLO

Editor-in-Chief of *Reader's Digest* and author of *The Digest Diet!*

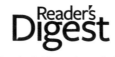

The Reader's Digest Association, Inc.
New York, NY/Montreal

A READER'S DIGEST BOOK

Copyright © 2013 The Reader's Digest Association
All rights reserved. Unauthorized reproduction, in any manner, is prohibited.
Reader's Digest is a registered trademark of The Reader's Digest Association, Inc.

Library of Congress Cataloging-in-Publication Data

Vaccariello, Liz.

 Digest diet cookbook : 150 all new fat releasing recipes to lose up to 26 lbs in 21 days!
/ Liz Vaccariello.

      p. cm.

 Includes index.

    Summary: "FEATURES 150 ALL-NEW MOUTHWATERING RECIPES: The
diet calls for 21 days of easy, delicious, home-cooked meals. The cookbook offers
dieters 150 all-new easy-to-make recipes, identified by diet phase so that it's simple
to mix and match according to their favorites. INCLUDES SAMPLE MENUS FOR
DIFFERENT LIFESTYLES: To show how readers can put the recipes together into
daily menus that fit within the diet, the book will include all-new sample meal plans
tailored to specific needs, such as a family-friendly, cooking for one, or on-the-go
dieter"-- Provided by publisher.

 ISBN 978-1-62145-025-2 (hardback) -- ISBN 978-1-62145-026-9 (adobe) -- ISBN 978-1-
62145-027-6 (epub)

1. Reducing diets. 2. Reducing diets--Recipes. I. Title.

 RM222.2V2542 2013

 641.5'63--dc23

                                2012032017

We are committed to both the quality of our products and the service we provide
to our customers. We value your comments, so please feel free to contact us.

The Reader's Digest Association, Inc.
Adult Trade Publishing
44 South Broadway
White Plains, NY 10601

For more Reader's Digest products and
information, visit our website:
rd.com (in the United States)
readersdigest.ca (in Canada)

Printed in the United States of America
1 3 5 7 9 10 8 6 4 2

The information in this book should not be substituted for, or used to alter, medical
therapy without your doctor's advice. For a specific health problem, consult your
physician for guidance.

Eating eggs or egg whites that are not completely cooked poses the possibility of
salmonella food poisoning. The risk is greater for pregnant women, the elderly, the
very young, and persons with impaired immune systems. If you are concerned about
salmonella, you can use reconstituted powdered egg whites or pasteurized eggs.

The Digest Diet

Go online for **EXCLUSIVE** success tools and tricks… **and it's all FREE!**

- **Guaranteed motivation** with community and support

- **Inspiring videos** full of savvy tips and insider advice from other Digest Diet participants

- **The latest news and studies** on fat releasing foods, moves, and attitudes, plus updates from the experts

- **Even more delicious recipes** starring your favorite fat releasers to keep you feeling full and fabulous

- **Food and fitness journals** to help you reach your goal

- **The best jokes** and funny stuff to get you to "laugh it off" when you need it

readersdigest.com/digestdiet

facebook.com/digestdiet

Coming Soon: The Digest Diet Dining Out Guide

Contents

Introduction

One year ago, as I sat down to write the original Digest Diet manuscript, I could never have imagined the lives it would change. As the months rolled along, and my e-mail box filled with letters of gratitude, I realized that we had created something special: a weight loss solution that was both fast and healthy.

As editor-in-chief of *Reader's Digest*, my job is to find the best stories on living a happy, enriched life. That's what *Reader's Digest* magazine and books have been doing for more than 90 years. Readers trust us to sort through the latest information on the subjects they care about most, choose the most interesting and useful nuggets, and condense them into articles and books that are easy to use.

Throughout my entire career—as a journalist, author, and editor—I've made it my mission to help people like you get healthy because I know it's one of your greatest concerns. Personally, I define good health as being able to live life to the fullest for as many years as possible. And when I'm healthy, I have the energy to do the things I love to do. You can, too!

Health is also a big part of my other important job—being the mother of two daughters. Our family embraces health. We hike, ride bikes, and swim together. Every summer, we build and tend a garden together. And as often as possible, we gather in the kitchen to cook (everyone participates!). I want to show my girls healthy behavior rather than just talk about it. I want them to know that if you eat wholesome foods, you will be on the path to good health. I want them to enjoy the food at the core of our most pleasurable moments—not only holiday celebrations, but everyday dinners together, meals and snacks shared over laughs and inside jokes. Eating well—and eating together—is fundamental to a good and happy life.

Body weight goes hand in hand with this. When you bring your weight into a healthy range by eating good food that's good for you, and being active on a daily basis, you improve your overall health. The Digest Diet make it easy.

To develop the Digest Diet, the *Reader's Digest* staff and I talked to researchers and read articles on the science of body weight and looked for cutting-edge medical breakthroughs. We tossed out the weight loss gimmicks and were astonished to discover how seemingly healthy habits—and even our very environment—cause fat to creep on. We were also encouraged to find actionable strategies that actually work in your body to help release fat from cells, resulting in a slimmer you.

I want you to have more energy to do the things you love to do.

In the Digest Diet, we put these findings into a fast and effective eating plan based on healthy, natural foods that have been scientifically proven to aid you to shed fat quickly and safely. When we first developed the plan, I was so excited about the potential that I selected 12 men and women to take a sneak peak. They followed the Digest Diet for 3 weeks with incredible results. One dieter lost 26 pounds (altogether they lost a collective 151 pounds!), along with 2 inches of belly fat. You'll find a few of their success stories in this book, along with others who have lost weight, improved their health, and feel happier and more energetic.

Since we first released the book in March 2012, thousands have laughed, danced, and eaten their way to their happy weight. Many of them, including members of our Digest Diet online and Facebook communities, asked for new recipes, more menu ideas, and guidance for continuing. I created this cookbook in response.

I wanted to develop a cookbook for another reason, as well. A growing body of research says that cooking and eating at home with loved ones is better for your health than dining out. In a Minnesota study, families that had at least one weekly dinner away from home were more likely to be overweight. Why is eating at home so good for your health? It's easier to control how much you eat and balance your meals nutritionally when you prepare your own food. Also, when you take the time to make your own meals, you're more likely to find them satisfying—and, as you'll see later, joy is a key component of the Digest Diet.

I understand how busy you are—and I know that a sit-down dinner every night isn't always practical—so the recipes in this book are quick and easy to make, like Pan-Seared Sirloin with Red Wine Sauce (page 116), Pomegranate-Glazed Salmon (page 145), and Romaine with Guacamole Dressing (page 199). Plus the Digest Diet recipes are so delicious and un-diet-like that you won't feel deprived.

If you are new to the Digest Diet, be sure to read through Chapter 1, which will give you an overview of the diet. Chapter 2 will show you how to make over your kitchen and grocery cart so that they can help you release fat. And in Chapter 3, you'll learn how to create your own 21-day meal plan.

Those of you who have already done the diet and want to maintain your results or keep losing may find these chapters helpful, too, as a refresher on the diet "rules." Plus, we've packed these chapters with new tools to help you save time and money, as well as shed pounds. Or, if you choose, you can dive right into the recipes starting in Chapter 4.

Remember: It *is* possible to be happy and successful on a diet, and you don't need to spend hours in the kitchen to do it. Set goals that are realistic, attainable, and anchored in improving your health, and avoid trying to reach for perfection.

Cooking and eating at home with loved ones is **better for your health** than eating out.

The Digest Diet is designed to be flexible so you can make it work for you. Whether you love to cook or not, are allergic to peanuts or can't stand plain yogurt, cooking for one or feeding your whole family, just follow the Digest Diet principles as best you can, add more fat releasers to your next meal, and enjoy the journey, because this is your first step to lifelong good health. Cheers!

Chapter 1

Fat Increasers and Fat Releasers

Avoid the surprising culprits that make you fat—and shift your body into fat release mode with these fun and easy secrets to frustration-free weight loss.

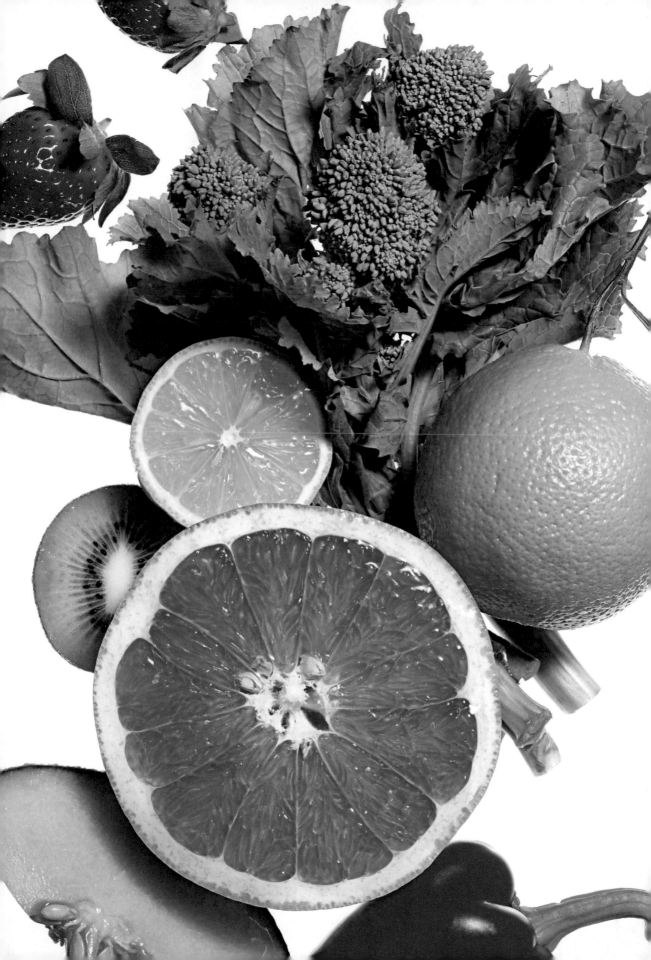

Too much body fat can make us feel unattractive, unhealthy, and unhappy. That is why this book focuses on fat and specifically the factors that either increase or release it. Body fat is different from the fat in your diet. Your body turns extra calories you eat into fat. It doesn't matter if those calories come from having too much fat, protein, or carbohydrate. And where the fat goes is up to your body. (Mine goes straight to my thighs!) But what I learned in researching this book is that some types of dietary fat are bad for your health and waistline while others can help both.

We make choices every day that can either increase or decrease our fat stores. When I decided to create the Digest Diet, my team of editors and I culled through everything in our database of research and were excited to discover foods and activities that actually help you release fat. These "fat releasers" form the foundation of the Digest Diet and are featured prominently in the recipes in this book. At the same time, we help you reduce the number of "fat increasers," those foods and behaviors that consistently cause body fat to accumulate. We show you why being overweight is more of a whole-life experience than just a matter of calories in and calories out.

● REDUCING FAT INCREASERS

The decisions we make can have a major impact on our weight. But we're not always aware that a lot of the choices we make are sabotaging our efforts to lose weight or maintain a healthy weight. Fat increasers fall into three groups—eating, environment, and exercise.

Fat Increaser #1: Eating

Of course, we all have to eat. But that doesn't mean we're doomed to be fat. Eating only becomes a fat increaser if you eat the wrong things at the wrong times in the wrong quantities. I am referring to more than just calories. Being deficient in certain nutrients for instance, can actually increase your body's fat stores. Once you know what increases body fat, you can make simple shifts in your everyday choices that will add up to big benefits.

> We **make choices every day** that can either increase or decrease our fat stores.

For starters, we eat too much food in the form of fuel, fakes, and fads. Fuel is calories, and it's no surprise that we take in more than we use. But it's not necessarily because we're all pigging out. We also are being faked out by new, tastier versions of processed foods that have additional fat, sugar, and salt to make them even more appealing. Former FDA commissioner David A. Kessler points out in his book *The End of Overeating* that eating such appealing foods changes brain chemistry, creating a cycle of addiction. The time-saving nature of these foods is even more alluring. But the problem is that they don't provide a lot of nutrition in their calories, so our bodies and brains literally hunger for more.

The next problem: Fad diets cause us to eat too much by denying us the foods and calories our bodies need. How often have you been on an overly restrictive diet and then rebounded by overeating those forbidden foods? The reality is that whole foods, real foods of all sorts, are what your body wants, needs, and should be getting.

Eating too little food also can increase fat. Surprised?

SUCCESS STORIES
from Our Facebook Community

▶ "Starting round 2 of Fast Release today—have lost 37 pounds in 9 weeks!!! Motivation? The new look in my hubby's eye…;)"

—CARLYE ELM GLASER

When you eat too few calories, your body slows down and hangs on to what it has—this is called *homeostasis*—and stores more fat as a result. Even worse is trying to cut calories by skipping breakfast. In a Korean study, people who didn't eat breakfast ate more fat and desserts later in the day. Breakfast skippers in Minnesota experienced big drops in late-morning blood sugar, which can increase hunger. Other studies show that going without breakfast leads to increased appetite, worse food choices later in the day, poor diet quality overall, and a heightened risk of diabetes and cardiovascular disease.

Another fat increaser: Eating enough calories but not enough micronutrients of the type found in whole and plant-based foods. Specifically, calcium deficiencies are associated with more body fat and less appetite control. So are deficiencies in nutrients such as zinc, magnesium, and vitamin E. Researchers in Quebec, Canada, call these "unsuspected determinants of obesity" because they increase your chances of being overweight and having belly fat. And I'm all for getting enough vitamin C—who wants the extra weight and bigger waist that Arizona researchers say are linked to low levels of vitamin C? Or the difficulties in losing fat when the body does not have enough? I know I don't!

That being said, I am not telling you to go out and buy supplements. We made sure that the Digest Diet includes plenty of real foods rich with these micronutrients. Real food is really good for you, really tasty, and chock-full of vitamins, minerals, phytochemicals, and other micronutrients that work for health and a healthy weight.

And, as I alluded to in my introduction, not getting enough satisfaction from food also can increase fat. People who are not satisfied physically and emotionally are more likely to

 LAUGH IT OFF

Over dinner, I explained the health benefits of a colorful meal to my family. "The more colors, the more variety of nutrients," I told them. Pointing to our food, I asked, "How many different colors do you see?"

"Six," volunteered my daughter. "Seven if you count the burned parts."

—ALLISON BEVANS

reach for food, especially sugary foods, to make them feel better. But the happy feeling you get from eating a cinnamon bun is only temporary. That's why eating mindfully—taking your time and relishing every bite—is a fundamental must-do on this plan.

Fat Increaser #2: Environment

Our daily environment also sets the stage for fat accumulation. We sit in chairs and at desks instead of hunting for our food as nature intended, and that deprives us of something called *NEAT*—non-exercise activity thermogenesis. NEAT is the term for calories burned by daily activities such as bending, walking, fidgeting, doing a favorite hobby, or standing in the kitchen cooking. A person can burn as many as 700 calories a day this way! In addition to making us burn fewer calories, Canadian researchers say sitting at a desk also causes us to eat more calories and fat because we have a tougher time controlling our appetites. The amount you sleep also matters. Too much—more than 7 or 8 hours a night—and you're at higher risk of becoming overweight because you're not being active enough. Too little—less than 4 to 6 hours per night—interferes with hormones that regulate appetite, leaving you hungrier and looking for "energy" in the form of unhealthy snacks!

In addition, the environment around us can be problematic. Study after study shows that organochlorine compounds found in plastics, herbicides, and pesticides, as well as chlorine-based household products, interfere with your body's ability to burn fat. And exposure to air pollution has been shown by researchers at the Ohio State University to increase inflammation and change metabolism in fat cells, causing problems in handling blood sugar and increasing risk for diabetes.

FAT INCREASERS

Eating
▶ Too much food
▶ Too little food
▶ Too little satisfaction

Environment
▶ Too much sitting
▶ Too much thinking
▶ Too much or too little sleep
▶ Too much pollution
▶ Too little joy

Exercise
▶ Too little variety
▶ Too little effort
▶ Too little enjoyment

Finally, personal happiness matters. You don't need a researcher to tell you about the link between stress and obesity. Many of us turn to food when we're feeling blue or stressing out, and the effects are worsened by the link between anxiety and an increase in belly fat accumulation. Feedback to the brain from fat cells can actually increase your risk of depression. This is one more reason to stop fat creep before it affects your emotional health and well-being.

Fat Increaser #3: Exercise

Don't get me wrong—exercise is wonderful! It relieves stress, boosts mood, helps prevent disease, and burns calories. And exercise is a key factor in maintaining a healthy weight in the long term. But if you've ever tried to drop the pounds by spending a little more time on the treadmill, you won't be surprised to learn that exercise by itself (especially if you're doing the same aerobic workout over and over) doesn't do much for weight loss. In fact, since aerobic exercise can make you hungrier, sometimes it can actually increase your body fat.

Also, to get the most benefit, you need to mix up your exercise regimen rather than doing the same workout each time. I do not doubt your effort, but I encourage you to be realistic about how hard you really are working. When I look around the gym, I see lots of people who think they're pushing but really are not working very hard. Even if you are sweating up a storm, you'll find that your body adapts, so it's important to surprise your body with different types of exercise. Don't let your workout become a routine. (More on that later.)

Lastly, exercise has to be important to you. I understand

that formal exercise is not fun for some people and never will be. If this is you, focus instead on exercise-related personal goals like getting stronger or having more energy as a result of exercising. And explore different activities to find ones that you like. Personally, I spend 2 hours a week lifting weights; it makes me feel like Superwoman! I enjoy feeling strong so much that few things ever keep me from my gym time. Once you find a routine you like (A walking commute? A pet who can run alongside you? A garden you like to tend?), you'll be more likely to stick with it and benefit from your efforts.

Laughing **actually burns calories** and can boost energy expenditure by up to 20 percent!

● ADDING FAT RELEASERS

Have you heard the lyrics from the 1940s Bing Crosby song, "Accentuate the positive, eliminate the negative"? Now that you know how to eliminate the negative "fat increasers," let's turn our attention toward accentuating the positive "fat releasers." These are simple foods and behaviors that will help the fat fade away. Ironically, the fat releasers I'm going to tell you about fall in the same categories as the fat increasers: eating, environment, and exercise.

Fat Releaser #1: Eating

When I was researching the *Flat Belly Diet!*, I remember getting goose bumps when I read about the research showing that monounsaturated fatty acids (MUFAs) were nutrients that helped the body shed fat. Finally, here was a "magic ingredient" for weight loss that was natural, healthy, and delicious—and very easy to find and incorporate into my busy life. So imagine how much more excited I was when I realized that MUFAs were not the only foods that could release fat.

In the Digest Diet, I bring you 12 more such releasers. They are in the very foods that probably already fill your shopping

Joe Rinaldi
26 Pounds and 7.75 Inches Lost!

Even though he's always been active, Joe Rinaldi has been struggling with his weight for some time. Over the past 2 years, it began to seriously interfere with his life. He could no longer ice-skate with his four children. "It's hard to tie my skates. I'm in tons of pain. I have to take breaks."

So he was highly motivated to try again. "I don't know what you can lose in 21 days, but it will be a good start," he said before Day 1. Well, he lost 26 pounds in 3 weeks!

"I honestly love the diet. If you follow it, it really works. . . . As we started eating more, my cravings went away." After 3 short weeks, he finds it easier to breathe when he's walking up steps, and his right knee feels less pain.

But that's not all. "I have more energy. I feel like I have control of my eating. I even feel more confident at work. My clothes fit better, and I'm looking forward to taking the rest of my weight off. I feel like I am out of the rut I was in." At this pace, he'll be skating rings around his youngsters in no time.

cart every week. They make up the foundation of the 21-Day Fat Release Plan, sample meals, and recipes in this book. You'll learn more about these foods later in the chapter.

Fat Releaser #2: Environment

As with their role in increasing fat, environmental factors can help release fat, too. But it takes a bit of rebellion against convenience. Remember NEAT, those extra calories you burn by just moving around? Every day, I actually look for ways to pump up NEAT by being inefficient, especially when I cook. This means chopping instead of using the food processor, making several trips to the fridge to gather ingredients, stirring by hand, and even washing dishes.

Here are a few other easy ways to tackle body fat.

Focus on exercise-related personal goals like **getting stronger** or having more energy.

▶ **Snack it off** by arming yourself with Digest Diet snacks—they're packed with at least three satiety-inducing fat releasers—as an alternative to the chips, candy bars, and other calorie-loaded, nutrient-poor choices you might otherwise make.

▶ **Sleep it off** by clocking enough hours in bed unhampered by caffeine or sugar. Studies show that getting too little sleep can be a fat increaser.

▶ **Clean it off** by shopping for organic foods and cleaning supplies wherever and whenever you can. Remember those pesky organochlorine compounds that mess up cell metabolism in a way that increases fat? Every switch you make to organic means fewer organochlorines.

▶ **Laugh it off** every day. It actually burns calories and can boost energy expenditure by up to 20 percent! Look for the "Laugh It Off" boxes throughout these chapters for a few jokes to start.

FAT RELEASERS

Eating
- Vitamin C
- Calcium and dairy
- Protein
- PUFAs and MUFAs
- Coconut oil
- Resveratrol
- Fiber
- Vinegar
- Quinoa
- Honey
- Cocoa

Environment
- Fidget it off
- Snack it off
- Sleep it off
- Clean it off and up
- Laugh it off

Exercise
- Lift it off
- HIIT it off
- Love it off

Fat Releaser #3: Exercise

As I noted earlier in the chapter, while exercise may not help you drop the pounds, it's instrumental in helping to keep fat away once you have. Exercise also helps keep you young—literally! Telomeres, tiny caps on the ends of our DNA strands, serve as a reliable marker of our cells' age. The shorter our telomeres are, the older and more tired our bodies' cells are. In one German study, middle-aged subjects who were sedentary had telomeres that were on average 40 percent shorter than those of active subjects.

Remember that it's important to switch up your workout so that you keep surprising your body. I like to alternate between strength training to build and tone muscle—more muscle means more fat burning—and intervals of aerobics to burn calories. Plus, my secret strategy for bashing fat is to stand and walk around whenever I can rather than sitting. It really makes a difference!

You don't have to spend an hour a day at the gym to get results, unless that makes you happy. Give this simple approach a try:

▶ Lift it off with strength training with as little as three 11-minute intense strength-training sessions each week. The Department of Kinesiology at Southern Illinois University found that this increases fat and calorie burn all day long, and even during sleep!

▶ HIIT it off by doing a type of aerobics called high-intensity interval training (HIIT). When you alternate intense bursts of activity with short periods of rest, you release fat, build muscle, and boost heart health. You'll start with a 4-minute warm-up, push hard for 30 seconds at your favorite activity—rowing, working out on a stationary bike, elliptical, treadmill, or stair-stepper—

and then rest for 30 seconds. Alternate between intense activity and rest six times. Now slow it down for 2 minutes with shorter bursts and rests. Just 12 minutes to chase away fat!

▶ **Love it off** by doing what makes you happiest. Maybe solo sports like running and swimming are your favorites. Or you like the camaraderie of exercise classes. You might enjoy baseball, soccer, and other team sports best. Taking the dog for a walk counts, too! Go with the activity that gets you moving, makes you smile, and lifts your mood for the entire day.

● FAT RELEASING FOODS

By now, you're probably wondering, "So what can I eat on this diet, anyway?" The answer is: almost anything! The 13 nutrients and foods we've sleuthed out for their fat busting properties include a wide variety of fruits, vegetables, grains, meats, and other foods. You may notice that some lists appear to be missing certain foods, such as chocolate/cocoa in the healthy fats list. That's because they also qualify for a different category of fat releaser. For the purposes of these lists, we placed foods with multiple fat releasers where they had the most of a particular nutrient. If it's a close

> ### SUCCESS STORIES
> #### from Our Facebook Community
>
> ▶ "I have been on the Digest Diet since March. I love, love, love the smoothies. I buy fresh fruit when it goes on sale and freeze it in small bags. I am growing a small herb garden in my yard with the most frequently used herbs. Every Sunday I make one of the soup recipes and freeze it in 1-cup containers. I have frozen cooked turkey burgers and oatmeal breakfast cakes ready to use when I need a quick, on-the-go item. My main motivation comes from the comments I am receiving from co-workers, friends, and my husband. I just got back from the beach and wore a bathing suit in public for the first time in 6 years. I love this diet because I don't feel like I am on a diet at all; I feel healthy and great about myself." —**NANCY H. BROWN**

call, then you may see them in more than one place. You may also notice that some of your favorite foods are missing from these lists. That doesn't mean you can't eat them or that they don't contain some fat releasing nutrients, just that they're not among the top sources. Finally, if you're familiar with the original Digest Diet fat releaser food lists, you'll see that we've made a few additions as we've uncovered new research about the top sources for each fat releasing category.

Fat Releaser #1: Vitamin C

People who have low blood levels of vitamin C burn less fat during exercise, according to research at Arizona State University. The good news is that people with adequate vitamin C levels burn more fat and tend to weigh less.

Fat Releasers #2 and #3: Calcium and Dairy

When your mom told you to drink milk because its calcium was good for your bones, I doubt she knew that calcium was also great for controlling hunger. Also, for reasons that are not yet understood, people who have deficiencies in calcium often have

TOP SOURCES OF VITAMIN C

Vegetables
Asparagus
Bell peppers, red and green
Broccoli
Broccoli rabe
Brussels sprouts
Cabbage
Cauliflower
Escarole
Garlic
Greens (collards,
  mustard, turnip)

Kale
Kohlrabi
Onions
Peas, sugar snap
Spinach
Squash, summer and winter
Sweet potatoes

Fruits
Cantaloupe
Grapefruit and fresh juice
Kiwifruit

Lemons
Limes
Mango
Oranges and fresh juice
Papaya
Pineapple
Raspberries
Strawberries
Tomatoes

TOP SOURCES OF CALCIUM AND DAIRY

Dairy
Buttermilk
Cheese (Cheddar, cottage,
cream, feta, Gruyère,
mozzarella, Parmesan,
provolone, ricotta, Swiss)
Milk
Yogurt

Nuts and seeds
Almonds or almond butter
Brazil nuts
Roasted sesame seeds or
sesame butter

Vegetables
Bok choy
Broccoli

Broccoli rabe
Greens (collards,
dandelion, turnip,
and mustard)
Kale
Spinach
Watercress

a greater fat mass and experience less control of their appetite. Dairy sources of calcium such as milk have been shown to be markedly more effective than other sources in speeding up fat loss when they are part of a calorie-restricted diet. This may be because dairy foods stimulate enzymes in fat cells that metabolize fat, according to research at the University of Tennessee. Dairy foods also appear to block the types of hormone responses that increase fat storage and boost the use of energy from fat cells. If you can't tolerate dairy, be sure to get calcium from other foods or supplements.

What can you eat on this diet? Almost anything!

Fat Releaser #4: Protein

This macronutrient powerhouse promotes healthy skin, hair, nails, bones, and muscle. As a fat releaser, it increases satiety—that feeling of fullness and satisfaction that you get after a really good meal. Because protein is harder to metabolize than fat or carbohydrate, it takes up to three times more calories to digest and absorb protein after meals. Researchers also found that people on higher-protein diets naturally ate less food as compared to those who ate a high-carbohydrate diet.

To avoid unwanted calories tagging along with protein, choose lean proteins that don't have much marbling, trim excess fat from

TOP SOURCES OF LEAN PROTEIN

Beans and legumes
Baby lima beans
Black beans
Chickpeas
Lentils
Soybeans
White beans

Dairy
(see Dairy section on page 13)

Grains
Barley
  Bread and tortillas, whole-wheat and multigrain
Couscous, whole-wheat
Oats
Quinoa

Nuts and seeds
Almonds and almond butter
Hazelnuts
Peanuts and peanut butter
Pistachios
Pumpkin, sunflower, squash, or watermelon seeds, roasted

Poultry and eggs
Chicken
Eggs
Turkey

Meats (lean cuts)
Beef
Pork
Veal

Fish
Anchovies, fresh
Cod
Crab
Halibut
Lobster
Salmon, canned and fresh
Sardines, canned and fresh
Shrimp
Tuna, canned and fresh

meat before cooking, and always remove the skin from poultry before eating. Vegetarians should include beans, tofu, nuts, or other plant sources of protein at each meal to ensure they get enough of this important fat releaser.

Fat Releasers #5 and #6: PUFAs and MUFAs (Healthy Fats)

Are you surprised to see fats listed as fat releasers, especially since they're so highly concentrated in calories? Back in the 1980s, much of America jumped on the antifat bandwagon to shed body fat. Guess what happened? We didn't lose weight because we replaced fat with carbohydrates. So the answer isn't to get rid of fat but instead to include certain healthy fats and manage total calories. Healthy fats bring out flavors and make foods taste good, help the body absorb certain vitamins, and supply the essential fatty acids that are necessary for normal body functioning.

There are two types of essential fatty acids that support health: monounsaturated and polyunsaturated fatty acids (MUFAs and PUFAs). If you've read my earlier books or seen me on TV, you know that I am solidly behind foods rich in monounsaturated fatty acids (MUFAs). Eating a diet rich in olives, olive oil, nuts and seeds, dark chocolate, and avocado has kept my belly flat and my energy up for years! MUFAs also promote heart health and help cool inflammation.

Of the different types of PUFAs, the one you've probably heard the most about is omega-3, and with good reason. Did you know that omega-3 fatty acids can make you happy? They have been shown to boost mood, lessen anxiety, and alleviate depression, as well as protect your heart, protect against cancer, and maybe even aid weight loss by revving up metabolism and postmeal calorie burn. That's a lot to be happy about! These healthy fats are a mainstay of my diet and an essential part of this plan as well.

The U.S. government recommends that 20 to 35 percent of your total daily calories come from fat. Most of that should come in the form of MUFAs and PUFAs. You also should limit saturated fat, found in red meat and full-fat dairy, to less than 10 percent of total calories and totally avoid trans fats, the "fake" fat in partially hydrogenated oils found in processed food.

TOP SOURCES OF MUFAS AND PUFAS

Avocado
Coconut milk
Nuts, seeds, and nut butters, particularly flax, walnut, and sunflower
Olive oil
Salmon
Sardines
Soybean oil
Sunflower oil

Fat Releaser #7: Coconut Oil

Coconut oil is the one type of saturated fat that you can enjoy on the Digest Diet. In a Brazilian study, it helped a group of abdominally obese women decrease belly fat, increase blood levels of HDL "good" cholesterol, and improve their ratio of "bad" to good cholesterol.

Did you know that omega-3 fatty acids can **make you happy?**

Fat Releaser #8: Resveratrol

Let's give a toast to having a glass of red wine when you're trying to lose weight! In addition to studies on its overall health benefits, research on animals suggests that red wine holds great promise as a fat releaser. And studies on women show that those who are light to moderate drinkers gain less weight and are less likely to become overweight, as compared to women who do not drink at all. The not-so-secret compound in red wine is resveratrol, an antioxidant also found in red grapes and Spanish peanuts, a small peanut eaten with the red skin coating.

Fat Releaser #9: Fiber

Nothing fills you up—and prevents overeating—quite like fiber, a nutrient found in vegetables, fruits, beans, whole grains, and nuts and seeds. That is why diets often recommend starting a meal with a salad to stave off hunger and ensure that you don't overeat.

Fat Releaser #10: Vinegar

Top your salad with vinegar for added fat releasing benefits. Vinegar may help boost satiety through its potential for smoothing out spikes in blood sugar after meals. When you feel more satis-

TOP SOURCES OF FIBER

Fruits
Avocado
Blackberries
Plums
Raspberries
Tomatoes (fresh
  and sun-dried)

Nuts and seeds
Almonds
Brazil nuts

Flaxseed and
  flaxseed meal
Pecans
Pistachios
Sesame seeds
Sunflower seeds

Grains
Barley
Couscous,
  whole-wheat

Oats
Rice, brown

Legumes
Beans
Chickpeas
Lentils
Peas, dried, fresh,
  snow, and sugar
  snap

Vegetables
Artichoke
Broccoli rabe
Lettuce
Mustard greens
Radishes
Turnip greens

fied, you eat less. Animal studies suggest that vinegar may also prevent body-fat accumulation. All types of vinegars have similar fat releasing effects, but different types add different flavors to your cooking. So have an assortment of vinegars on hand to use whenever you feel the need to tame your appetite and turn on fat burning.

Fat Releaser #11: Quinoa

I would eat this ancient grain for its powerhouse nutrition profile, with plenty of protein, phytosterols, and vitamin E, even if it wasn't a fat releaser. And there's more. Studies published in 2011 and 2012 revealed that animals supplemented with an extract made from quinoa seeds showed less body fat, smaller fat cells, and lower body weight, and they also cut down on their eating.

Fat Releaser #12: Honey

I love the fact that my favorite sweetener might help me keep my weight in check. Compared to sugar, honey's effects on appetite

SUCCESS STORIES
from Our Facebook Community

▶ "After struggling with many diets over countless years, I finally found the one that works for me. I no longer crave sugar—the shakes and red grapes take care of that issue. I am down 8.5 pounds and still going strong. Even eating out has been easier than I imagined. Without thinking, I just keep picturing what foods will be best for me. I began this journey at the end of April, and although I haven't lost as much as some, I know this way of flavorful eating will help me continue to shed the pounds."

—DIANNE FORTH

hormones are much more positive. A laboratory study found that animals whose diets included honey gained less weight and had less body fat than animals on a diet with sugar. Honey has been highly regarded throughout history for its wide-ranging antibacterial, antiviral, and antifungal properties. All types of honey have similar fat releasing effects, so you might want to experiment with different types to find your favorite!

Fat Releaser #13: Cocoa

Like most of you, I can't imagine life without chocolate. Fortunately, I don't have to. Researchers in Korea and Japan showed that extracts of beneficial compounds in cocoa reduced weight gain and accumulation of fat in laboratory animals. Add this great news to what we already know about cocoa and heart health. Can you see the smile on my face? Just remember to opt mostly for dark chocolate, with higher cocoa content.

 LAUGH IT OFF

Every 10 years, the monks in the monastery are allowed to break their vow of silence to speak two words. Ten years go by and it's one monk's first chance. He thinks for a second before saying, "Food bad."

Ten years later, he says, "Bed hard."

It's the big day, a decade later. He gives the head monk a long stare and says, "I quit."

"I'm not surprised," the head monk says. "You've been complaining ever since you got here."

—ALAN LYNCH

Adrienne Farr
18 Pounds and 9.5 Inches Lost!

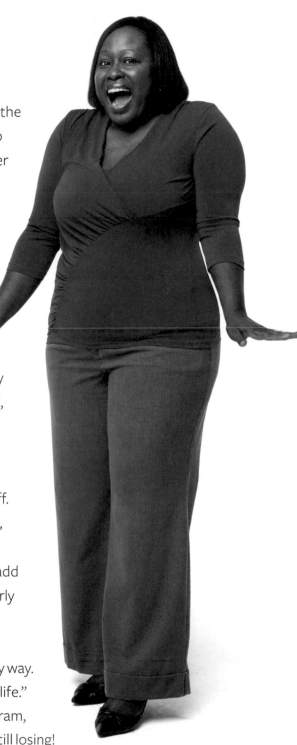

Adrienne's busy lifestyle as an executive assistant has made it difficult for her to find the time for healthy habits. But she was ready to change when the scale climbed past 200. Her back and knees hurt, and she was worried about her high cholesterol. A former high school gymnast, Adrienne, 36, yearned to be fit again.

Within days of starting the plan, her energy was soaring. "I literally jumped out of bed at 5 a.m. I have never done that." She also found that her food tastes naturally shifted. "I craved greens—spinach, broccoli, fennel. That's new for me."

At her first weigh-in, Adrienne had lost an amazing 7 pounds in 4 days. Bringing more fun into each day helped the pounds melt off. "I loved watching old TV programs—*Rhoda, Good Times, 227, All in the Family, Three's Company*—it made me laugh out loud." To add more movement to each day, she woke up early each morning and danced in her living room.

"I never thought it was possible to lose so much weight so quickly and in such a healthy way. This is something I can do for the rest of my life." Six months after the official end of the program, Adrienne is down a total of 50 pounds and still losing!

Chapter 2

Cooking with Fat Releasers

Turn your kitchen into a hub for fat releasing of meals and activity with these simple tips on how to make over your pantry, shop smart, and cook to release fat.

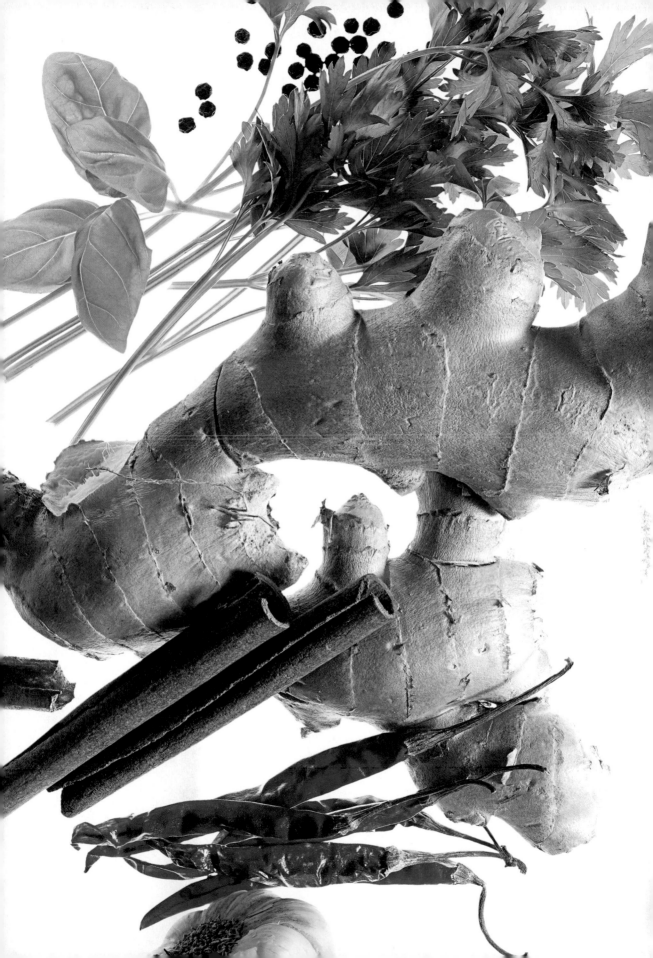

When I first learned about all the fat increasers in our environment, I was overwhelmed. It seemed like the deck was stacked against healthy eating, and I was afraid that shifting the balance toward fat releasers was going to require hours in the kitchen and hundreds of dollars in special foods. I didn't want the Digest Diet to be that kind of unsustainable plan.

Luckily, it turns out that fat releasers are all around us, too, so it only takes small shifts in habits to pack them in. Our recipes use foods that are probably in your fridge already and don't take a lot of time to prepare. To make it even easier, this chapter shows you how to set up your kitchen and pantry to make it a snap to cook your Digest Diet meals.

Chefs use the French term *mise en place* (putting in place) to describe the advance prep that is necessary in cooking. Mise en place involves gathering, measuring, and readying all ingredients; setting out equipment; preheating the oven; and doing whatever you can to make the actual cooking more organized. Now, I want you to think about mise en place in terms of your entire kitchen. We are going to work together to put things in place in your kitchen so that you can prepare delicious meals filled with fat releasers without getting tripped up by fat increasers along the way.

● YOUR FAT RELEASING KITCHEN

If you're like me, your kitchen drawers and cupboards are filled with gadgets and equipment that you never use. To be honest, I don't remember what some of the stuff I have is supposed to do!

If that sounds like you, do a kitchen purge. First, clean out the gear from every drawer and cupboard (and wipe out the crumbs and gunk while you're at it!). Then sort the items into two piles, those that you really plan to use and those that are broken, dull, or useless. You'd be amazed at how much you come up with. Toss the broken stuff, clean the keepers, and then put things back in logical places. For example, I keep all my wooden spoons and spatulas together and store fruit and veggie tools like peelers and ballers in the same drawer. Now that you've made some room, we can talk about what else you might need.

I've put together a list of basic equipment for making the recipes in this book. Depending on which recipes you choose, you might want everything that's on the list or you might feel that some items aren't essential for your kitchen. That's entirely up to you! To keep my kitchen from being overrun by gear and to help me stay organized, I've come up with a few personal food musts that you might find helpful:

1. Sharp knives

There's a reason all cooks will tell you that sharp knives are a must. Otherwise food prep is difficult and you're actually more likely to cut yourself. Sharpen knives yourself, get them sharpened regularly, or buy inexpensive knives that you can toss when they get dull.

SUCCESS STORIES
from Our Facebook Community

▶ "I loooove this diet! Never have I enjoyed the experience of dieting, but between the shakes and soups, it's very easy! I really look forward to eating both, and to top it off, the pounds are coming off so quickly! Unreal. If I weren't seeing it with my own eyes, I may not believe it! As of today I've lost 20 pounds!! Congratulations to anyone else feeling better about themselves, and thank you, Liz, for the book!" —RACHEL NAATZ

2. Multitasking kitchen gear

You can use a sharp peeler for shaving thin ribbons of Parmesan cheese or chocolate, as well as peeling carrots and other veggies. A melon baller comes in handy for scooping out seeds in other types of fruit. Some coffee grinders do a fine job grinding spices.

3. A digital scale and other portion-control tools

You need a good digital scale to know what you're putting in your mouths and how much you're actually eating. For the most versatility, choose one that allows you to switch from ounce measures to grams. In addition to my kitchen scale and measuring cups, I use food scoops of different sizes, from a tablespoon or so up to half a cup, to help me dish out right-size portions. And Tupperware or other food storage containers are a must to store leftovers in easy-to-grab single servings.

4. Easy-to-clean equipment

I don't mean just nonstick pans but also gear without nooks and crannies to trap bits of food. Also, I recommend cutting boards that can be scrubbed or go in the dishwasher.

5. Sturdy stuff

Nothing annoys me more than tools that break after just a few uses. I love Oxo for their durable kitchen tools that are designed to be comfortable and easy to use. Choose metal or plastic measuring spoons that don't bend easily. My favorite measuring cups are made from stainless steel and have handles that are firmly anchored to the cup. Any of the major knife companies—Wusthof, Henckels, Victorinox, and Shun, to name a few—make durable knives that will last for years.

6. Nonstick pots and pans

For me, nothing is more important than a surface that doesn't need a lot of extra oil to prevent food from sticking. Nonstick surfaces are much more durable and longer lasting than they used to be. They're also safe to use at everyday cooking temperatures. Make sure that your skillets are the right size—a 12-inch should be adequate for recipes that serve four and an 8-inch is handy for single servings or cooking small amounts.

7. Blender

A blender is a must for the Digest Diet so that you can prepare the various shakes. You don't need one with a lot of different speeds, but make sure you buy one that is sturdy.

● YOUR FAT RELEASING PANTRY AND FREEZER

You know what it's like when you come home from a long day of work, then have to help the kids with homework, take the dog for a walk, maybe even run a load of laundry. Then you have to find the time and energy to make dinner! This is when it's really tempting to call for takeout or just pop a frozen dinner in the microwave. But if you've stocked your pantry and freezer properly, you can get real healthy food on the table faster than the time it takes the pizza delivery guy to arrive.

That's why I really appreciate foods that will save me time in the kitchen. The good thing about these items is that most have a long shelf life, meaning that you can buy them and not have to replace them for a while. But that's also

 LAUGH IT OFF

At day care, my 4-year-old watched as a teacher pulled something hot from the oven.

"What's that on your hand?" he asked.

"An oven mitt," she said. "It keeps me from getting burned. Doesn't your mother use them?"

"No, my mom's just really careful when she opens the pizza box." **—JESSICA DODGE**

MUST-HAVE KITCHEN EQUIPMENT

FOR PEELING AND CUTTING

▮ **Knives**
  Paring knife for peeling and cutting
  Chef's knife for cutting and chopping
  Serrated or bread knife for slicing
▮ **Knife sharpener or steel**
▮ **Vegetable peeler**
▮ **Melon baller**
▮ **Kitchen/poultry shears**
▮ **Washable cutting boards**
  One for raw meats
  One for vegetables, fruits, and other foods
▮ **Grater**
▮ **Microplane or other zester**

FOR MEASURING

▮ **Kitchen scale**
▮ **Nested measuring cups for dry ingredients**
▮ **1- and 2-cup liquid measuring cups**
▮ **Set of measuring spoons**
▮ **Stackable, sealable containers in several sizes for holding ingredients, plus storing leftovers and single-serve portions**

FOR COOKING AND BAKING

▮ **Electric**
  Blender
  Food processor (mini and/or full-size)
  Electric mixer
  Slow cooker
▮ **Stovetop**
▮ **Nonstick ovenproof skillets**
  Wok
  Nonstick grill pan
  Saucepans with lids
    Large or Dutch oven for soups
    Medium for general cooking
    Small for sauce
    Nonstick
  Veggie steamer (metal basket or microwave-safe)
▮ **Oven**
  10 x 15-inch rimmed baking sheet
  Standard baking sheet
  Roasting pan
  Glass baking dishes
  Square metal baking pans
  9 x 13-inch baking pan
  8½- or 9-inch springform pan
  9 x 5-inch loaf pan
  12-cup muffin pan
  Paper muffin cup liners
  6-ounce ramekins
  Waxed paper, parchment paper, and/or a nonstick liner
  Foil
▮ **Miscellaneous**
  Wooden spoons
  Slotted spoon
  Whisk
  Mixing bowls
  Salad bowl
  Screw-top jar
  Tongs
  Spatulas that won't damage nonstick surfaces
  Skewers
  Instant-read thermometer

FOR GRINDING

▮ **Spice grinder**
▮ **Pepper mill**

FOR CLEANING AND DRAINING

▮ **Colander**
▮ **Salad spinner**

FOR STORAGE

▮ **Sealable sandwich and storage bags**
▮ **Plastic storage containers**

why so many of us have cupboards filled with flavorless spices, soggy bread crumbs, and oils that are past their prime, along with dried-out frozen foods. They're easy to buy, use once, and forget. I encourage you to clear old and stale items out of your pantry and freezer and give them a good cleaning before restocking with Digest Diet essentials. However, don't toss opened bottles of vinegar, a fat releaser that comes in lots of tasty varieties to brighten up the soups, salads, mains, and sides in this book. Although its color may change over time, vinegar can last in the cupboard for years after opening.

I always keep canned beans, tomato products, and tuna on my shelves. When packing your meal with fat releasers is as easy as opening a can, you can't go wrong. Just choose "no-salt-added" or "low-sodium" varieties. Dried fruit, the kind that hasn't been sweetened with sugar, is another favorite for adding color, flavor, and fiber to salads without having to peel and cut fresh fruit. Because dried fruit is high in calories and not very filling as a snack, use just small amounts in cooking to impart a lot of flavor. I always keep frozen unsweetened fruits and sauce-free veggies in my freezer because they're so easy to use and are at least as nutritious as fresh (and definitely a better option than canned veggies, which tend to be high in sodium). I also save time and money by buying the family-size package of meat or chicken and divvying it up into smaller packages that I wrap, label, and freeze. And, of course, different types of whole grains, a great source of fiber, occupy some of the real estate in my freezer (yes, the freezer; the natural oils in many whole grains can go rancid if left out in the pantry).

The list of fat releaser staples on pages 30–31 is intended as a guide to help you find the fat releasers in your grocery

OUR FAVORITE CRACKERS

To maximize fiber, beneficial plant compounds, and other nutrients, we picked crackers with whole ingredients, such as whole wheat, whole oats, etc., as the first ingredient. Our picks also have about 1.5 grams of fiber and 30 calories per cracker:

Finn Crisp Plus: 30 calories, 1.3g fiber

Kavli Five Grain: 30 calories, 1.5g fiber

RyKrisp Multigrain: 25 calories, 1.5g fiber

Wasa crackers: 45 calories, 2g fiber

store. Don't feel you need to go out and buy all of these foods in order to succeed on the Digest Diet. First, take a look at the recipes that appeal to you, and just start with the ingredients you'll need to make those. You'll soon figure out which of these will become staples in your household. I love that I can "thrive with five" (fiber, protein, vitamin C, calcium, and dairy—the top five fat releasers) just by opening my freezer and pantry. I hope you will, too!

Healthy Fats

If your local market is like mine, it stocks plenty of different oils, from everyday to exotic. I use soybean, sunflower, or olive oil for most of my cooking and drizzle specialty oils like almond and sesame onto salads and other dishes to punch up the flavor. Most oils are sensitive to heat and light; store them in a cool, dark cabinet or in the refrigerator to keep them fresh. They may harden in the refrigerator but will reliquefy when allowed to warm up on the counter for 15 minutes or so. Be sure to give oils a sniff before using and throw them away if you smell an "off" aroma.

While nuts, nut butters, and seeds can be stored unrefrigerated, they stay freshest when kept in the refrigerator. In fact, experts at the University of California at Davis say that nuts can be stored for a year in the fridge and even longer in the freezer—you can add them to recipes and dishes straight from the freezer. Light, heat, and air oxidize the oil in nuts, which is why they may start smelling funny after a month or two at room temperature.

Grains

Lots of grains and foods made from grains can be kept in the pantry. The assortment of whole-wheat and whole-grain pastas keeps on growing; I love their hearty, nutty flavor. Did you know that whole-wheat couscous is a type of pasta? My family also enjoys eating different whole grains, including quinoa, which comes in white, red, and black varieties; bulgur wheat; and barley. Wraps, breads, and rolls stay fresh at room temperature for just a couple of days but can be stored well wrapped in the freezer for a couple of months. If you don't use them that often, I'd also suggest storing brown rice, wheat berries, and other whole-grain kernels in the freezer to prevent their fat from going rancid.

Fat Releaser Seasonings

The recipes in this book call for a variety of different seasonings. Many do double duty by enhancing flavor and boosting the fat releasing properties of the dish. You'll certainly want to stock those that are called for in the recipes you plan to make, but also consider trying other less-familiar seasonings to spice up your meals. Remember to store dried herbs such as basil and oregano in a cool, dry place and replace them after about a year or when their vibrant aroma fades. Fresh herbs have to be refrigerated. Spices such as pepper, cinnamon, ginger, allspice, and others also belong in a cool, dry place. They can last ground for about 6 months and unground for up to a couple of years, depending on the spice.

We've tried to keep salt to a minimum in this book, but sometimes a pinch or two of salt is really what's needed to pull a

continued on page 32

FAT RELEASER STAPLES

FREEZER

- Frozen berries
- Frozen broccoli
- Frozen fruits
- Frozen greens
- Frozen shelled and in-shell edamame
- Frozen spinach
- Frozen vegetables and vegetable combos

BREADS

- Whole-wheat/grain breads (thin-sliced bread, English muffins, rolls, thins, tortillas/wraps)

OILS

- Coconut oil
- Vegetable oils (choose from almond, avocado, flaxseed, olive, peanut, pistachio, sesame, soybean, sunflower)

VINEGAR

- Assorted (choose from balsamic for drizzling; cider for veggie salads; red wine, white wine, and sherry for lettuce; rice for Asian dishes)

PANTRY

- Buttermilk powder
- Chickpea flour
- Cocoa
  Cocoa powder
  Mini chocolate chips
- Coconut powder
- Honey
  Light flavor for beverages— alfalfa, blueberry, clover, orange blossom, or tupelo
  Stronger flavor for baking or drizzling— avocado, buckwheat, or wildflower
- Nonfat dry milk powder
- Packaged dried legumes (black beans, black-eyed peas, chickpeas, lentils, split peas, white beans)
- Quinoa and quinoa pasta
- Raisins, dried currants, and dried fruit as needed for recipes
- Shredded unsweetened coconut
- Sun-dried tomatoes
- Whole grains (barley, bulgur, kasha [buckwheat], oats, quinoa, brown rice, wheat berries)
- Whole-wheat flour
- Whole-wheat/grain pasta (couscous, linguine, orzo, penne, spaghetti)

NUTS, NUT BUTTERS, AND SEEDS

- Almonds, almond flour, and almond butter
- Brazil nuts
- Cashews
- Flaxseeds and flaxseed meal
- Hazelnuts
- Peanuts and peanut butter
- Pecans
- Pine nuts
- Pistachios
- Pumpkin seeds
- Sesame seeds and sesame butter
- Spanish peanuts
- Sunflower seeds
- Walnuts

RED WINE

GROUND SPICES

- Allspice
- Cayenne
- Celery seeds
- Chili powder
- Cinnamon
- Coriander
- Cumin
- Curry powder
- Fennel seeds
- Garam masala
- Ginger
- Chile peppers
- Mustard seeds
- Nutmeg
- Paprika, regular and smoked
- Pepper, black, red, and white

DRIED HERBS

- Basil
- Bay leaves
- Marjoram
- Mint
- Oregano
- Rosemary
- Sage
- Tarragon
- Thyme

CONDIMENTS

- Agave syrup
- Anchovies
- Bread crumbs, whole-wheat
- Broth (low-sodium canned beef, chicken, vegetable)
- Capers
- Chipotle peppers, canned in adobo sauce or dried
- Gelatin, unflavored
- Horseradish, prepared
- Hot sauce
- Jalapeño peppers, pickled
- Maple syrup
- Mushrooms, dried
- Mustard (yellow, Dijon)
- Olives (black, green, Kalamata)
- Soy sauce, reduced-sodium
- Sugar, turbinado (raw)
- Worcestershire sauce

CANNED

- Evaporated fat-free milk
- Legumes (black beans, black-eyed peas, chickpeas, lentils, peas, white beans)
- Light coconut milk
- Salmon and sardines (canned with bones)
- Tomato products (diced, paste, puree, sauce)
- Tuna

LAUGH IT OFF

The local market has a bin where employees keep returned items. The bin is labeled "Spoils." I never thought much about it until one afternoon I heard an announcement over the loudspeaker: "Victor to the spoils. Thank you."

—CHRIS DEJONG

continued from page 29

recipe together. We've called for regular table salt throughout to make it easy, but if you can splurge a little, I'd encourage you to try sea salt instead. It tends to be more flavorful (so you might need less of it) and naturally contains the essential mineral iodine (which has to be added back in to iodized table salt), which is great for thyroid health. Regardless of which salt you choose, use fine grain for easy mixing into recipes. In a few instances, you'll see we've called for kosher salt, which is coarser than regular table salt and by volume has less sodium. Coarse salt is best in rubs or when sprinkled lightly on top of a dish before serving, because it distributes more evenly than regular table salt. But best of all is to skip the shaker and choose a fat releaser seasoning or a squeeze of lemon or lime juice instead.

WHAT ABOUT SWEETENERS?

Recipes that require a sweetener usually call for honey, our top choice and also a fat releaser. Honey has positive effects on appetite hormones, plus it helps fight bacteria, viruses, and fungi. All types of honey release fat. But there are a few other natural sweeteners we like:

Agave nectar or syrup is derived from the juice in the core of the agave plant. The juice is processed to create syrup. It is thinner than and not as sweet as honey.

Maple syrup comes from the boiled sap of the maple tree. Grade A has the lightest flavor, while grade B is best for cooking because its flavor is more prominent.

Turbinado sugar is a natural brown sugar with sugar crystals that are lightly coated in molasses. The crystals are larger than white sugar crystals and not sticky like brown sugar.

A lot of readers ask us about whether they can use noncaloric sweeteners on the Digest Diet. The answer is no. All but stevia are fake foods and hence are fat increasers. Even stevia, which is natural and derived from a plant, is usually processed in a way that makes them unacceptable for this diet.

Condiments

Like herbs and spices, condiments can liven up your cooking, and some, namely honey, vinegar, and cocoa, also are fat releasers. Most can stay in your pantry unopened for at least a year or two. Once they're opened, dry condiments like bread crumbs generally can remain on the cupboard shelf, but liquids usually should be refrigerated. Refer to the package label for guidance on proper storage.

SHOPPING AND STORAGE TIPS FOR FAT RELEASING FRESH FOODS

There are different ways to go about stocking your kitchen with the fat releasers you need to make recipes in this book. A lot of readers tell me that they pick out a bunch of recipes, prepare them on the weekend, and then either eat them during the week or freeze them in single portions. If this describes you, I recommend that you create one shopping list with all the ingredients you need for all the recipes you plan to make. Other readers prefer to cook every day or so; some of them make one big list for a single shopping trip and some go to the store more often with shorter lists. The more daring cooks go to the store first, buy what looks good, and then decide what to do with the ingredients!

However, if this is your first time on the Digest Diet, I'd caution you to be careful when shopping without a list because it's easy to be tempted by fat increasers. I recommend either following the 21-Day Plan in the original book or sticking to the meal plan and recipes in this book for the first 3 weeks. Once you've gone through the plan and are familiar with fat releasers, then you can start experimenting. By then, I predict that you'll have stopped craving junk food and started craving greens and other healthy foods, just like our test panel did!

The dairy products, fresh vegetables and fruits, and protein sources in the Digest Diet recipes tend to be highly perishable, so follow these storage guidelines for good food safety practices.

OUR FAVORITE MINI CHEESES

We love these single-serving reduced-fat cheeses, especially as part of a quick snack.

The Laughing Cow Mini Babybel Light:
50 calories

The Laughing Cow Light (any flavor):
35 calories

Les Petites Fermieres Reduced-Fat Cheddar Cheese Sticks:
60 calories

Sargento Reduced-Fat Colby-Jack Stick:
70 calories

Polly-O 2% Mozzarella & Cheddar Cheese Twist: 50 calories

Dairy

When you're shopping in the dairy aisle, always choose fat-free, low-fat, or reduced-fat products. Milk and yogurt should be fat-free for maximum fat release, but I like reduced-fat or low-fat cheeses for flavor and fun. For freshness, look for a "use by" date that is furthest into the future. However, most dairy products usually are okay to eat a few days past the date stamped on the package. Once you've opened the package or carton, keep milk, cottage cheese, and soft cheeses like feta in the fridge for up to about 5 days, yogurt for up to 10 days, and hard cheeses (Cheddar, Swiss, etc.) that are well wrapped for about 2 weeks.

Meat, Fish, Poultry, Eggs

Many markets now label meat, fish, and poultry with nutrition information, making it easier to shop for the lean proteins we recommend in Digest Diet recipes. There's no need to shop for extra lean. In fact, we find extra-lean cuts to be too dry. So we call for pork tenderloin or loin, sirloin or flank steak, and both light and dark meat poultry. Some recipes cook poultry with the skin on and then call for it to be removed before serving.

Pay close attention to the "use by" date for freshness and food safety, and plan your purchases carefully, since raw meat, fish, and poultry should be used within 2 days of purchase, or frozen. You may want to stock up on sale items, wrap them in recipe portions, and label and freeze them. Raw eggs can be kept in the fridge for about 4 weeks; unpeeled hard-boiled eggs last for a week refrigerated.

Fresh Vegetables and Herbs

Choose from a wide assortment of vegetables and herbs. To save money, pick recipes that call for veggies that happen to be on sale at your market. And experiment with unfamiliar veggies and herbs—the greater variety you eat, the more nutrients you get. Plus, you may discover some new favorites! Most vegetables should be refrigerated; tomatoes and some root vegetables can be stored in a cool, dry place without refrigeration. Always wash vegetables before using.

Fresh Fruits

We encourage you to enjoy fruits in recipes and for dessert. In general, flavor, nutrition, and price are best when fruits are in season in North America—citrus, apples, and pears

> I predict that you'll have **stopped craving junk food** and started craving greens.

in the fall and winter; melons, berries, and stone fruits (peaches, plums, cherries) in the spring and summer—but today you can buy most fruits year-round. (See www.fruitsandveggiesmorematters. org/what-fruits-and-vegetables-are-in-season to find out when particular fruits are in season.) Many fruits require a few days of ripening at room temperature before refrigerating. They're ripe when their fruit aroma gets stronger and they feel slightly soft when you press them gently. Eat ripe fruit immediately or store it in the fridge, and always wash fruits before using.

● COOKING TO RELEASE FAT

Here's the best news of all—you won't need any fancy cooking skills to prepare the delicious recipes in this book. In fact, recipes like Tropical Fruit & Berry Salad with Yogurt Dressing (page 87), Golden Gazpacho (page 99), Italian Tuna & Fennel Salad (page 214), and Frozen Berry Terrine (page 265) need no cooking at all! And our Homemade Instant Oatmeal (page 79) requires nothing more than a few minutes on the stove or a few button pushes on the microwave. I don't have a lot of time to spend in the kitchen, so I made sure that most of the dishes require no more than 20 minutes of hands-on time. A favorite of mine is the slow cooker. Ingredients can cook together all day while I'm off doing other things. What could be easier?

It shouldn't come as a surprise that we don't use fat increasing types of cooking. So you won't find us calling for frying, sautéing with lots of fat, or adding generous amounts of oil or butter to baked goods. Instead, we use a variety of different cooking methods and tools that reduce fat from recipes and therefore help release fat from your body:

▶ Cooking in a nonstick skillet or saucepan so there's no need for fat to prevent sticking; we can get away with adding just a touch for flavor

▶ Broiling or grilling, which browns meat and makes it more flavorful while allowing fat to drip off

▶ Spraying with cooking spray to add just a couple calories' worth of fat to prevent sticking

▶ Lining baking sheets with parchment paper or a nonstick liner—they make removing foods from the baking sheet a breeze and negate the need for more oil

▶ Slow-cooking for moist heat and gentle cooking to tenderize meat and poultry without added fat

▶ Roasting or braising (simmering) with moist ingredients to make foods flavorful, tender, and juicy without added fat

▶ Steaming in a vegetable steamer, which requires no fat and retains vitamin C and other vitamins and minerals

▶ Stir-steaming—steaming veggies first in water with a touch of oil and sizzling to finish when the water evaporates—to keep fat to a minimum

▶ Adding honey and moist ingredients to baked goods to provide more moisture with much less fat

Christina Ierace
11 Pounds and 7 Inches Lost!

Christina, 26, is the ultimate multitasker, working a full-time job as a secretary while also being a full-time student. Burning the candle at both ends definitely has its downsides— less time to be active, a slower metabolism, and weight gain. The stress is also affecting her life in other ways. "I can definitely use better sleep. Also, my right knee hurts, and I notice that once I lose weight, it goes away."

All of this motivated her to try again to make a change that would stick. She committed to and followed the diet closely and was pleasantly surprised to find that the foods fit her busy lifestyle. "I really found it easy when it was a shake for dinner," she says, referring to the Fast Release phase. She also found that moving every day was key to sticking with it. Some days were harder to exercise than others but worth it. "When I work out, I don't want to eat junk food because I just worked my butt off."

On the Digest Diet, she's flourished, losing the weight she aimed to shed and discovering a healthy life balance that works for her. "Instead of saying that I want to go on a diet, I can just say I want to stay the way I am."

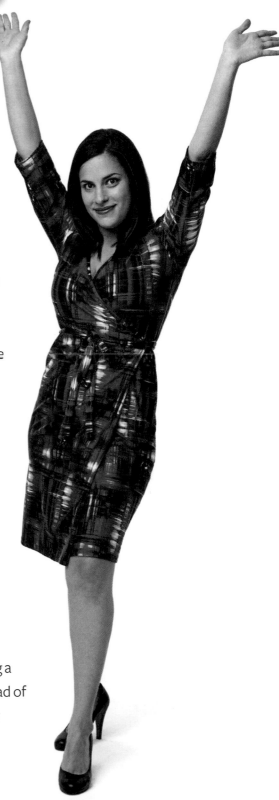

Chapter

3

Create Your Own 21-Day Fat Release Plan

Get ready to get cooking and lose weight fast with your favorite foods.

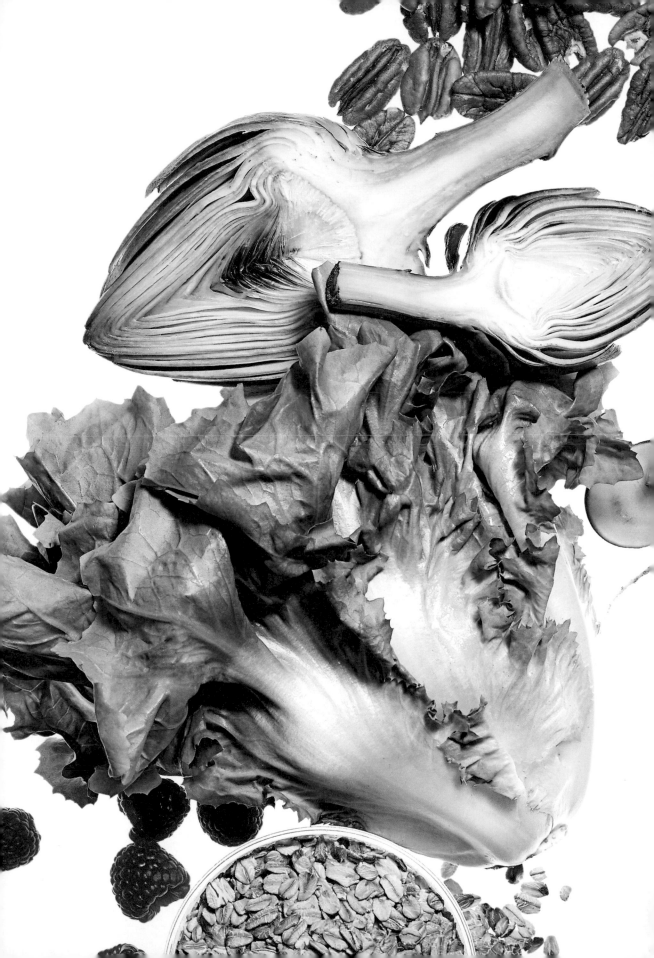

M

ost of us are creatures of habit, and I'm no exception. For years, I ate the same turkey sandwich every day for lunch. It was quick, it was easy, it kept me going through the day, and I didn't have to think about it. But after a while, that turkey sandwich stopped satisfying me, and I found myself reaching for candy bars after lunch just to add some variety. (Remember, not enough satisfaction in eating is a fat increaser!)

But with the Digest Diet, I never need to get bored with what I'm eating and neither do you. If you're one of the thousands of people who have already lost weight using the 21-Day Fat Release Plan in the original book, congratulations! You already have a repertoire of delicious and easy-to-prepare recipes in your weight loss arsenal and a good idea of how filling and, yes, satisfying the right balance of fat releasing foods can be. Now you're ready to start making your own Digest Diet menus. This chapter will give you all the information you need to maintain the fabulous success you've already had and even to keep losing if you want. You can still keep eating and making your favorite shakes, soups, and other dishes from the first 21 days, but now you'll have a whole new set of recipes to mix and match with them.

If you're new to the Digest Diet, this chapter will give you a peek behind the curtain to explain how we created the original 21-Day Fat Release Plan and how you can apply the same principles with the recipes in this book to create your own.

Before going into the three phases of the diet, I want to share with you a few handy guidelines to help you make smart fat releasing choices every day.

● THE DIGEST DIET "RULES"

Here are a few simple strategies to follow no matter where you are in the diet.

▶ Eat **breakfast.**

▶ Eat **real food**—that is, whole foods rather than processed. When you need to use packaged foods, pick those that have the fewest ingredients and have ingredient names you can pronounce.

▶ Choose **organic** when it's available.

▶ Include **fat releasers** at every meal and snack.

▶ **Thrive with five:** fiber, protein, vitamin C, calcium, and dairy. Try to include them at most meals.

▶ Eat **three servings** of fat-free, low-fat, or reduced-fat dairy each day.

If you've been down the weight loss path before, you know that shedding pounds involves more than just a diet. It's a lifestyle. Keep these basics in mind along the way.

▶ **Laugh daily** for at least 30 minutes with a loved one, watching a favorite show, visiting humor websites, or reading the Laugh It Off sidebars in this book.

▶ **Rethink convenience** to increase fat releasing activities (walk, bend, garden, stretch) and reduce fat increasers, those habits that give you reasons not to move around (such as e-mailing your colleagues down the hall or driving to the gym).

▶ Get a **good night's sleep.**

▶ **Find your middle place,** where moderation, balance, and good sense converge to bring you health and happiness.

▶ **Don't go it alone.** Surround yourself with people who will support and applaud your efforts, including our Digest Diet community at readersdigest.com/digestdiet and at facebook.com/digestdiet.

▶ **Make exercise** a part of your day, every day. I feel so good when I do. For best results, exercise first thing in the morning to start your day with an energy boost. (If you just can't get to it in the morning, though, do it whenever you can.) Go hard in short bursts and mix it up to keep your body guessing and your metabolism revved up. If a structured workout would help you, check out the 12-Minute Fat Release Workout in the original Digest Diet book. It incorporates simple, no-equipment-needed strength-training exercises (squats, step-ups, push-ups, and dips) into a superfast, supereffective HIIT routine. Combine that with some daily walks,

Surround yourself with people who will **support and applaud** your efforts.

and you'll be flexing your biceps and baring your toned tummy in no time. If you already have a workout regimen that's working for you, by all means keep it up! Just remember to switch it up from time to time. If you only have time to squeeze in a few 1-minute activity bursts (doing jumping jacks, climbing stairs, dancing around your living room, anything that gets your heart rate up), anything is better than nothing. And remember, when exercise is fun, the battle is won!

● THE 21-DAY FAT RELEASE PLAN

The Digest Diet includes three phases, each with its own calorie and macronutrient ratios to maximize fat release . . . and results. Although we're providing these guidelines to help you construct your own menus, please do not get hung up on counting calories or calculating protein or fiber grams. As long as you stick to the Digest Diet meals and fat releasing foods, you'll automatically come pretty close to meeting these goals. And it's much more important—and more fun—to think about what good foods you want to eat rather than how many calories you've consumed.

That said, there are a few things you should NOT eat for the duration of the diet. Avoid any fakes—that is, processed foods— especially artificial sweeteners and trans fats. Also, put down the salt shaker and reach for one of the Fat Releaser Seasonings instead. And no soda! (Coffee or tea is okay, though, as long as you stick to just one cup and be careful of using cream or sugar.)

You'll see that the recipes in the chapters that follow are free of fakes and full of fat releasers. To make it easy for you to figure out what to eat on any given day, we've organized them by phases. In each chapter, you'll find Phase 1 Fast Release recipes (if any) first; then Phase 2 Fade Away recipes; and finally Phase 3 Finish Strong recipes. You'll notice that there aren't many Fast Release recipes; as you'll see, that phase is the most restrictive, so you get the least variety during those 4 days. Once you get into Phases 2 and 3, though, you'll see that you have a lot of choices.

In Phases 2 and 3, each meal should total around 400 to 450 calories. You'll see that most of the recipes (even the One-Dish Mains) provide fewer than that. This is to give you maximum flexibility so that you can mix and match different recipes (within the same phase) to make your meals. For instance, you might choose to pair the Indian-Spiced Shrimp, a Phase 2 Main Dish that comes in at 227 calories per serving, with the Warm Broccolini Salad with Cashew Pesto, a Phase 2 Salad at 124 calories per serving. That still leaves you plenty of room for a 4-ounce glass of red wine (about 100 calories). That adds up to 451 calories for a flavorful Fade Away meal. In the sections below, we'll give you some other ideas on how you can combine the different recipes. And in the appendix, you'll find some sample daily menus that

continued on page 46

SUCCESS STORIES
from Our Facebook Community

▶ "I wanted to let you know what a wonderful thing the Digest Diet has been for me! Over the past couple of years, I have had problems with my thyroid. During this time, I gained 35 pounds. The Digest Diet caught my attention because it didn't use sugar or white flour and it used healthy foods. This is Day 21 on the diet and I've lost 10 pounds! This is HUGE considering my fight with my thyroid and parathyroid! I love, love, love the shakes and most of the recipes. I will use some of these the rest of my life!" —**TAMMY WELLER**

CREATE YOUR OWN DIGEST DIET SNACK

AT A GLANCE

Each Digest Diet snack should weigh in at around 100 to 150 calories and ideally deliver a combo of fiber, protein, and vitamin C. (Don't worry, though, if you can't get all three nutrients into every snack; you're sure to get plenty from your meals.

If you followed the original Digest Diet meal plan, you no doubt have a few go-to snacks in your repertoire already. By all means, feel free to stick with those if they work for you. In the recipes that follow, you'll also see "Save for a Snack" tips so that you can make tasty snacks from your leftovers. And in the menus in the appendix, you'll find lots of quick snack ideas that anyone can try.

Or, if you're on the go a lot, here's a list of portable snack choices that are easy to tuck into a small cooler bag and bring with you:

1. 1 mini cheese, ¼ cup peanuts, 3 mini bell peppers (any color)
2. One 5.3- to 6-ounce carton 0% plain Greek yogurt, 1 teaspoon sliced almonds, 10 grape tomatoes
3. 2 teaspoons almond butter on 1 high-fiber cracker, ½ cup snap peas
4. 10 almonds, 1 single-serve packet of baby carrots (about 10), ½ cup steamed, chilled in-pod edamame
5. 1 mini cheese, 1 high-fiber cracker, 1 cup broccoli
6. ¼ cup hummus, 4 mini bell peppers
7. 4 teaspoons natural peanut butter on cucumber wedges
8. One 5.3- to 6-ounce carton 0% plain Greek yogurt, 5 almonds, ½ cup green beans
9. One 6-ounce carton plain fat-free yogurt, 1 single-serve packet of celery sticks (about 10)
10. ¼ cup hummus, 1 cup broccoli florets

If you get tired of these combinations, use the guidelines below to make your own, using the portable and meal plan snacks as a guide. Some foods do double duty by providing both fiber and vitamin C; that's why snacks may have two foods instead of three.

CHOOSE ONE
OF THE FOLLOWING FOR
FIBER

1. 1 cup broccoli florets
2. 4 mini bell peppers
3. 4 cucumber wedges
4. 1 cup green beans
5. 1 single-serve packet of baby carrots or celery sticks
6. 1 small vegetable snack tray (no dip)
7. 1 high-fiber cracker (see the list on page 27)
8. 1 small apple (PHASE 3 ONLY)
9. 1 small pear (PHASE 3 ONLY)

THEN ADD
ONE OF THE FOLLOWING FOR
PROTEIN

1. 1 mini cheese (see the list on page 33)
2. One 5.3- to 6-ounce container plain fat-free yogurt
3. 1 tablespoon nuts, seeds or nut butter
4. 2 tablespoons hummus
5. ½ cup in-pod edamame

FINISH WITH
ONE OF THESE FOR
VITAMIN C

1. 10 grape or cherry tomatoes
2. 1 cup broccoli florets
3. 1 cup cauliflower florets
4. ½ cup sugar snap peas
5. 4 mini bell peppers
6. 1 cup mixed vegetable juice
7. 2 clementines (PHASE 3 ONLY)
8. 1 kiwifruit (PHASE 3 ONLY)
9. 1 orange (PHASE 3 ONLY)
10. ½ cup cantaloupe (PHASE 3 ONLY)
11. ½ grapefruit (PHASE 3 ONLY)
12. ½ cup mango chunks (PHASE 3 ONLY)
13. ½ cup papaya chunks (PHASE 3 ONLY)
14. ½ cup berries (PHASE 3 ONLY)

continued from page 43

show you how to adapt the recipes for just about any lifestyle. Plus, in the recipes themselves, you'll see notes on how to easily adjust the recipes to make them complete meals or snacks.

Phase 1: Fast Release (Days 1 through 4)

This phase sheds fat quickly to give you a jump start. In reviewing research for the Digest Diet, I learned that losing weight quickly not only boosts motivation, but it may also help you keep the pounds off. The results of a study conducted in Florida suggest that fast weight loss leads to greater short- and long-term weight loss. I'm sold, as were the members of our test panel: Adrienne Farr and Diane Rohan each lost 7 pounds in Phase 1, and they felt great!

During Phase 1, you'll be flooding your body with nutrition from two shakes each day. You'll find the recipe on page 67. As you'll see, the basic ingredients—nonfat yogurt, light coconut milk, nonfat milk powder, and honey—load you up with protein, calcium, and healthy fats. Then you can mix and match your choice of fruit/fiber, healthy fats, and flavorings to get as much variety as you'd like. (If you have blender issues, try blending everything except the frozen ingredients first; then add the ice cubes and frozen fruit, if using, push to the bottom, and blend.) Be sure to refrigerate your shake if you've made it in advance. Then give it a good shaking to remix; otherwise it might be too thick to drink.

Soup it up with our fiber- and protein-rich meals in a bowl once

DAILY CALORIE AND NUTRIENT GUIDELINES

Calories	**Phase 1: 1,200 calories; Phases 2 and 3: 1,400 to 1,600 calories for women; 1,600 to 1,800 calories for men**
Protein	46 to 58g
Vitamin C	75mg
Fiber	35g or more
Calcium	1,000mg, from three servings of dairy foods
Fat	20 to 35 percent of total calories; no more than 10 percent of calories from saturated fat; no trans fats
Sodium	Use reduced-sodium, low-sodium, and no-salt-added products when available

Diane Rohan

11 Pounds and 8.5 Inches Lost!

"I've been battling my weight all my life," says this energetic 48-year-old event planner and mother of a teenage son. She eats well and exercises because it makes her feel good. That's why it's all the more frustrating that since entering her early forties, losing weight has felt like an unwinnable challenge. "The last 4 or 5 years, nothing is working. The doctor tells me I'm 'middle-aging.' Well, I just don't accept that, the whole 'You're getting older, you're spreading out, and that's the way it is.'"

The Digest Diet was just the jump start she needed—Diane lost 7 pounds in just 4 days and more than 11 pounds in 3 weeks. Around Day 15, she began to experience doubt: The menus provided such a bounty of food, she thought, that she couldn't possibly continue to lose. But the fat releasing menu surprised her and proved its power.

"I stuck to this diet. I was determined to lose weight. And I did." Not only did she succeed in releasing the pounds, she also feels and looks amazing. "I am less sluggish and can zip my size 10 jeans!" When asked what's next for her, the answer is simple: "The size 8s at the back of my closet!"

a day. Be sure to stick with the Phase 1 soup recipes that you'll find on pages 90–95 of Chapter 5 (or any of the soups from the original Digest Diet book). But no doubt you'll want to eat some of the soups more often than others, so feel free to swap them as you like. You also can swap ingredients from the same fat releaser category, for example, chicken rather than beef for protein or cauliflower in place of broccoli for vitamin C. The soup recipes make big enough batches to share with family members and friends or to pack into single servings for yourself.

A snack a day is essential during Phase 1. I find crunchy snacks to be particularly satisfying on the days when most of my calories are liquid. They give my teeth something to sink into and help keep hunger at bay between meals. Each snack contains fiber for crunch and satisfaction, plus protein and vitamin C. See pages 44–45 for details.

Be sure to drink plenty of water in addition to the liquids you're getting in the shakes and soups to keep you well hydrated. There's nothing good in soda, so definitely do without. But if you're craving the bubbles and don't mind the bloat, limit yourself to one glass of seltzer per day with a generous squeeze of lemon or lime.

So, to recap, here's what you need to do on Phase 1 Fast Release:

▶ Drink two shakes a day. Use the recipe on page 67.

▶ Have soup for one of your meals. Choose from the recipes on pages 90–95.

▶ Eat one crunchy snack a day. Choose from the list on pages 44–45.

▶ Drink plain or sparkling water throughout the day. Add lime or lemon for flavor, if you prefer.

Phase 2: Fade Away (Days 5 through 14)

Liquids remain a big part of your diet in Phase 2 Fade Away. First, have a big glass of water with a few generous squeezes of fresh lemon, lime, or orange before each meal or snack. This boosts hydration, amps up your vitamin C, and helps curb your appetite. Then, continue to shake it up with one shake a day. You'll notice that the Fade Away Shake (on page 69) is a bit different from the Fast Release Shake, with more fat releasing protein and less fat. I suggest having the shake as your breakfast to kick off your morning with fat releasing calcium, dairy, and protein. For those mornings when you're in the mood for one of our protein-rich breakfast dishes on pages 70–77, you can have your shake at lunch instead.

Now, think lean and green. This phase emphasizes lean protein and micronutrient-rich greens to help your body flush out fat and build muscle. We were inspired by the lean meats, green veggies, and healthy fats in traditional Mediterranean-style diets, so we crafted our Fade Away recipes around these nutrition-packed foods but changed up the spicing with seasonings and flavors from around the world. In the recipe chapters, look for your Fade Away recipes at the beginning of most of the chapters. Check out our simple combinations of chicken, fish, beef, or pork with a rainbow array of different veggies, prepared with healthy MUFAs and PUFAs. A nightly glass of wine—4 ounces for women and 6 ounces for men—is an added bonus for its fat releasing resveratrol! If you don't drink wine, red grapes are a sweet alternative.

Add an extra snack to bring your total to two for the day. As in Phase 1, snacks should offer a combination of protein, fiber, and vitamin C.

 LAUGH IT OFF

It was an absolutely crazy evening at our emergency clinic. The doctor on duty was being bombarded with questions, given forms to fill out, and even asked for his dinner order. I was in the next room, cleaning up a sutured wound, when I realized the doctor hadn't given instructions for a bandage.

"What kind of dressing do you want on that?" I shouted through the door.

"Ranch," he yelled back. —BRENDA TODD

So, here's what you need to remember on Phase 2 Fade Away:

▶ Drink water first, eat second.

▶ Have one shake a day. Use the recipe on page 69.

▶ Go lean (proteins) and green (veggies) at meals. Each meal should be around 425 to 450 calories, but be sure to leave some room for your red wine (about 100 calories for 4 ounces, 150 for 6 ounces or 20 to 30 red grapes. You can do this in several ways:

- Mix and match Phase 2 recipes in the following chapters to reach the appropriate calorie count. For instance, you may pair a Phase 2 Main Dish with a Phase 2 Salad and a Phase 2 Side Dish.

- Choose from the Phase 2 One-Dish Mains on pages 152–167. Toss 2 cups of salad greens with 1 tablespoon Digest Diet Vinaigrette (see below) and serve on the side.

- Pair a Phase 2 Main Dish (from pages 112–131) with 2 cups steamed (or microwaved) nonstarchy vegetables (broccoli, cauliflower, green beans, peppers, eggplant, fennel, jicama, kale, spinach, collards, etc.).

Digest Diet Vinaigrette

To make the Digest Diet Vinaigrette, grate 1 clove garlic on a citrus zester into a small screw-top jar or any tight-sealing container. Add ½ cup fresh lemon juice, fresh lime juice, or vinegar (red wine, white wine, sherry, rice, red balsamic, white balsamic); 2 tablespoons Dijon mustard; ½ teaspoon dried tarragon, oregano, mint, or dill (if you'd like); and ½ teaspoon ground black pepper. Shake well to combine. Then add ¼ cup + 1 tablespoon extra-virgin olive oil and shake to emulsify. If you have the time, let the dressing sit for a while. This should yield 1 cup of dressing. Each tablespoon of Digest Diet Vinaigrette is 41 calories.

Keep this simple fat releasing vinaigrette on hand to dress up salads and plain steamed greens. It's easy to whip up a batch—it only takes 5 minutes—and you can store it in the refrigerator for up to a week. The oil might solidify in the fridge, though; just leave it out at room temperature for a few minutes before using.

- Pair 4 ounces of broiled, grilled, or roasted lean protein (chicken, beef, pork) or 6 ounces of broiled, grilled, or poached lean fish or shrimp with a Phase 2 Side Dish (from pages 224–236). Or look for the "Make It a Main" tips on some of the recipes for more creative ways to round out those side dishes or salads into a meal.

▶ In most cases, you'll see that the recipes already contain healthy MUFAs and omega-3 PUFAs, so you don't need to add more.

▶ Snack twice a day. Choose from the list on pages 44–45, any of the snacks in the appendix or the original Digest Diet book, or create your own.

▶ Enjoy a glass of red wine or a bunch of red grapes at dinner.

Phase 3: Finish Strong (Days 15 through 21)

This last week is filled with balanced, healthy, whole foods that also are rich in fat releasers. By this point in the plan, you should be looking and feeling pretty great. Now's the time to fully embrace balance in a way that brings you through this final week while also readying you to continue moving forward. What do I mean by balance? Balancing your protein, fat, and carbohydrates. Balancing your plate with a variety of different foods at each meal. Balancing your fat releasers at each meal. Balancing your life so there's room for enjoyment.

Continue your good Phase 2 habits. Drink water first and eat second. In this phase, you can add a serving of carbs to your meals; in most cases, we recommend that you stick to just ½ cup of brown rice, quinoa, or other whole grain. Snack twice a day, adding fruit on occasion. (You'll also see fruit in some of the Phase 3 recipes.) Raise a glass or pop some grapes every evening. And enjoy a dessert or favorite treat once each week to avoid feeling deprived. After all your efforts, there's no need to let deprivation sabotage your success.

SUITABLE SWAPS

What if you are allergic to particular foods, just don't like them, or want to mix it up a bit? In general, most types of protein are interchangeable, as are most types of nuts or seeds and most types of whole grains. Here are some specific swaps to try but keep in mind that changing ingredients in recipes may require adjusting cooking times. Have fun experimenting!

Instead of . . .	Try . . .
Fat-free milk	Calcium-fortified soy milk; calcium-fortified almond or other nut milk
Coconut milk	Coconut oil plus water
Plain yogurt	Kefir; fat-free milk; 0% plain Greek yogurt (but not in the shakes)
Fish and shellfish	4 ounces lean chicken, turkey, beef, or pork; tofu; beans
Sandwich thins	Thin-sliced, whole-grain bread
Zucchini	Yellow squash
Leeks	Onions
Escarole	Kale; spinach
Broccoli	Cauliflower
Broccoli rabe	Broccoli; broccolini
Butternut squash	Carrot
Serrano chile pepper	Jalapeño pepper
Ancho chile powder	Other types of powdered chiles or chili seasoning
Raw almond butter	Regular almond butter; natural peanut butter
White beans	Black, red kidney or pinto beans; chickpeas
Flaxseed (in the shakes)	Oat bran; Chia seeds
One type of nut or seed	Another nut or seed
One type of whole grain	Any other type of whole grain

This is what you need to do on Phase 3 Finish Strong:

⟩ Drink first, eat second.

⟩ Balance lean proteins, healthy fats, and whole grains with each meal. Each meal should be around 425 to 450 calories. You can do this in several ways:

- Mix and match recipes in the following chapters to reach the appropriate calorie count. For instance, you may pair a Phase 2 or 3 Main Dish with a Phase 2 or 3 Side Dish.

- Choose from any of the One-Dish Mains on pages 152–187. Toss 2 cups of salad greens with 1 tablespoon Digest Diet Vinaigrette (see page 50) and serve on the side.

- Pair a Phase 3 Main Dish (from pages 132–149) with 2 cups steamed (or microwaved) nonstarchy vegetables (broccoli, cauliflower, green beans, peppers, eggplant, fennel, jicama, kale, spinach, collards, etc.).

- Pair 4 ounces of broiled, grilled, or roasted lean protein (chicken, beef, pork) or 6 ounces of broiled, grilled, or poached lean fish or shrimp with a Phase 3 Side Dish (from pages 237–251). Or look for the "Make It a Main" tips on some of the recipes for more creative ways to round side dishes out into a meal.

- Add a ½-cup serving of couscous or brown rice or 2 ounces of whole-grain bread to any Phase 2 Main Dish.

⟩ Snack twice a day. Choose from the list on pages 44–45, any of the snacks in the appendix or the original Digest Diet book, or create your own.

⟩ Enjoy a dessert once a week. Choose from the recipes on pages 254–277.

● MAKING THE DIGEST DIET YOUR DIET

Each of us is an individual, so what works for me and what works for you may be very different. For instance, because caffeine is dehydrating, I encourage you to give it up if you can. I was surprised to find I didn't miss it when I did. But if you really need a little pick-me-up in the morning, feel free to drink up to one cup a day of coffee or tea, but not soda. If you need your drink sweetened, honey is the first choice because it's a fat releaser. If you don't like honey, use up to 1 teaspoon of raw or turbinado sugar. Artificial sweeteners are off limits. To whiten your drink, add a splash of nonfat or skim-plus milk. But no fake creamers or fat-free half-and-half—they make up for the fat by adding a lot of corn syrup.

Eat foods *you* like:

If a recipe or meal includes a food that you are allergic to or don't enjoy eating, swap it for something else within the same phase. See the list of suitable swaps on page 52.

If you find recipes or meals you particularly like, feel free to keep repeating them as long as you stay within the right phase of the diet. Make a big batch of a favorite recipe and enjoy it for a few days, or divide it into single servings and freeze.

Give dairy a try—most of us don't get enough of it. But if you truly can't tolerate milk, even after taking a lactase tablet, switch to soy, almond, or other nut milks. Make sure you choose brands that are fortified with calcium to replace the calcium in cow's milk. And add as many nondairy sources of calcium as you can. See the list of top nondairy sources of calcium, opposite.

Adjust the diet to fit *your* lifestyle:

If your weeknights are always busy, plan and prep ahead. Spend Sunday afternoon chopping vegetables, precooking meats, making soups ahead of time, and freezing portions. If it works within your budget, buy vegetables and meat that are already trimmed and cut.

If you're frequently on the go, invest in sturdy containers to carry food with you—an insulated lunchbox, single-serve containers and plastic bags, freezable gel packs, utensils.

Top Nondairy Sources of Calcium	Serving size	Calcium (mg)	% of daily needs
Almond milk (calcium-fortified)	1 cup	450	45
Almonds	1 ounce	75	7
Black-eyed peas, cooked	1 cup	211	21
Bok choy, cooked	2 cups	316	32
Broccoli, cooked	2 cups	125	12
Canned salmon	3 ounces	181	18
Canned sardines	3 ounces	325	33
Coconut milk yogurt	4 ounces	200	20
Collard greens, cooked	1 cup	266	27
Edamame, shelled	1 cup	261	26
Mixed vegetable juice (calcium-enhanced)	1 cup	295	30
Orange juice (calcium-fortified)	1 cup	350	35
Rice milk (calcium-fortified)	1 cup	283	28
Soy yogurt	1 cup	300	30
Soy milk (calcium-fortified)	1 cup	299	30
Spinach, cooked	1 cup	291	29
Tofu, firm	3 ounces	163	16
Turnip greens, cooked	1 cup	197	20
White beans, cooked	1 cup	191	19

If you're on a budget, buy ingredients in bulk, portion them into smaller packages, and freeze for later use. Also, feel free to substitute less-expensive ingredients in the recipes (frozen shrimp instead of fresh, for instance; regular peanut butter instead of raw almond butter). See the list of suitable swaps on page 52.

continued on page 58

THE 21-DAY PLAN

PHASE 1: DAYS 1–4
FAST RELEASE

Flood your body with nutrition:
Phase 1 fills you up on liquid shakes and soups that are rich in vitamins, minerals, and protein, to gently coax your body into quick, safe weight loss. (Our top tester lost 10 pounds during this phase!)

Eating Rules

▶ Drink two Fast Release Shakes a day (see recipe on page 67). One at breakfast, to start the day off right; the second, you can choose to have as your lunch or dinner meal.

▶ Snack once a day.

▶ Have a 2-cup serving of soup for lunch or dinner. See pages 90–95 for a variety of soup recipes.

▶ Space meals according to your needs, but try to go no longer than 4 hours between eating.

PHASE 2: DAYS 5–14
FADE AWAY

Go lean and green: That's the theme of this 10-day phase in which you'll continue to enjoy steady weight loss, while enjoying a Mediterranean-style diet rich in lean protein, healthy fats, and a bounty of vegetables. And yes: You get to enjoy a glass of red wine with dinner, if you like.

Eating Rules

▶ Drink water first, eat second.

▶ Have 1 Fade Away Shake a day (see recipe on page 69).

▶ Think lean and green when making choices.

▶ Eat healthy fats (MUFAs and PUFAs).

▶ Snack twice a day.

▶ Enjoy a glass of wine or a handful of red grapes at dinner.

PHASE 3: DAYS 15–21 FINISH STRONG

Eat a balanced diet for life: That's what Phase 3 teaches you as you enjoy a wider variety of foods (such as pizza, pasta, and bread), while consuming proper portions of carbs, proteins, and healthy fats. And, of course, every meal will contain a number of healthy fat releasing foods! This phase helps you both reach your goal weight and maintain what you've lost.

Eating Rules

▶ Continue to drink water first, eat second.

▶ Continue to snack twice a day.

▶ Continue to enjoy a glass of red wine with dinner.

▶ Enjoy a dessert or favorite treat once a week.

▶ Bring a balanced eye.

HELPFUL HINT
FOLLOW OUR SERVING SIZES

Pay careful attention to serving sizes as you plan your meals. Most of the recipes serve 4 (and in the case of soups, up to 8). This is so those of you cooking for families or who wish to make and freeze meals ahead can do so. To be sure you are eating single servings, follow the portion guide at the bottom of the recipes (where the nutritional information is given). Also, if you are cooking for one, you'll see tips on many of the recipes to help you scale them to size.

continued from page 55

If you're cooking for one, pay careful attention to serving sizes as you read through the recipes. Most of the recipes make 4 or more servings. This is so those of you cooking for families or who wish to make and freeze meals ahead can do so. To be sure you are eating single servings, follow the portion guide at the bottom of the recipes (where the nutritional information is given). And look for the "Cooking for One" tips on some of the recipes to help you scale down the ingredients.

In the appendix, you'll find sample menu plans for some common diet challenges like these. There you'll also find more tips and advice on how to tailor the recipes and the plan for people who are: Vegetarian, Dairy-free, On a Budget, Cooking for One, and in need of a Quick Fix.

Finally, make the Digest Diet *your* diet for life:

If you've reached your goal weight or are close to it, keep following Phase 3 after the 21 days.

If you still have some weight to lose, cycle between Phase 2 Fade Away for 10 days and Phase 3 Finish Strong for 2 weeks. We recommend waiting 1 or 2 months before repeating Phase 1 and limiting repeats to no more than four times a year. Here's why: We chose, and science supports, the 1,200-calorie level in Phase 1 to quickly jump-start weight loss. But it's too limited and not sustainable long term. Plus, your body may think it's being deprived and react by holding on to, rather than releasing, fat. So keep on cycling between Phases 2 and 3 until you've reached your goal weight.

 LAUGH IT OFF

"When I married Donna, I could get both hands around her waist," said my husband's grandfather. Pointing at his full-figured wife, he boasted, "Now look how much I got. That's what I call an investment!"

—KATHERINE EBY

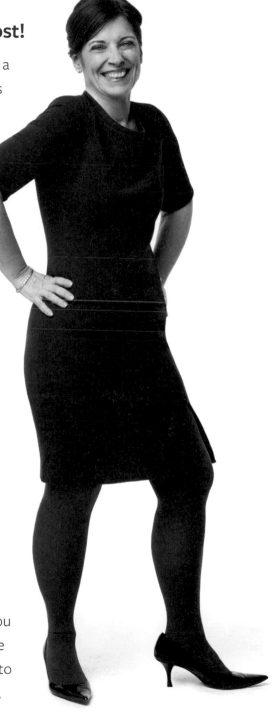

Annette Procida

11 Pounds and Almost 6 Inches Lost!

This busy working mom of three had come to a full stop. After losing 50 pounds, her weight loss had come to a standstill. She believed that the plateau was due to the hormonal changes going on in her body. "I felt that this diet came at the right time, to help me put my body back in losing mode."

According to Annette, "In the beginning, I was a little freaked out when I saw those shakes and soups. I thought I would be starving. But to tell you the truth, that was my favorite part! It was filling; it was delicious; it was easy."

One major factor in Annette's success: her 23-year-old daughter, Dana, who did the Digest Diet with her mother and lost 8 pounds in 3 weeks. Says Dana: "We enjoyed making the recipes together, putting love into the food." What else added to their success? They both exercised every day.

Annette intends to reach her goal weight by continuing with the Digest Diet. And her advice to those who fall off the path is simple: "Sure, you are going to want to eat something you love, like pizza or pasta, but that's okay. You have a guide to get right back and keep on going with your new, healthy way of eating."

FREQUENTLY ASKED QUESTIONS

We've received great feedback from readers like you, along with questions and comments about the Digest Diet details, stages, menus, and recipes. I've been collecting them to share with you to make your Digest Diet experience easier and more successful.

Will I still lose weight during Phase 2 Fade Away, even though I'm eating more food than in Phase 1 Fast Release?

No worries. We've designed the Digest Diet to help you release fat in each of the three phases. During Fade Away, your lunch and dinner switch from the shakes and soups of Fast Release to lean proteins and micronutrient-rich greens. The protein and vegetables provide your body with what it needs to help you release fat and build muscle. You'll also be drinking a big glass of water with a few generous squeezes of fresh lemon, lime, or orange before each meal or snack for hydration and to help curb your appetite.

If I get hungry, what should I do?

We've designed the Digest Diet with meals and snacks that help manage hunger. And it may take a day or so for your body to adjust to a new way of eating. But if you do feel an occasional pang or two, first enjoy a big glass of water or seltzer with a squeeze of fresh lemon or lime juice. Still hungry? Have an all-veggie salad with a teaspoon of Digest Diet Vinaigrette (page 50).

I'm a big guy. Are you sure that the Digest Diet provides me with enough food?

If you consistently feel weak or shaky, you may need more food. First, add a snack (see pages 44–45 for ideas). If that's still not enough, increase your meal portions by a half cup or so. Also, see if drinking a big glass of water with a squeeze of lemon juice or eating raw veggies plus a teaspoon of Digest Diet Vinaigrette might help you manage your hunger.

Can I wait to eat if I'm not hungry?

We'd like you to follow the meal and snack plan as closely as possible. It has been designed to help you manage your hunger in a way that helps you avoid the urge to overeat. In particular, snacks help keep you full, ward off cravings, and provide a satisfying crunch to your day.

What should I do if I can't give up coffee?

You don't have to! Because caffeine is a diuretic and dehydrating, though, we recommend limiting yourself to one cup of coffee or tea a day. Remember to leave out fat increasers such as creamers and artificial sweeteners.

Where can I find flaxseed meal and some of the other less common ingredients?

Your supermarket or local natural foods store likely carries flaxseed meal (sometimes labeled "ground flaxseed"), whole-grain products, and a wide assortment of vegetables. For top flavor, freshness, and nutrition, buy from a store that keeps its stock fresh. The oil in flaxseed meal and whole grains can turn rancid after more than a couple of months on the shelf. If your store doesn't carry certain grain products, visit the website for Bob's Red Mill, at bobsredmill.com, or for Hodgson Mill, at hodgsonmill.com.

I fell off the diet for a few days. Now what? Do I start over?

No need to start from Day 1. Just pick up where you left off and go from there. If you know ahead of time that you're going to have trouble following the diet for a few days—because you're going on vacation, have a big party to attend, or just have a busy stretch at work—plan ahead as much as possible. Prepare some portable snacks, freeze some Digest Diet meals, and study up on fat releasers so you can recognize them wherever you are. Then just do the best you can during those days—do your best to avoid fake foods, get as many fat releasers into your meals as possible, and remember to drink water before each meal.

My weight loss has stalled. What's going on?

Everybody loses weight at different rates; and frequently, especially after losing several pounds quickly, your body wants to hang on to the fat it has left. Don't panic, and especially don't cut back on the number of calories you're eating. That will just make your body hang on tighter to its protective fat. Instead, keep following the plan, enjoy the food, add some more movement to your day, and trust that safe and lasting weight loss will follow. If you don't start losing weight again after a week or so, though, you may want to start tracking your meals and activity more closely to see if you're unconsciously sabotaging your efforts in any way.

Could the diet be the cause of my headache and stuffed nose that started on Day 2?

Giving up drinks with caffeine—coffee, tea, soda—may be the cause. It's okay to have one daily cup of coffee or tea, just no soda. Make sure you're drinking enough water by sipping throughout the day to stay hydrated. Eat no more than 4 hours after your last meal or snack, as hunger can cause headaches. Your body also might be detoxing now that you're eating a healthy diet. Our test panel found that they felt great after a day or two. And consider stress as a possible cause; then destress by taking a walk or doing something positive and healthy that helps you relax.

Can I use fat-free creamer or fat-free half-and-half in my coffee or tea? What about aspartame, stevia, or other calorie-free sweeteners?

No. They are "fakes," a type of fat increaser that is filled with artificial additives. Instead, try skim-plus milk. It has a rich and creamy flavor and supplies two fat releasers—dairy and calcium. For a sweetener, try a teaspoon of honey, another fat releaser. Homegrown stevia would be okay, but steer clear of store-bought stevia. Although it says it is "natural," the way it is processed is not.

A lot of the snacks and meals are served with fat-free milk. I understand it's important to get my dairy, but I hate the taste of fat-free milk! Any suggestions?

I love to boost milk's fat releasing properties with a teaspoon of unsweetened cocoa powder per cup of milk. Or you could try ½ teaspoon honey for sweetness. Another alternative to plain milk is nonfat yogurt (see page 34 for a list of our favorites), to which you can add any Fat Releaser Seasonings (page 31) you'd like.

Is it okay to add coconut oil to my shakes as a healthy fat?

No. The coconut milk in the shakes supplies coconut oil, a proven fat releaser, so adding more would be too much. If you really want to use coconut oil, add ½ tablespoon plus water in place of coconut milk and then choose a different healthy fat.

Can I use Greek yogurt or kefir in my shakes?

In general, Greek yogurt has less calcium and more calories than regular yogurt, so it's not appropriate for the shakes. Feel free to substitute it for regular yogurt in other recipes, though; just keep in mind that it's thicker than regular yogurt. Kefir is okay to use in your shakes, though it will make for a thinner shake; just read the ingredient label to make sure the brand you choose has a comparable amount of calcium as regular yogurt, at least 30 percent of the Daily Value per 1-cup serving.

I'm lactose intolerant. How can I follow the diet?

Dairy is a key fat releaser, so it's worth trying to get as much as you can. Enzymes like those in Lactaid can help. Also, many people find that hard cheese gives them less trouble than milk, cream, and soft cheeses. But if you truly can't tolerate it, look for soy, almond, and other nondairy substitutes. See the appendix for sample meal plans to show you how to follow the Digest Diet dairy-free.

Does the Digest Diet work for vegetarians?

Vegetarians can follow the Digest Diet by sticking to the eating plan while substituting plant options as needed, such as beans, tofu, or nuts as a protein source and fortified nut milk for calcium. See the appendix for sample meal plans to show you how to do that. Be sure to consult your doctor, dietitian, or nutritionist if you have specific questions.

Can I use meals from one phase in a different phase?

In Phase 1 and 2, we suggest only swapping shakes and foods that are in the same phase. Once you're in Phase 3 Finish Strong, you can use recipes from any of the phases, but we do suggest trying some of the breakfast recipes in place of the shakes to get the right balance of carbs and protein.

I have type 2 diabetes. Can I follow the Digest Diet? Some of the fat releasers are very high in carbs.

While it's true that a few of the fat releasers are high in carbs, we do emphasize whole grains and complex carbohydrates that break down more slowly and have a less severe impact on your blood sugar levels. Plus, many of the fat releasers, such as dairy and fiber, have been shown to be beneficial for keeping blood sugar under control, so most of the meals on the Digest Diet are very healthy for someone with diabetes. But consult with your doctor, dietitian, or certified diabetes educator to be sure you're getting the right nutrition for your specific condition.

Is it okay to add more seasoning?

Yes, you can choose from the variety of seasonings listed on page 31. However, we suggest that you limit salt and use lemon or lime juice instead to brighten flavor and boost fat release.

How can I make the meals gluten-free?

Most fat releasing foods, recipes, and meals already are gluten-free. You can substitute comparable gluten-free ingredients for any gluten-containing ingredients in recipes.

I don't see peaches, watermelon, or cucumber on the list of fat releasing foods or anywhere in the diet. Does that mean I can't have them?

Not all fruits are fat releasers, but that doesn't mean you can't eat them! Because some fruits are high in sugar, in Phases 1 and 2, you'll find fruit only in the shakes. But we didn't have room to list all the possible fruit combinations, so feel free to try some different ones in the shakes. In Phase 3 Finish Strong, you can also have fruit as a snack or dessert.

Similarly, if your favorite vegetable isn't on the list, that doesn't mean it's unhealthy, just that it doesn't have as many fat releasing properties as the ones that are on the list. So feel free to add them to your diet when appropriate.

Should I be taking a multivitamin?

When you're eating a well-balanced diet of real foods like the Digest Diet, you shouldn't need a multivitamin. But check with your doctor to make sure you don't have a condition that may warrant supplementation.

What types of exercise should I be doing?

If you have a steady exercise routine, stick with it as long as it works for you and offers a combo of strength training and aerobic calorie burning. You can help protect yourself against injury by avoiding strength training 2 days in a row, maintaining proper form during exercise, and taking it easy when your body says it needs a rest.

If you don't already have a regular routine or if you want to shake things up, you may want to try the 12-Minute Fat Release Workout in the original *The Digest Diet* book. A simple strength-training regimen that incorporates HIIT, it can really help jump-start your weight loss when combined with daily walks. You may want to work with a trainer if you're new to exercise, have a high body weight, or have injured or painful joints. You may not see a difference on the scale right away, but you'll notice how much better you look and feel!

Is there someone I can ask if I have more questions about the Digest Diet?

Visit us at readersdigest.com/digestdiet or facebook.com/digestdiet. Not only can you ask questions about the diet there, but you'll also find a built-in support group in the many other readers around the country who are doing the Digest Diet with you! Remember, one of the key tenets of the diet is to buddy up; here's a good way to do it!

Chapter

4

Breakfasts

Start your day right with these
delicious grab-and-go recipes!

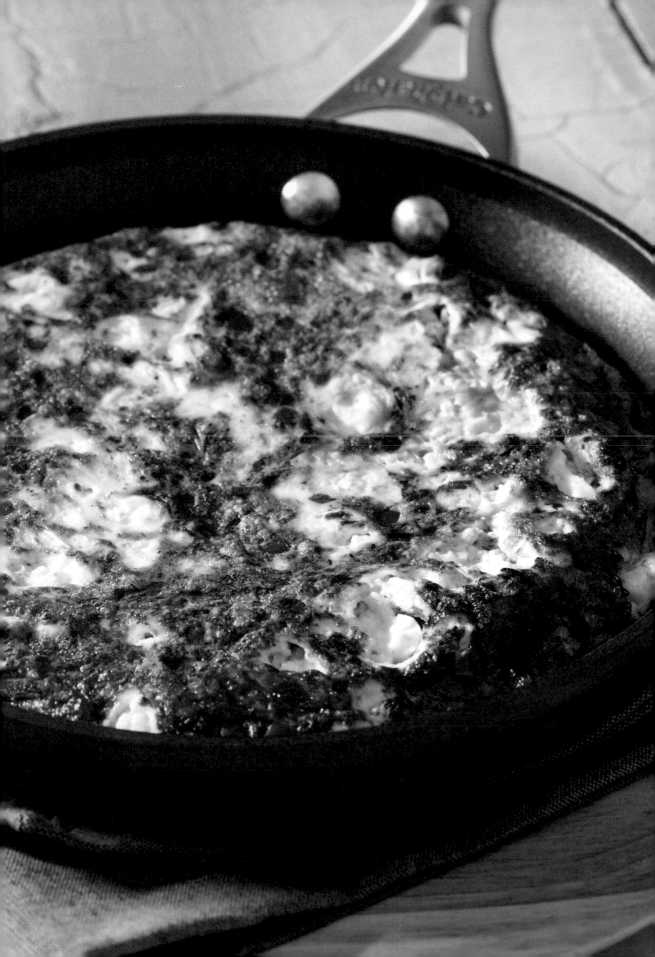

Strawberry Almond Shake

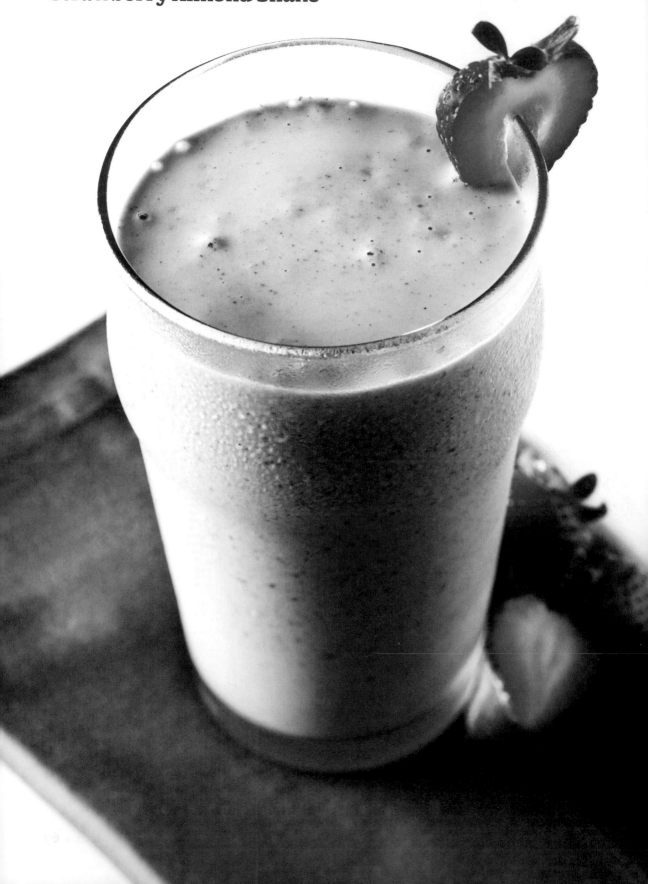

Fast Release Shake (Days 1–4)

Hands-On Time: 10 minutes • **Total Time:** 10 minutes • **Makes:** 1 shake

Pick your favorite shake and stick with it for simplicity, or if you're feeling adventurous, plan a different flavor combination for every day. Remember, during this stage of the diet, you'll be drinking two shakes a day (see Chapter 3, pages 46–48). Note that the shake is minimally sweet on purpose to keep you from getting hungry too soon. Please don't be tempted to add more honey.

Fat Releasers
Yogurt, coconut milk, fruit/fiber, healthy fats, honey

MASTER RECIPE

- ¾ cup (6 ounces) nonfat yogurt
- ¼ cup light coconut milk
- 3 tablespoons nonfat milk powder

FRUIT/FIBER

HEALTHY FATS

- 2 teaspoons honey
- ½ teaspoon vanilla extract

FLAVORINGS (optional)

- 4 ice cubes

Combine all the ingredients in a blender and blend until nice and frothy.

A typical shake:

- 395 calories • 16g protein
- 18g fat (5g saturated)
- 9.5g fiber • 430mg calcium
- 40mg vitamin C
- 50g carbohydrate
- 210mg sodium

FRUIT/FIBER (choose 1)

1 banana

1 apple (peeled and cored) + 1 tablespoon flaxseed meal

8 strawberries (fresh or frozen) + 1 tablespoon flaxseed meal

4 ounces mixed frozen berries* (¾ to 1 cup, depending on the berries' size) + 1 tablespoon flaxseed meal

¾ cup seedless red grapes* (10 large) + 1 tablespoon flaxseed meal. Omit the honey.

1 tangerine or small orange* + 1 tablespoon flaxseed meal

HEALTHY FATS (choose 1)

½ avocado

1 tablespoon natural peanut butter

1 tablespoon raw or regular almond butter

1 tablespoon tahini

1 tablespoon sunflower seed butter

FLAVORINGS (choose none, 1, or both)

1 teaspoon unsweetened cocoa powder

¼ teaspoon ground cinnamon

*See Tasty Tips, page 68.

Peanut Butter and Grape Shake

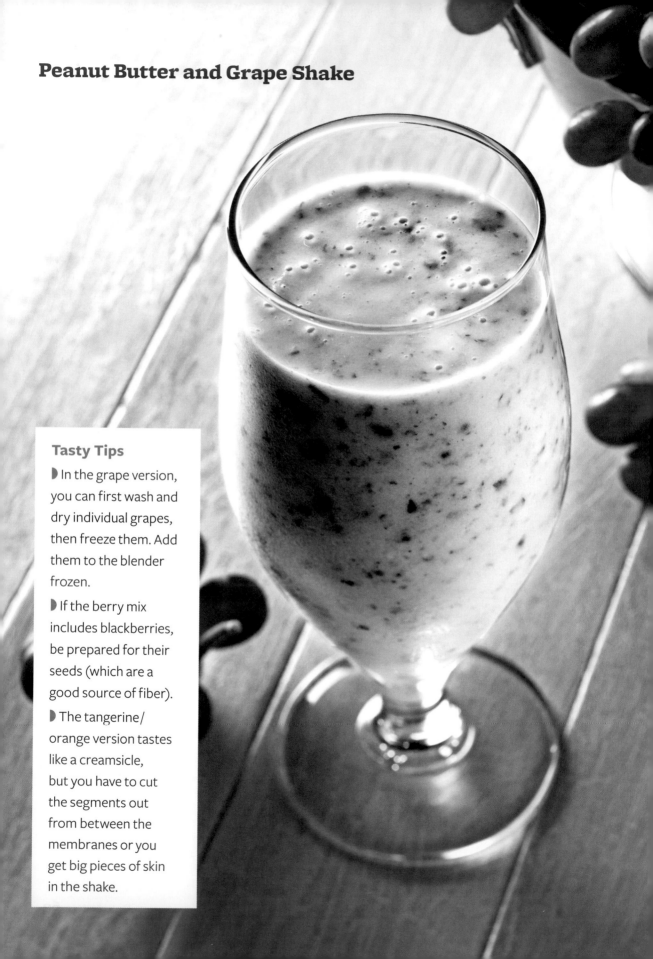

Tasty Tips

▶ In the grape version, you can first wash and dry individual grapes, then freeze them. Add them to the blender frozen.

▶ If the berry mix includes blackberries, be prepared for their seeds (which are a good source of fiber).

▶ The tangerine/orange version tastes like a creamsicle, but you have to cut the segments out from between the membranes or you get big pieces of skin in the shake.

Fade Away Shake (Days 5–14)

Hands-On Time: 10 minutes • **Total Time:** 10 minutes • **Makes:** 1 shake

This is principally the same as the Fast Release Shake (page 67), but the amount of fat has been cut back, since the focus in this phase is on lean protein and including more macronutrients in your meals. Remember, at this stage, you will be drinking a shake once a day, while snacking twice a day see Chapter 3, pages 49–51.

Fat Releasers
Yogurt, coconut milk, fruit/fiber, healthy fats, honey

MASTER RECIPE

- ¾ **cup (6 ounces) nonfat yogurt**
- 2 **tablespoons light coconut milk**
- 2 **tablespoons water**
- 3 **tablespoons nonfat milk powder**
- **FRUIT/FIBER**
- **HEALTHY FATS**
- 2 **teaspoons honey**
- ½ **teaspoon vanilla extract**
- **FLAVORINGS (optional)**
- 4 **ice cubes**

Combine all the ingredients in a blender and blend until nice and frothy.

A typical shake:
- 320 calories • 15g protein
- 11g fat (2.5g saturated)
- 7g fiber • 425mg calcium
- 40mg vitamin C
- 45g carbohydrate
- 205mg sodium

FRUIT/FIBER (choose 1)

1 banana

1 apple (peeled and cored) + 1 tablespoon flaxseed meal

8 strawberries (fresh or frozen) + 1 tablespoon flaxseed meal

4 ounces mixed frozen berries* (¾ to 1 cup, depending on the berries' size) + 1 tablespoon flaxseed meal

¾ cup seedless red grapes* (10 large) + 1 tablespoon flaxseed meal. Omit the honey.

1 tangerine or small orange* + 1 tablespoon flaxseed meal

HEALTHY FATS (choose 1)

¼ avocado

1 teaspoon natural peanut butter

1 teaspoon raw or regular almond butter

1 teaspoon tahini

1 teaspoon sunflower seed butter

FLAVORINGS (choose none, 1, or both)

1 teaspoon unsweetened cocoa powder

¼ teaspoon ground cinnamon

*See Tasty Tips, opposite.

Breakfast Egg Salad

Hands-On Time: 5 minutes • **Total Time:** 35 minutes • **Makes:** 2 servings

To keep the fat levels reasonable in this breakfast egg dish, a hard-boiled egg yolk is used to make a mayonnaise-style dressing using fat-free Greek yogurt, pureed sun-dried tomatoes, and a little vinegar. Any kind of vinegar will work here; white wine vinegar or cider vinegar would be nice, or choose your favorite. If you're in the Finish Strong phase, you can serve the salad on a slice of whole-grain toast.

Fat Releasers
Eggs, sun-dried tomatoes, yogurt, vinegar, black pepper

6 **large eggs**

3 **sun-dried tomatoes**

3 **tablespoons 0% Greek yogurt**

2 **teaspoons water**

1 **teaspoon vinegar**

Ground black pepper

3 **ounces low-sodium smoked ham, in one piece, cut into chunks to match the eggs**

1 **tablespoon chopped fresh herb, such as parsley, dill, basil, or cilantro (optional)**

1. In a medium saucepan, bring the eggs with water to cover to a low boil. Boil for 3 minutes, throw in the sun-dried tomatoes, turn off the heat, cover, and let sit for 17 minutes.

2. Fish out the sun-dried tomatoes and transfer to a mini food processor.

3. Peel the eggs and halve them. Discard 4 of the yolks and transfer 1 yolk to the mini food processor. Cut the remaining egg whites and yolk into large chunks and place in a bowl.

4. Add the yogurt, water, vinegar, and a large pinch of pepper to the mini food processor and process to a smooth dressing.

5. Add the dressing, ham, and herb (if using) to the eggs and toss to combine.

Per 1-cup serving: 187 calories • 25g protein • 7.5g fat (2.5g saturated) 0.5g fiber • 54mg calcium • 1mg vitamin C • 4g carbohydrate • 608mg sodium

Scrambled Eggs Piperade

Hands-On Time: 25 minutes • **Total Time:** 25 minutes • **Makes:** 4 servings

The combo of eggs, egg whites, cottage cheese, and a touch of reduced-fat cream cheese is rich without being overly fatty. You'll find a little bit of liquid remaining in the pan after it's cooked; just drain it off. If you're in Finish Strong, fold the eggs into a whole-grain flour tortilla and top it with a little salsa.

Fat Releasers
Olive oil, bell peppers, eggs, cottage cheese, cream cheese

- 4 teaspoons extra-virgin olive oil
- 1 small red bell pepper, cut into ½-inch squares
- 1 small green bell pepper, cut into ½-inch squares
- 4 large eggs
- 4 large egg whites
- ½ cup no-salt-added 1% cottage cheese
- 2 tablespoons ⅓-less-fat cream cheese
- ½ teaspoon salt

1. In a large nonstick skillet, heat 2 teaspoons of the oil over medium heat. Add the bell peppers and cook, stirring frequently, until tender, about 5 minutes. Transfer to a bowl.

2. In a food processor, combine the whole eggs, egg whites, cottage cheese, cream cheese, and salt and puree until smooth.

3. Add the remaining 2 teaspoons oil to the pan and cook the egg mixture over low heat, stirring all the while, until large soft curds form and the egg mixture is almost set, about 7 minutes. Stir in the peppers until combined, about 1 minute longer. Drain any liquid and serve.

COOKING FOR ONE: Use 1 teaspoon oil, 1 each whole egg and egg white, 2 tablespoons cottage cheese, and 1½ teaspoons cream cheese. Use half of a small bell pepper and ⅛ teaspoon salt.

Per ¾-cup serving: 176 calories • 14g protein • 11g fat (3.5g saturated) 0.5g fiber • 59mg calcium • 39mg vitamin C • 4g carbohydrate • 445mg sodium

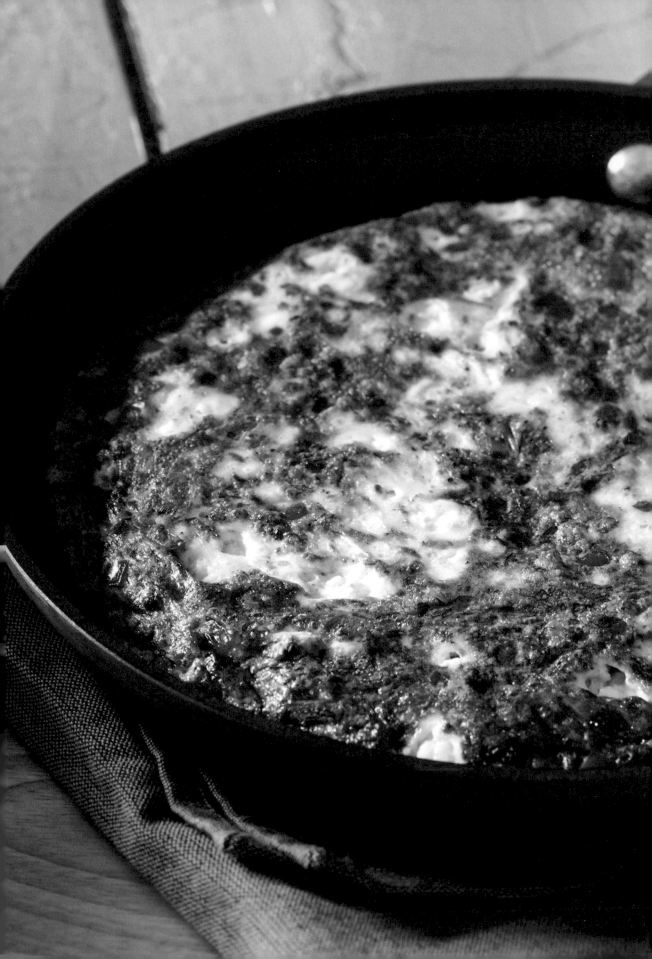

Savory Mediterranean Egg Cake

Hands-On Time: 10 minutes • **Total Time:** 25 minutes + standing time

Makes: 8 wedges

You can have the egg cake hot out of the pan, at room temp, or chilled. It's a great grab-and-go breakfast. Just pop 2 wedges in a sandwich bag—and if you'd prefer them warm, reheat gently in a toaster oven (about 10 minutes at 250°F) or the microwave (about 2 minutes at 50% power). Because the egg cake is made with a lot of egg whites, it will get wet as it sits, so you need to store the wedges (in the fridge) separated by sheets of waxed paper to absorb any excess liquid.

Fat Releasers
Olive oil, bell peppers, black pepper, eggs, parsley, cheese

- 4 teaspoons extra-virgin olive oil
- 1 tablespoon water
- 1 large red bell pepper, diced
- Salt
- Ground black pepper
- 5 large eggs
- 6 large egg whites
- ½ cup chopped parsley
- 2 teaspoons crumbled dried mint
- 2 teaspoons grated lemon zest
- ½ cup crumbled reduced-fat feta cheese

1. In a large nonstick skillet, heat 1 teaspoon of the oil and the water over medium-high heat. Add the bell pepper and a pinch each of salt and pepper, and cook until the water evaporates and the pepper is starting to sizzle. Scrape out of the skillet and set aside to cool slightly.

2. In a large bowl, beat together the whole eggs and egg whites. Stir in the parsley, mint, lemon zest, a pinch of salt and a generous pinch of pepper. Stir in the cooled bell pepper.

3. In the same skillet (no need to clean), heat the remaining 1 tablespoon oil over medium heat. Add the egg mixture and cook until set around the edges, about 1 minute. Reduce the heat to medium-low, cover, and cook until about halfway cooked, about 3 minutes.

4. Sprinkle on the feta, cover, and cook until mostly firm but still a little moist on top, 6 to 8 minutes. Remove from the heat and let sit covered for 10 minutes. (If the top is still too wet, place the skillet under broiler 6 inches from the heat for 1 or 2 minutes; make sure the handle of the skillet is wrapped in aluminum foil if it's not broilerproof.) Cut into 8 wedges.

Per 2-wedge serving: 207 calories • 18g protein • 13g fat (4g saturated) 1.5g fiber • 107mg calcium • 64mg vitamin C • 5g carbohydrate • 486mg sodium

Scallion Frittata

Hands-On Time: 10 minutes ● **Total Time:** 25 minutes ● **Makes:** 4 servings

A frittata is basically a giant omelet that can be served hot, warm, or even chilled. It's the perfect opportunity to use up leftover cooked vegetables such as chopped broccoli, asparagus, diced green beans, or chopped cooked greens. Add them to the pan with the scallions before adding the eggs.

Fat Releasers
Eggs, Parmesan cheese, black pepper, olive oil, scallions, cream cheese, tomato

- 3 **large eggs**
- 5 **large egg whites**
- ½ **cup grated Parmesan cheese**
- ¼ **teaspoon salt**
- ¼ **teaspoon ground black pepper**
- 1 **tablespoon plus 1 teaspoon extra-virgin olive oil**
- 1½ **cups thinly sliced scallions (about 6 large)**
- 2 **tablespoons ⅓-less-fat cream cheese, cut into small pieces**
- 1 **large tomato, diced**

1. Preheat the oven to 400°F. In a large bowl, whisk together the whole eggs, egg whites, Parmesan cheese, salt, and pepper.

2. In a large nonstick ovenproof skillet, heat the oil over medium heat. Add the scallions and cook, stirring occasionally, until tender, about 3 minutes. Add the beaten egg mixture and dollop the cream cheese on top. Reduce the heat to low and cook until the frittata starts to set around the edges, about 3 minutes.

3. Transfer to the oven and bake until set, 5 to 7 minutes. Run a spatula around the edges and slide the frittata onto a platter or serve from the pan; cut into 4 wedges. Serve topped with the tomato.

SAVE FOR A SNACK: If you have leftover frittata, cut a wedge in half (⅛ of the frittata) and have as a snack with ½ cup fat-free milk or 1 high-fiber cracker.

Per serving: 189 calories ● 14g protein ● 13g fat (4.5g saturated) ● 1g fiber 159mg calcium ● 9mg vitamin C ● 4g carbohydrate ● 448mg sodium

Homemade Breakfast Sausage

Hands-On Time: 25 minutes • **Total Time:** 25 minutes • **Makes:** 4 servings

It's super easy to make your own sausage patties when you use lean pork tenderloin and a food processor. Ancho chile powder is smoky with just a little bit of heat; feel free to swap in your favorite chili powder. If you'd like, double the ingredients and freeze for later. Form the patties and freeze them on a parchment-lined tray, then transfer them to freezer containers; freeze up to 3 months. Thaw in the refrigerator before cooking.

Fat Releasers
Pork, onion, garlic, chile powder, oregano, thyme, black pepper

1 **pound pork tenderloin, cut into chunks**

1 **onion, finely chopped**

2 **cloves garlic, finely chopped**

¾ **teaspoon grated orange zest**

1 **teaspoon ancho chile powder**

½ **teaspoon dried oregano**

½ **teaspoon dried thyme**

½ **teaspoon salt**

¼ **teaspoon ground black pepper**

1. Place half of the pork in the bowl of a food processor and pulse until coarsely ground. Transfer to a large bowl and repeat with the remaining pork. Add the onion, garlic, orange zest, ancho chile powder, oregano, thyme, salt, and pepper.

2. Shape into 8 patties, each about 1 inch thick.

3. Preheat the broiler with the rack 4 inches from the heat. Broil the sausages 3 minutes, then turn them over and broil until just cooked through, about 1 minute more.

Per 2-patty serving: 140 calories • 24g protein • 2.5g fat (1g saturated) 0.5g fiber • 21mg calcium • 3mg vitamin C • 4g carbohydrate • 352mg sodium

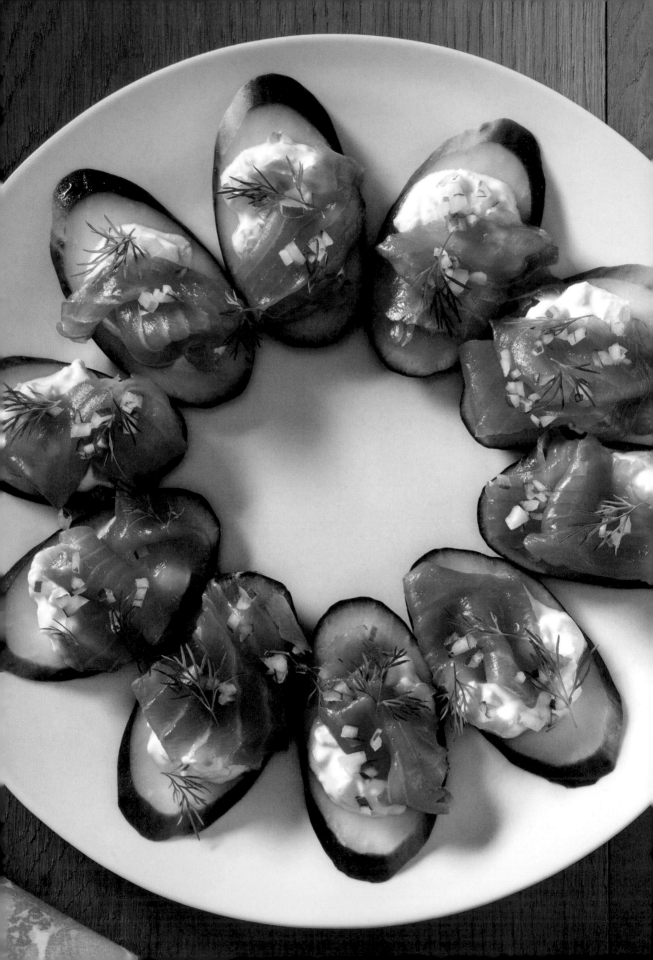

Smoked Salmon Breakfast Canapés

Hands-On Time: 30 minutes • **Total Time:** 30 minutes • **Makes:** 20 canapés

While these are great for breakfast (think bagels, cream cheese, and smoked salmon), they're also perfect for parties or a snack. In Finish Strong, you could assemble the canapés on slices of multigrain or pumpernickel cocktail bread instead.

Fat Releasers
Yogurt, cheese, salmon, onion

¾ cup 0% Greek yogurt

1½ ounces reduced-fat feta cheese, crumbled

2 small ribs celery, quartered lengthwise and thinly sliced (½ cup)

2 cucumbers, cut crosswise on the diagonal into long ovals (a total of 20 slices)

5 ounces sliced smoked salmon

2 tablespoons minced red onion

Sprigs of fresh dill

In a small bowl, stir together the yogurt, feta, and celery. Place the 20 cucumber slices on a platter and top with the feta mixture, smoked salmon, red onion, and dill.

Per 5-canapé serving: 124 calories • 14g protein • 3g fat (1.5g saturated) • 1.5g fiber • 124mg calcium • 7mg vitamin C • 11g carbohydrate • 457mg sodium

Fluffy Cottage Cheese Pancakes

Hands-On Time: 20 minutes • **Total Time:** 20 minutes • **Makes:** 12 pancakes

If you're making your own almond flour (which is just ground up almonds), there's always the risk you'll take it too far and end up with almond butter. Here we're grinding raw almonds with just a little whole-wheat flour to keep the almonds dry and fluffy when you grind them. Of course you could just use ½ cup store-bought almond flour if you happen to have it on hand, but keep the whole-wheat flour in the recipe to help bind the pancakes.

Fat Releasers
Almonds, whole-wheat flour, cottage cheese, honey, cinnamon, eggs, olive oil

½ cup raw almonds
¼ cup whole-wheat pastry flour
1 cup 1% cottage cheese
3 tablespoons honey
½ teaspoon ground cinnamon
½ teaspoon vanilla extract
1 large egg
3 large egg whites
¼ teaspoon salt
3 teaspoons extra-light olive oil

MAKE AHEAD: Make the whole batch and freeze what you aren't serving. Freeze the pancakes individually on a tray, then wrap in foil and store in a plastic storage bag. To reheat, leave in the foil and place in a toaster oven for 3 to 4 minutes, or unwrap completely and place on a microwave-safe dish and microwave in 30-second increments until heated through.

1. In a food processor, process the almonds and flour until the almonds are finely ground. Transfer to a large bowl and stir in the cottage cheese, honey, cinnamon, and vanilla. Stir in the whole egg.

2. In a large bowl, with an electric mixer, beat together the egg whites and salt until the whites form stiff but not dry peaks, about 2 minutes. Fold the whites into the batter until just combined with some streaks remaining.

3. In a large nonstick skillet, heat 1 teaspoon of the oil over medium-low heat. Drop the pancake batter into the pan in ¼ cupfuls, and cook until the tops of the pancakes are speckled with bubbles and some bubbles have popped and the underside of the pancake is golden brown, about 2 minutes. Using a thin-bladed spatula, carefully turn the pancakes over (they're delicate but will hold their shape) and cook until golden brown on the second side and set, about 1 minute. Repeat with the remaining oil and batter.

Per 3-pancake serving: 282 calories • 16g protein • 14g fat (2g saturated) 3.5g fiber • 100mg calcium • 0mg vitamin C • 25g carbohydrate • 435mg sodium

Homemade Instant Oatmeal

Hands-On Time: 3 minutes ● **Total Time:** 6 minutes ● **Makes:** 1 serving

Make up a whole bunch of these instant oatmeal packets to have on hand for a quick breakfast at home or at the office. The cooked oatmeal can be sweetened to taste with honey, agave nectar, or maple syrup. Start with 1 teaspoon sweetener and see if you can manage with a minimum. You can also make this in the microwave (especially helpful if you're planning on taking this to work): Place the oatmeal mixture in a 2-cup microwave-safe bowl or mug and stir to combine. Add 1 cup water and stir well. Cook on high for 45 seconds. Stir. Cook on high for 30 seconds. Stir and let sit for 1 minute.

Fat Releasers
Oats, coconut, cinnamon

½ **cup quick-cooking oats**
1 **tablespoon powdered coconut milk or buttermilk powder**
1 **tablespoon chopped dried fruit**
1 **tablespoon chopped nuts (optional)**
⅛ **teaspoon ground cinnamon**

1. Combine all the ingredients in a sandwich bag and seal. Store in an airtight container or in the refrigerator. Label it so you know what you put in it. If making oatmeal for multiple days, mix up each portion separately to ensure that you get the right distribution of ingredients.

2. When ready to cook, bring 1 cup water to a boil in a small saucepan. Stir in the oatmeal mixture and cook for 30 seconds. Remove from the heat, cover, and let sit for 1 minute.

Per serving: 228 calories ● 7g protein ● 4g fat (1g saturated) ● 7.5g fiber 39mg calcium ● 0mg vitamin C ● 41g carbohydrate ● 16mg sodium

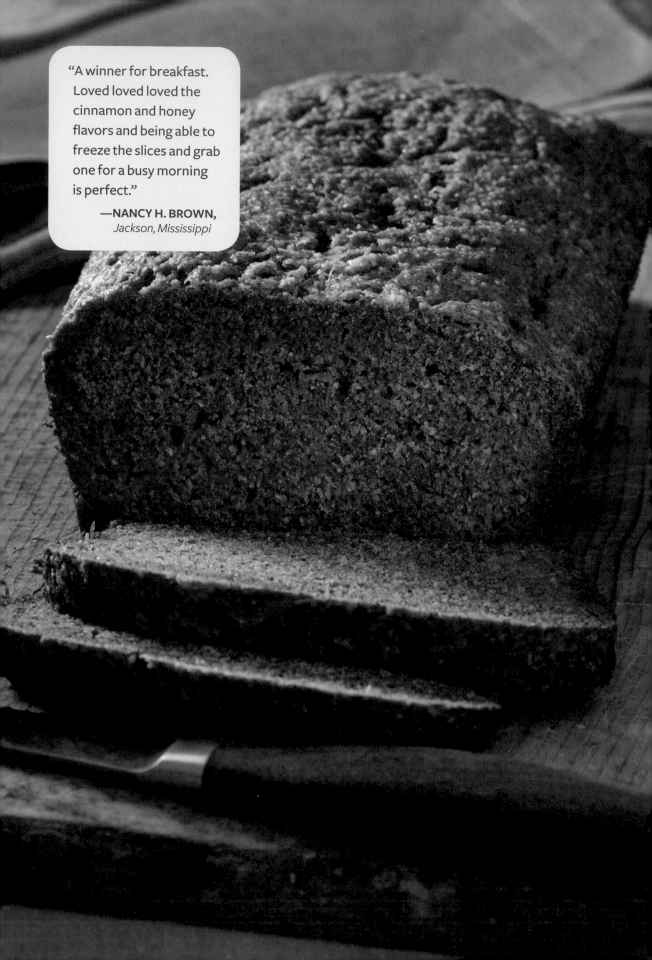

"A winner for breakfast. Loved loved loved the cinnamon and honey flavors and being able to freeze the slices and grab one for a busy morning is perfect."

—NANCY H. BROWN,
Jackson, Mississippi

Butternut Breakfast Bread

Hands-On Time: 10 minutes • **Total Time:** 50 minutes + cooling time

Makes: one 9-inch loaf

This is a dense, moist, and only lightly sweetened bread. It's brimming with beta-carotene and good fats, and it has over 4 grams of protein per slice. To make this a complete breakfast, have 2 slices (toasted, if you want) and top each with 2 tablespoons 0% Greek yogurt or 1 tablespoon fat-free cream cheese.

Fat Releasers
Almond flour, cinnamon, coconut oil, honey, eggs, butternut squash

2 cups white whole-wheat flour, spooned into the cup and then leveled

1 cup almond flour

2 teaspoons ground cinnamon

1½ teaspoons baking soda

½ teaspoon salt

⅓ cup coconut oil, melted

⅓ cup water

¼ cup honey, preferably dark

1 large egg

2 large egg whites

3 cups grated butternut squash (10 ounces)

1. Preheat the oven to 350°F. Lightly coat a 9 x 5-inch loaf pan with olive oil spray.

2. In a large bowl, combine the flours, cinnamon, baking soda, and salt and blend well. Beat in the oil, water, honey, whole egg, and egg whites. Fold in the squash.

3. Scrape the batter into the pan and smooth the top. Bake until a wooden pick inserted in the center of the loaf comes out clean, 35 to 45 minutes.

4. Let cool in the pan on a rack for 5 minutes, then turn out onto the rack to cool completely.

SAVE FOR A SNACK: After the bread is completely cooled, cut the loaf into ½-inch slices. Lay them on a tray or baking sheet and freeze solid. Once they are frozen, pack them into a large freezer storage bag. Then you can microwave or toast individual slices when you want one for breakfast.

Per ½-inch slice: 143 calories • 4g protein • 7.5g fat (4g saturated) • 3g fiber 35mg calcium • 3mg vitamin C • 17g carbohydrate • 191mg sodium

Quinoa & Walnut Muffins

Hands-On Time: 15 minutes • **Total Time:** 35 minutes • **Makes:** 12 muffins

To get 1½ cups of cooked quinoa, cook ½ cup raw in 2 cups of boiling water until tender, about 12 minutes; drain well. If you plan on making more of these muffins, make up a double batch of quinoa and store it in the freezer, where it will keep for 3 months. You can also bake extra muffins and store them in the freezer. Pop a frozen muffin, wrapped in foil, into a 350°F oven for 10 minutes to thaw.

Fat Releasers
Buttermilk, honey, oranges, flaxseed meal, olive oil, whole-wheat flour, quinoa, walnuts

¾ cup light (1.5%) buttermilk

⅓ cup honey

1 teaspoon grated orange zest

¼ cup fresh orange juice

3 tablespoons flaxseed meal

3 tablespoons extra-light olive oil

2 cups whole-wheat pastry flour

1½ teaspoons baking powder

¼ teaspoon baking soda

¼ teaspoon salt

1½ cups cooked quinoa

½ cup coarsely chopped walnuts (2½ ounces)

1. Preheat the oven to 350°F. Line a 12-cup muffin tin with paper liners.

2. In a large bowl, stir together the buttermilk, honey, orange zest, orange juice, flax meal, and oil.

3. In a separate bowl, stir together the flour, baking powder, baking soda, and salt. Pour the wet ingredients into the dry and stir just until moistened. Fold in the quinoa and walnuts.

4. Divide the batter among the muffin cups and bake until a wooden pick inserted in the center of a muffin comes out clean, 17 to 20 minutes. Cool in the pan for 5 minutes, then transfer the muffins to a wire rack to cool completely.

Per muffin: 210 calories • 5g protein • 8g fat (1g saturated) • 4g fiber
57mg calcium • 2mg vitamin C • 31g carbohydrate • 146mg sodium

Buttermilk Pancakes with Cherries

Hands-On Time: 30 minutes • **Total Time:** 30 minutes • **Makes:** 12 pancakes

You can make these pancakes ahead. Spread them out on a tray or cooling rack and place in the freezer. When frozen solid, pack a portion (2 pancakes) into individual plastic resealable bags. Pop them into the toaster oven (to "light" toast) or microwave (in 20-second bursts until heated through) to reheat for breakfast.

Fat Releasers
Pecans, oats, buttermilk powder, cinnamon, eggs, olive oil

- ¼ **pound fresh or thawed frozen cherries**
- 2 **teaspoons turbinado sugar**
- 1 **cup white whole-wheat flour**
- ½ **cup all-purpose flour**
- ¼ **cup finely ground pecans (the texture of cornmeal)**
- ¼ **cup quick-cooking oats**
- ⅓ **cup buttermilk powder or nonfat dried milk**
- 1 **tablespoon baking powder**
- ½ **teaspoon ground cinnamon**
- ½ **teaspoon salt**
- 2 **large eggs**
- 1 **tablespoon plus 1 teaspoon extra-light olive oil**
- 1⅓ **cups water**

1. At least 30 minutes before you plan on making the pancakes, finely mince ¼ cup of the cherries and set aside. Thinly slice the remaining cherries and toss in a bowl with 1 teaspoon of the sugar. Let the sliced cherries sit to develop some juiciness. (You can do this well ahead if you'd like; the longer you let the cherries sit, the more juice you'll get.)

2. In a medium bowl, stir together the flours, pecans, oats, buttermilk powder, baking powder, 1 teaspoon of the sugar, the cinnamon, and salt.

3. Make a well in the middle of the flour mixture. Add the eggs and lightly beat with a fork. Add the oil and water and blend to make a batter. Stir in the minced cherries. (If the batter seems too thick, add a touch more water.)

4. Lightly coat a large nonstick skillet or griddle with cooking spray and heat over medium-high heat. Ladle in ¼ cupfuls of the batter and cook until the tops of the pancakes are speckled with bubbles and some bubbles have popped and the underside of the pancake is golden brown; then flip the pancakes and cook until browned on the second side. The second side will take about half as long as the first side did.

5. To serve, spoon the sliced cherries and some of the accumulated juices over each 2-pancake portion.

Per 2-pancake serving: 251 calories • 9g protein • 9g fat (1.5g saturated)
4.5g fiber • 173mg calcium • 1mg vitamin C • 35g carbohydrate • 544mg sodium

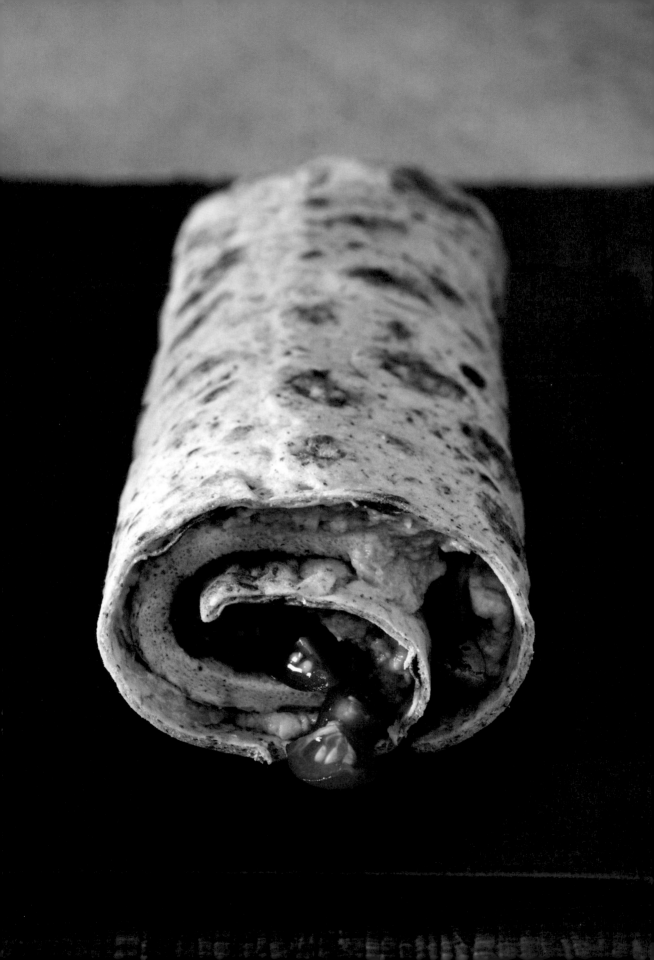

California Breakfast Wrap

Hands-On Time: 15 minutes • **Total Time:** 30 minutes + cooling time

Makes: 4 wraps

You can make the egg pancake well ahead and store in the fridge. Separate the pancakes with sheets of waxed paper and cover well. You can also make up entire breakfast wraps ahead of time: Wrap them tightly in plastic and keep them in the fridge until you're ready for them. If you're in Fade Away, skip the wraps and just spread the avocado, cheese, and tomatoes over the baked egg.

Fat Releasers
Avocado oil, eggs, oregano, black pepper, cheese, avocado, limes, multigrain bread, tomatoes

- 2 **teaspoons avocado oil or extra-light olive oil**
- 4 **large eggs**
- 8 **large egg whites**
- 1 **tablespoon water**
- ¾ **teaspoon dried oregano**
- ¾ **teaspoon ground cumin**
- ¼ **teaspoon ground black pepper**
- ½ **cup shredded reduced-fat Mexican blend cheese**
- 4 **rectangular multigrain (with flax, if possible) sandwich wraps (2 ounces each)**
- 1 **Hass avocado**
- 2 **teaspoons fresh lime juice**
- 6 **ounces grape tomatoes, chopped (about 1 cup)**

1. Preheat the oven to 350°F. Line a 10 x 15-inch rimmed baking sheet (or jelly-roll pan) with waxed paper or parchment paper or use a nonstick pan. Brush the bottom and sides of the paper (or pan) with the oil.

2. Place the pan in the oven to preheat for 3 minutes.

3. Meanwhile, in a large bowl, beat the whole eggs and egg whites with water. Beat well to fully incorporate the whites and yolks. Beat in the oregano, cumin, and pepper.

4. Pull out the oven rack with the pan on it and carefully pour the egg mixture into the pan, covering the bottom evenly. Sprinkle evenly with the cheese. Bake until the egg puffs up and is cooked through (don't worry if there are cracks), about 15 minutes.

5. Let the egg cool in the pan. Halve the egg pancake lengthwise and then halve crosswise. Loosen the pancake around the edges and carefully remove each egg quarter.

6. In a small bowl, mash the avocado with the lime juice. Spread each sandwich wrap with one-quarter of the avocado mash, top with an egg pancake, then one-quarter of the chopped tomatoes (drain them if they're too wet) and roll up the short way.

Per wrap: 348 calories • 30g protein • 18g fat (4.5g saturated) • 12g fiber 238mg calcium • 17mg vitamin C • 24g carbohydrate • 652mg sodium

Smoked Turkey & Swiss Breakfast Sandwiches

Hands-On Time: 10 minutes • **Total Time:** 20 minutes • **Makes:** 4 sandwiches

Here's a lighter take on a *croque monsieur,* the classic French open-face ham and cheese sandwich. This version uses sandwich thins, which have only 100 calories each. They're readily available, but if you prefer, swap in thin sandwich bread. Just be sure it's a whole-grain bread.

Fat Releasers
Milk, whole-wheat flour, cayenne, cheeses, whole-grain bread, turkey

1 **cup 1% milk**

1½ **tablespoons whole-wheat flour**

⅛ **teaspoon salt**

⅛ **teaspoon grated nutmeg**

⅛ **teaspoon cayenne pepper**

4 **slices (¾ ounce each) reduced-fat Swiss cheese**

2 **tablespoons grated Parmesan cheese**

4 **honey-wheat sandwich thins, split and toasted**

1 **tablespoon Dijon mustard**

3 **ounces sliced reduced-sodium smoked turkey**

1. Preheat the oven to 400°F.

2. In a small saucepan, gradually whisk the milk into the flour until smooth. Cook over low heat, whisking constantly, until the sauce has thickened, about 3 minutes. Remove from the heat and stir in the salt, nutmeg, and cayenne. Tear 1 slice of Swiss cheese into smaller bits and add it to the sauce with the Parmesan cheese.

3. Place the sandwich thin halves on a baking sheet and brush 4 of them with mustard. Top the mustard sides with the smoked turkey and the remaining Swiss cheese. Top with the remaining bread and slather the cheese sauce on top. Bake until the cheese sauce is bubbling, about 8 minutes.

4. Turn the oven to broil and move the rack 4 inches from the heat. Broil for 1 minute to brown the tops.

Per sandwich: 238 calories • 19g protein • 7g fat (3.5g saturated) • 5.5g fiber 330mg calcium • 0mg vitamin C • 29g carbohydrate • 618mg sodium

Tropical Fruit & Berry Salad with Yogurt Dressing

Hands-On Time: 15 minutes • **Total Time:** 15 minutes • **Makes:** 4 servings

Berries, kiwifruit, and pineapple get tossed in orange juice and served with a sauce of Greek yogurt, honey, and spicy cinnamon. You can use fresh or juice-packed canned pineapple wedges. If using the canned, use the pineapple juice instead of the orange juice.

Fat Releasers
Yogurt, honey, cinnamon, raspberries, kiwifruit, pineapple, oranges

- 1 container (7 ounces) 0% Greek yogurt
- 1 tablespoon plus 1 teaspoon honey
- 2 teaspoons grated orange zest
- ½ teaspoon ground cinnamon
- 1 cup blueberries
- 1 cup raspberries
- 1 kiwifruit (4 ounces), peeled, quartered lengthwise, and thickly sliced
- 2 cups pineapple wedges (½ inch thick)
- ⅓ cup fresh orange juice

1. In a small bowl, stir together the yogurt, honey, orange zest, and cinnamon.
2. In a separate bowl, toss together the blueberries, raspberries, kiwifruit, and pineapple. Add the orange juice and toss to combine. Spoon the berry mix into glasses or bowls and drizzle with the yogurt.

Per serving: 154 calories • 6g protein • 0.5g fat (0g saturated) • 5g fiber 70mg calcium • 88mg vitamin C • 34g carbohydrate • 22mg sodium

Chapter

5

Soups

Load up on fat releasing liquid
nutrition with these comforting
meals any time of the year.

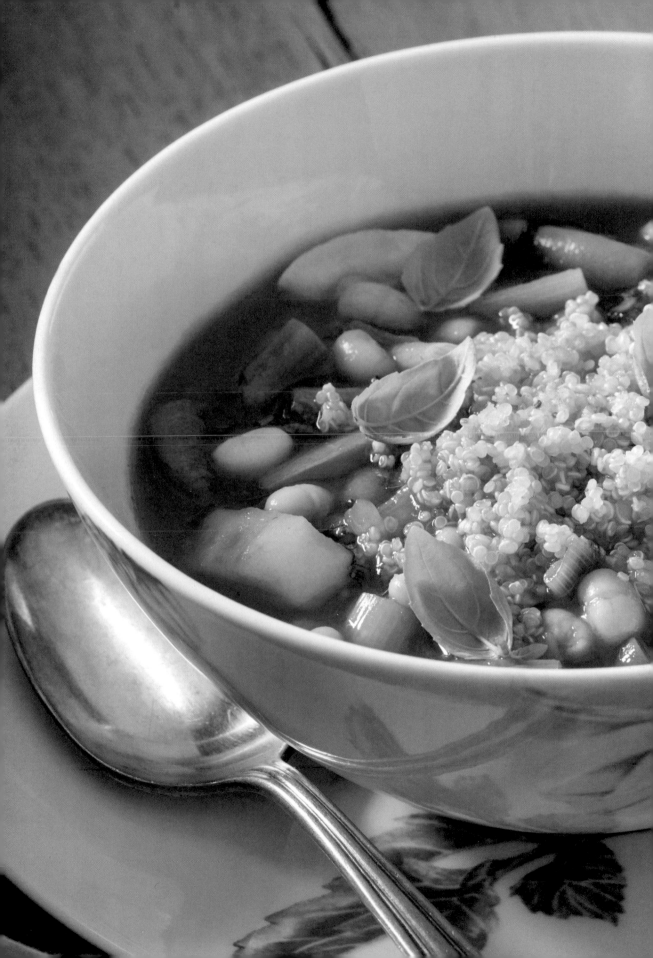

Spicy Garlic-Tomato Soup with Chicken

Hands-On Time: 20 minutes • **Total Time:** 35 minutes • **Makes:** 10 cups

This may seem like a lot of garlic cloves, but cooking them in broth mellows their bite. Not only does garlic contribute a tremendous amount of flavor to the soup, it may also have some important health benefits, ranging from promoting cardiovascular health to fighting the common cold. Since the recipe makes more than you need for the Fast Release phase, just freeze the leftovers in 1-cup portions; it freezes well.

Fat Releasers
Garlic, chicken, tomatoes, bell peppers, cayenne, limes, jalapeño

- 4 **cups low-sodium chicken broth**
- 16 **cloves garlic, peeled but whole**
- 1½ **pounds skinless, boneless chicken breast**
- 2 **cans (14.5 ounces each) no-salt-added diced tomatoes**
- 1 **red bell pepper, cut into small squares**
- 2 **green bell peppers, cut into small squares**
- 1½ **teaspoons ground cumin**
- 1 **teaspoon salt**
- ¼ **teaspoon cayenne pepper**
- ½ **cup minced cilantro plus extra for garnish**
- 3 **tablespoons fresh lime juice (about 2 limes)**
- 1 **tablespoon minced pickled jalapeño**

1. In a large saucepan, combine the broth and garlic and bring to a boil. Add the chicken, reduce to a simmer, cover, and cook until the chicken is just cooked through, 8 to 10 minutes. Remove the chicken and set aside.

2. With a slotted spoon, transfer the garlic to a food processor or blender along with ⅓ cup of the broth, and puree until smooth.

3. Return the garlic puree to the saucepan along with the tomatoes, bell peppers, cumin, salt, and cayenne. Bring to a boil, reduce to a simmer, cover, and cook until the peppers are tender, 4 to 5 minutes.

4. Meanwhile, when the chicken is cool enough to handle, cut into bite-size pieces.

5. Return the chicken to the pan along with the ½ cup cilantro, lime juice, and jalapeño, and cook just until heated through, about 1 minute. Serve garnished with more cilantro.

Per 2-cup serving: 242 calories • 33g protein • 4g fat (1g saturated) • 3g fiber 61mg calcium • 103mg vitamin C • 16g carbohydrate • 606mg sodium

Per 1-cup serving: 121 calories • 17g protein • 2g fat (0.5g saturated) 1.5g fiber • 31mg calcium • 51mg vitamin C • 8g carbohydrate • 303mg sodium

Lemon & Escarole Soup with Turkey

Hands-On Time: 20 minutes • **Total Time:** 20 minutes • **Makes:** 12 cups

A combo of eggs and lemon juice is added to the simmering soup both to flavor and give richness. If you like, add some fresh dill to the soup at the end. In the Finish Strong phase, add ¼ cup cooked whole-wheat orzo or couscous to each 2-cup serving of soup; add it to the soup bowl, and then ladle the soup over it.

Fat Releasers
Rosemary, black pepper, turkey, escarole, edamame, eggs, lemons

- 6 cups low-sodium chicken broth
- 1 teaspoon crumbled dried rosemary
- ¼ teaspoon ground black pepper
- 1 pound turkey breast meat, cut into bite-size pieces
- 1 small head escarole (8 ounces), cut into bite-size pieces (4 cups)
- 1½ cups frozen shelled edamame
- 3 large eggs
- ⅓ cup fresh lemon juice

1. In a large saucepan or Dutch oven, bring the broth, rosemary, and pepper to a boil over medium heat. Reduce to a simmer. Add the turkey, escarole, and edamame and cook until the turkey is cooked through and the escarole is tender, about 7 minutes.

2. Meanwhile, in a medium bowl, whisk together the eggs and lemon juice. Whisking all the while, ladle about 2 cups of the hot broth into the egg mixture and then stir the egg mixture into the saucepan of soup. Cook, stirring for 2 minutes; serve immediately.

SAVE FOR A SNACK: A 1-cup serving of the soup makes a nice snack. Have it with a mini cheese and 4 baby carrots.

Per 2-cup serving: 174 calories • 27g protein • 4.5g fat (1g saturated) • 2.5g fiber 60mg calcium • 11mg vitamin C • 6g carbohydrate • 147mg sodium

Per 1-cup serving: 87 calories • 13g protein • 2g fat (0.5g saturated) • 1.5g fiber 30mg calcium • 5mg vitamin C • 3g carbohydrate • 73mg sodium

"Bacon," Lettuce & Tomato Soup

Hands-On Time: 25 minutes • **Total Time:** 35 minutes • **Makes:** 12 cups

All the flavors of a BLT (with smoked turkey replacing the high-fat bacon) in a soup. To give the soup some heft (not to mention protein), we've added chickpeas.

Fat Releasers
Olive oil, onions, turkey, lettuce, tomatoes, chickpeas, vinegar, rosemary, thyme, ground black pepper

- 2 **tablespoons extra-virgin olive oil**
- 1 **large onion, coarsely chopped**
- ¾ **pound reduced-sodium smoked turkey, cut into thin matchsticks**
- 1 **large head romaine lettuce (12 ounces), quartered lengthwise and cut into 1-inch-wide strips (8 cups)**
- 3 **cans (14.5 ounces each) no-salt-added diced tomatoes**
- 1 **can (15 ounces) no-salt-added chickpeas, rinsed and drained**
- 3 **cups water**
- ¼ **cup red wine vinegar**
- ¾ **teaspoon crumbled dried rosemary**
- ½ **teaspoon dried thyme**
- ½ **teaspoon ground black pepper**
- ¼ **teaspoon salt**

1. In a large saucepan or Dutch oven, heat the oil over medium heat. Add the onion and cook, stirring frequently, until tender, about 7 minutes.

2. Add the smoked turkey and lettuce and cook, stirring occasionally, until the lettuce has wilted, about 3 minutes.

3. Add the tomatoes, chickpeas, water, vinegar, rosemary, thyme, pepper, and salt and bring to a boil. Reduce to a simmer; cover and cook for 10 minutes to blend the flavors.

Per 2-cup serving: 235 calories • 19g protein • 5.5g fat (0.5g saturated) 5.5g fiber • 87mg calcium • 37mg vitamin C • 25g carbohydrate • 507mg sodium

Per 1-cup serving: 117 calories • 10g protein • 3g fat (0.5g saturated) 3g fiber • 43mg calcium • 19mg vitamin C • 13g carbohydrate • 253mg sodium

Hot & Sour Soup with Tofu

Hands-On Time: 20 minutes • **Total Time:** 45 minutes • **Makes:** 8 cups

This soup can be made ahead of time. Store the broth-vegetable mixture and the tofu separately. Reheat the broth mixture and top with the tofu when ready to serve.

Fat Releasers
Tofu, vinegar, sesame oil, scallions, garlic, ginger, red pepper flakes, watercress, snow peas, bell pepper, egg

- 1 package (14 ounces) extra-firm tofu
- 3 tablespoons cider vinegar
- 2 tablespoons reduced-sodium soy sauce
- 1 tablespoon sesame oil
- 4 cups low-sodium chicken broth or vegetable broth
- 1 bunch scallions, coarsely chopped, white and green parts kept separate
- 3 cloves garlic, grated on a zester
- 1 inch of fresh ginger, grated
- ½ teaspoon red pepper flakes
- ½ teaspoon salt
- 1 bunch watercress, thick stems trimmed, coarsely chopped
- 4 ounces snow peas, thinly sliced on the diagonal
- 1 large red bell pepper, diced
- 1 egg

1. Slice the block of tofu in half horizontally into 2 slabs. Place the tofu slabs on a double layer of paper towels on a cutting board and top with another double layer of paper towels and a small baking pan with heavy weights in it (like canned goods). Drain for at least 15 minutes.

2. Combine the vinegar, soy sauce, and sesame oil in a shallow container big enough to hold both slabs of tofu in a single layer. Transfer the slabs of tofu to the container and use a knife to cut them into ½-inch cubes right in the container.

3. In a large saucepan, combine the broth, scallion whites, garlic, ginger, red pepper flakes, and salt. Bring to a boil and let cook 5 minutes to develop flavor.

4. Stir in the watercress, snow peas, and bell pepper and cook 2 minutes to soften the vegetables.

5. In a small bowl, lightly beat the egg. Ladle in ½ cup hot broth and whisk quickly to combine. Stir the egg mixture back into the soup and cook for 30 seconds.

6. Drain the marinade out of the tofu container and into the soup. Divide the broth and vegetables among soup bowls, top with the tofu, and garnish with the scallion greens.

Per 2-cup serving: 213 calories • 17g protein • 10g fat (1.5g saturated) • 4g fiber 177mg calcium • 94mg vitamin C • 13g carbohydrate • 696mg sodium

Per 1-cup serving: 106 calories • 9g protein • 5g fat (1g saturated) • 2g fiber 89mg calcium • 47mg vitamin C • 7g carbohydrate • 348mg sodium

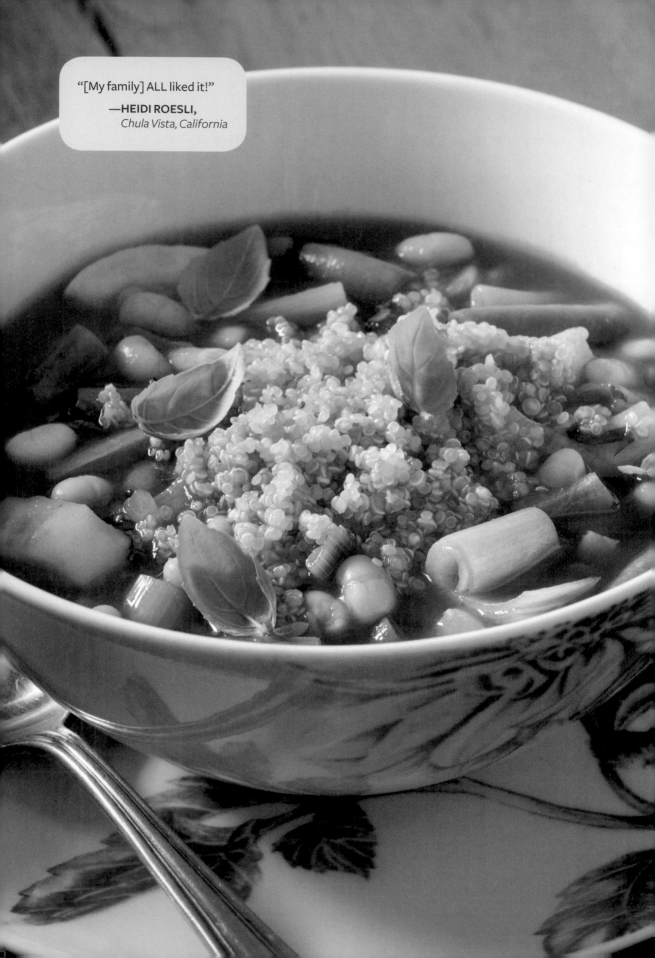

"[My family] ALL liked it!"
—HEIDI ROESLI,
Chula Vista, California

Hearty Minestrone with Quinoa

Hands-On Time: 20 minutes • **Total Time:** 50 minutes • **Makes:** 10 cups

This soup is very versatile: If you don't have any leeks, swap in onions. Got a ton of zucchini in the garden? Use it instead of yellow squash. Swap in snap peas for the green beans (but add them during the final 5 minutes of cooking time), and use any canned bean you like. A tablespoon or two of Parmesan cheese added at the end makes it even more flavorful.

Fat Releasers
Olive oil, leeks, garlic, squash, beans, tomato paste, basil, quinoa

- 2 tablespoons plus 2 teaspoons extra-virgin olive oil
- 1 pound leeks, halved lengthwise and sliced inch wide
- 5 cloves garlic, thinly sliced
- 1 pound yellow squash, quartered lengthwise and thickly sliced
- 8 ounces green beans, cut into 1-inch lengths
- ⅓ cup no-salt-added tomato paste
- 2 cans (15 ounces each) no-salt-added white beans, rinsed and drained
- 4 cups low-sodium vegetable broth
- 1 cup fresh basil leaves, half thinly sliced, half torn or left whole
- 1 teaspoon salt
- ½ cup quinoa, rinsed

1. In a large nonstick saucepan or Dutch oven, heat the oil over medium-low heat. Add the leeks and garlic and cook, stirring frequently, until the leeks are tender, about 10 minutes.

2. Add the yellow squash and green beans and cook, stirring frequently, until the squash starts to soften, about 5 minutes.

3. Stir in the tomato paste, white beans, broth, the sliced basil, and salt, and bring to a simmer. Cover and cook until the green beans are tender, about 15 minutes.

4. Meanwhile, in a medium pot of boiling water, cook the quinoa until tender, 10 to 12 minutes.

5. To serve, stir the quinoa into the soup and sprinkle with the torn or whole basil leaves. (If making the soup ahead, stir the basil in before refrigerating or freezing.)

Per 2-cup serving: 335 calories • 13g protein • 10g fat (1g saturated) • 11g fiber 144mg calcium • 31mg vitamin C • 50g carbohydrate • 650mg sodium

Per 1-cup serving: 167 calories • 7g protein • 5g fat (0.5g saturated) • 5.5g fiber 72mg calcium • 16mg vitamin C • 25g carbohydrate • 325mg sodium

Turkey, Black Bean & Winter Squash Soup

Hands-On Time: 15 minutes • **Total Time:** 1 hour 35 minutes • **Makes:** 10 cups

By making your own turkey stock, you not only save some money, but you also get a nice sodium-controlled homemade soup base. However, if you're pressed for time, make the soup with low-sodium canned chicken broth (you'll need 4½ cups) and 1 pound cooked roast turkey. Simmer the canned broth with the flavoring ingredients from step 1 for about 15 minutes, then jump to step 3.

Fat Releasers
Turkey, scallions, lemons, chili powder, bell pepper, basil, winter squash, cinnamon, black beans

2½ **pounds skin-on, bone-in turkey thighs, skinned**

6 **cups water**

4 **scallions, sliced**

Grated zest and juice of 1 lemon

2 **tablespoons mild chili powder**

1 **green bell pepper, cut into ½-inch squares**

1 **cup chopped fresh basil or cilantro**

2 **packages (10 ounces each) frozen winter squash puree, thawed**

1 **teaspoon ground cinnamon**

½ **teaspoon salt**

2 **cans (15 ounces each) no-salt-added black beans, rinsed and drained**

1. In a saucepan just big enough to fit the turkey thighs side by side, combine the water, turkey, scallions, lemon zest, chili powder, half of the bell pepper, and half of the basil or cilantro. Cover and bring to a boil. Reduce to a simmer, partially cover, and cook until the turkey is tender but still a little pink at the bone, 45 to 50 minutes. Turn the turkey in the broth once or twice.

2. Remove from the heat. Remove the turkey thighs from the soup; and when cool enough to handle, cut the meat from the bones and cut into bite-size pieces.

3. Stir the remaining bell pepper, the winter squash, cinnamon, and salt into the soup, bring to a simmer and cook 5 minutes. Add the turkey, black beans, and lemon juice and simmer briefly to heat through. Stir in the remaining basil or cilantro.

Per 2-cup serving: 386 calories • 38g protein • 7g fat (2g saturated) • 12g fiber 185mg calcium • 33mg vitamin C • 45g carbohydrate • 380mg sodium

Per 1-cup serving: 193 calories • 19g protein • 3.5g fat (1g saturated) • 6g fiber 93mg calcium • 16mg vitamin C • 23g carbohydrate • 190mg sodium

Manhattan Fish Chowder

Hands-On Time: 15 minutes • **Total Time:** 30 minutes • **Makes:** 8 cups

The puree made with roasted red pepper, almonds, tomato paste, and olive oil is based on a Spanish sauce called *romesco* that is often used for a vegetable dip. Here the sauce is used to give richness and body to the soup.

Fat Releasers
Bell pepper, almonds, tomato paste, olive oil, cayenne pepper, scallions, garlic, beans, cod, lemons

- 1 red bell pepper, cut vertically into flat panels
- 14 raw almonds (½ ounce)
- ¼ cup no-salt-added tomato paste
- 1 tablespoon plus 1 teaspoon extra-virgin olive oil
- 1 teaspoon paprika
- ⅛ teaspoon cayenne pepper
- 1½ cups bottled clam juice
- 1 cup water
- 4 scallions, thinly sliced
- 3 cloves garlic, thinly sliced
- 1 can (15 ounces) no-salt-added white beans, rinsed and drained
- ¾ pound skinless, boneless cod fillet, cut into 1-inch chunks
- 4 lemon wedges, for serving

1. Preheat the broiler. Place the flat pepper panels, skin-side up, on the broiler pan and broil 4 inches from the heat until the skin is charred all over, about 10 minutes.

2. Remove the pan from the oven, flip the pepper pieces over on the pan, and let sit until cool enough to handle. Peel and transfer to a food processor. Add the almonds, tomato paste, oil, paprika, and cayenne, and puree until smooth.

3. In a medium saucepan, combine the clam juice and water and bring to a boil. Add the scallions and garlic and cook until tender, about 2 minutes. Add the beans, cod, and roasted pepper puree and reduce to a simmer. Cover and cook until the fish is just cooked through, 3 to 5 minutes. Serve with lemon wedges.

SAVE FOR A SNACK: Make the red pepper puree (steps 1 and 2) and serve it as a dip for ½ cup steamed broccoli or cauliflower in Fade Away. Or, in Finish Strong, have 2 tablespoons of the puree on 3 high-fiber crackers.

Per 2-cup serving: 210 calories • 19g protein • 8g fat (1g saturated) • 5g fiber 64mg calcium • 49mg vitamin C • 17g carbohydrate • 500mg sodium

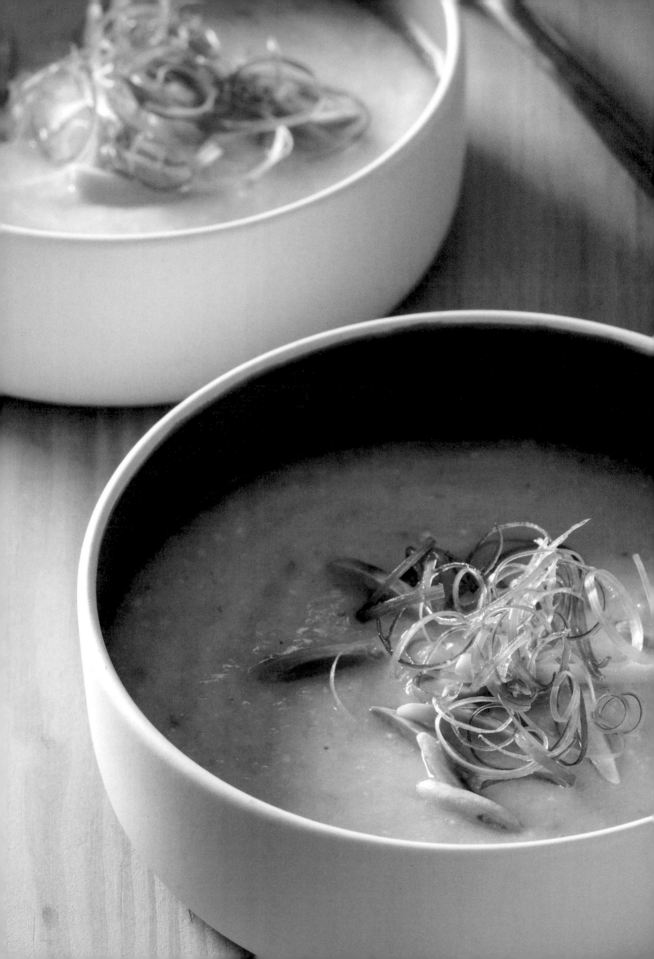

Golden Gazpacho

Hands-On Time: 15 minutes • **Total Time:** 15 minutes + chilling time

Makes: 4 servings

Gazpacho is typically made with red tomatoes, but yellow or orange tomatoes make a beautiful, vibrant, and equally tasty soup. This should be served icy cold in chilled glasses or bowls. To chill the soup quickly, place it in a bowl and set that bowl into a bowl of ice water; stir occasionally.

Fat Releasers
Tomatoes, squash, bell peppers, almonds, vinegar, olive oil, scallions

- 2 **pounds yellow tomatoes, cut into large chunks**
- 1 **yellow squash (6 ounces), halved lengthwise and thickly sliced**
- 1 **yellow bell pepper, cut into large chunks**
- ¼ **cup raw almonds**
- ¼ **cup cider vinegar**
- 1 **tablespoon plus 1 teaspoon extra-virgin olive oil**
- ½ **teaspoon salt**
- ¼ **cup water**
- 1 **scallion, thinly sliced**
- 4 **teaspoons slivered almonds, for garnish**

1. In a blender or food processor, combine the tomatoes, squash, bell pepper, almonds, vinegar, oil, salt, and water and puree until chunky. Refrigerate until very cold.

2. Garnish the soup with scallions and slivered almonds.

Per 1¾-cup serving: 159 calories • 5g protein • 11g fat (1g saturated) • 4g fiber 68mg calcium • 112mg vitamin C • 13g carbohydrate • 342mg sodium

Vegetarian Double-Pea Soup

Hands-On Time: 15 minutes • **Total Time:** 1 hour 5 minutes • **Makes:** 8 cups

A traditional split pea soup has chunks of ham; in this vegetarian rendition, chunks of portobello mushrooms and smoked paprika take its place. Have 2 cups of the soup as a dinner entrée, or have 1 cup for lunch and pair it with a glass of milk or 2 mini cheeses.

Fat Releasers
Olive oil, scallions, garlic, black pepper, split peas, tomatoes, green peas

2 tablespoons extra-virgin olive oil

1 bunch scallions, chopped, whites and greens kept separate

6 cloves garlic, minced

Ground black pepper

1 cup green split peas (about 8 ounces)

4½ cups water

½ teaspoon salt

1 can (15 ounces) no-salt-added crushed tomatoes

12 ounces portobello mushroom caps

½ teaspoon smoked paprika

2 cups frozen green peas, thawed

1. In a large saucepan, heat 1 tablespoon of the oil over medium heat. Add the scallion whites, garlic, and a generous pinch of pepper and cook until softened and just beginning to turn color, 2 to 3 minutes.

2. Add the split peas, water, and ¼ teaspoon of the salt. Bring to a boil, then reduce to a simmer, cover, and cook until mostly softened, 45 minutes. Add the crushed tomatoes and simmer, covered, until the split peas are tender, about 15 minutes.

3. Meanwhile, scrape the black gills out of the mushrooms and cut into cubes. In a large nonstick skillet, heat the remaining 1 tablespoon oil over medium-high heat; sprinkle the remaining ¼ teaspoon salt over the oil. Add the portobellos and cook, without stirring, for 3 minutes. Then stir the mushrooms, sprinkle with the paprika, and cook until the mushrooms are tender but not collapsed.

4. Add the green peas, scallion greens, and mushrooms (and all the juices from the skillet) to the saucepan and stir to combine.

Per 2-cup serving: 373 calories • 22g protein • 8g fat (1g saturated) • 22g fiber • 110mg calcium • 29mg vitamin C • 56g carbohydrate • 360mg sodium

Per 1-cup serving: 187 calories • 11g protein • 4g fat (0.5g saturated) • 11g fiber • 55mg calcium • 14mg vitamin C • 28g carbohydrate • 180mg sodium

Mexican Fajita Soup

Hands-On Time: 20 minutes • **Total Time:** 40 minutes • **Makes:** 4 servings

Tossing the cut-up strips of tortilla with the lime juice not only flavors them but also keeps them from becoming tough and crumbly. If you like, the tortilla strips can be seasoned with ½ teaspoon chili powder (in addition to the lime juice) before baking. If you have leftover tortillas, freeze and save them for Southwestern Turkey Tacos (page 179), or make chips for a snack (see Save for a Snack, below).

Fat Releasers
Whole-wheat tortillas, limes, olive oil, onion, bell peppers, oregano, lean beef

2 whole-wheat tortillas (taco size), halved and cut into thin strips

3 tablespoons fresh lime juice

4 teaspoons extra-virgin olive oil

1 onion, coarsely chopped

1 small red bell pepper, cut into thin strips

1 small green bell pepper, cut into thin strips

1 teaspoon dried oregano

4 cups low-sodium chicken broth

8 ounces sirloin or flank steak, very thinly sliced

¼ cup cilantro leaves

SAVE FOR A SNACK: Use leftover tortillas to make baked tortilla chips for a snack. For a single snack serving, cut ½ tortilla into strips and toss with ¾ teaspoon fresh lime juice and ¼ teaspoon oil and bake as directed. Serve with ¼ cup tomato salsa.

1. Preheat the oven to 400°F. In a medium bowl, toss the tortilla strips with 2 tablespoons of the lime juice and 2 teaspoons of the oil. Transfer to a baking sheet and bake until crisp, tossing once, about 20 minutes.

2. Meanwhile, in a large nonstick saucepan or Dutch oven, heat the remaining 2 teaspoons oil over medium heat. Add the onion, bell peppers, and oregano and cook, stirring frequently, until the vegetables are tender, about 7 minutes.

3. Add the broth, bring to a simmer, and cook for 5 minutes to blend the flavors. Add the steak and cook until just cooked through, about 2 minutes. Add the remaining 1 tablespoon lime juice.

4. Divide the tortilla strips and cilantro among 4 soup bowls and ladle the soup on top.

Per 1½-cup serving: 169 calories • 16g protein • 8g fat (1.5g saturated) • 5g fiber 35mg calcium • 44mg vitamin C • 12g carbohydrate • 210mg sodium

Russian Cabbage & Beef Soup

Hands-On Time: 30 minutes • **Total Time:** 55 minutes • **Makes:** 4 servings

Kohlrabi is a root vegetable often described as a cross between a cabbage and a turnip. If you can't find a kohlrabi, swap in turnip or even jicama. Serve this main-course soup with 2 thin slices of pumpernickel bread spread with 1 teaspoon unsalted butter (½ teaspoon per slice) or mustard.

Fat Releasers
Olive oil, onions, garlic, cabbage, kohlrabi, tomato paste, vinegar, beef, yogurt

- 1 tablespoon extra-virgin olive oil
- 1 large onion, halved lengthwise and thinly sliced
- 3 cloves garlic, thinly sliced
- 1 pound green cabbage, thinly sliced (8 cups)
- 1 kohlrabi or white turnip (5 ounces), peeled, halved, and thinly sliced (1 cup)
- 3 tablespoons no-salt-added tomato paste
- 3 tablespoons cider vinegar
- 3 cups low-sodium chicken broth
- 1½ cups carrot juice
- ½ teaspoon salt
- 10 ounces flank steak, thinly sliced
- ½ cup 0% plain Greek yogurt

1. In a large saucepan or Dutch oven, heat the oil over medium heat. Add the onion and garlic and cook, stirring frequently, until the onion is tender, about 7 minutes. Add the cabbage and cook, stirring occasionally, until it's beginning to wilt, about 5 minutes.

2. Stir in the kohlrabi, tomato paste, and vinegar. Add the broth, carrot juice, and salt and bring to a boil. Reduce to a simmer, cover, and cook until the cabbage is tender, about 20 minutes.

3. Add the flank steak and cook until no longer pink, about 1 minute. Serve topped with the yogurt.

Per 2¼-cup serving: 265 calories • 24g protein • 8g fat (2g saturated) 6.5g fiber • 149mg calcium • 95mg vitamin C • 27g carbohydrate • 493mg sodium

Winter Vegetable Soup with Smoked Pork

Hands-On Time: 20 minutes • **Total Time:** 45 minutes • **Makes:** 6 cups

It's well worth seeking out smoked pork chops: They have the great smoky flavor of a smoked ham, but they haven't been cured with sugar and salt. However, if you can't find them, you can swap in a low-sodium smoked ham. Have this for lunch with a toasted cheese sandwich: Toast a slice of multigrain sandwich bread, top with 1 tablespoon shredded reduced-fat cheese (your favorite), and put under the broiler or in the toaster oven just long enough to melt the cheese.

Fat Releasers
Olive oil, onion, garlic, pork, spinach, vinegar

- 1 tablespoon olive oil
- 1 medium onion, diced
- 3 cloves garlic, minced
- 2 cups low-sodium chicken broth
- 1 cup water
- ½ pound well-trimmed boneless smoked pork chops, cut into ½-inch cubes
- ½ pound parsnips, peeled and cut into ½-inch chunks
- ½ pound turnips, cut into ½-inch chunks
- ½ pound red potatoes, peeled and cut into ½-inch cubes
- ½ package frozen chopped spinach, thawed, or 5 ounces baby spinach
- 1½ tablespoons red wine vinegar

1. In a large saucepan, heat the oil over medium heat. Add the onion and garlic and cook, stirring frequently, until tender, 5 to 7 minutes.

2. Add the broth and water and bring to a low boil. Add the pork cubes, parsnips, turnips, and potatoes and return to a boil. Cover and cook until the vegetables are just firm-tender, 10 to 12 minutes.

3. Stir in the spinach and vinegar and cook for 1 minute to heat through.

Per 1½-cup serving: 248 calories • 16g protein • 7g fat (1.5g saturated) 7g fiber • 83mg calcium • 34mg vitamin C • 31g carbohydrate • 697mg sodium

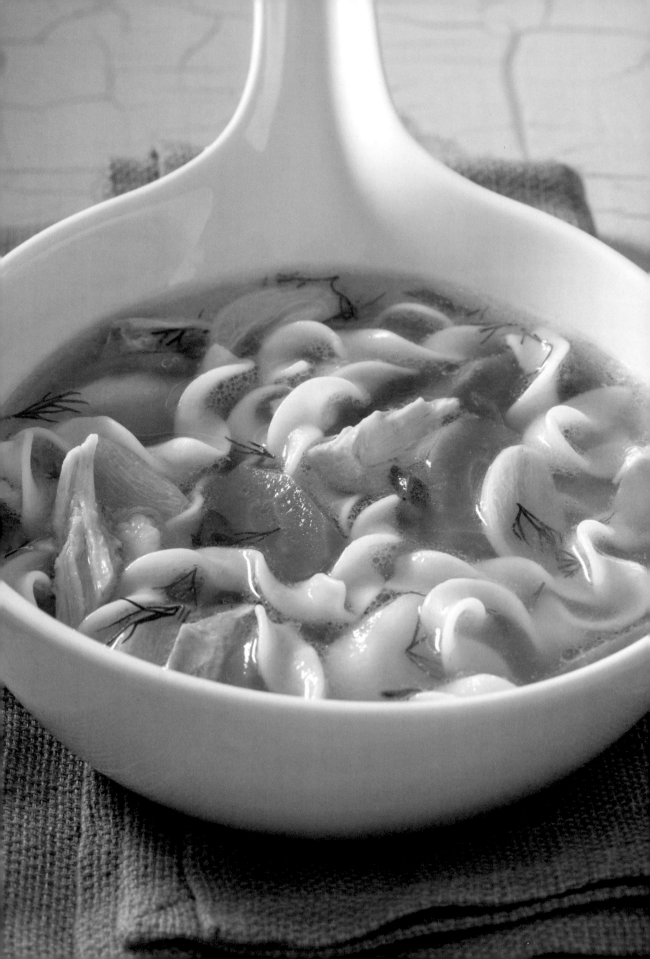

Mom's Chicken Noodle Soup

Hands-On Time: 15 minutes • **Total Time:** 1 hour 5 minutes • **Makes:** 8 cups

Chicken soup just the way Mom used to make it—with carrots, parsnips, and dill. Adding some dill just before serving makes this taste especially fresh. We've used chicken thighs because they can cook longer than breast and still be tender, and they also add more flavor to the broth.

Fat Releasers
Chicken, garlic, scallions

1 **pound skinless, bone-in chicken thighs**

7 **cups water**

2 **large carrots (8 ounces total), thinly sliced**

1 **large parsnip (6 ounces), thinly sliced**

3 **cloves garlic, thinly sliced**

4 **scallions, thinly sliced**

½ **cup chopped fresh dill**

½ **teaspoon salt**

4 **ounces no-yolks broad egg noodles**

1. In a large saucepan, combine the chicken and water and bring to a boil over medium heat, skimming any foam that rises to the surface. Reduce to a simmer, cover, and cook until the chicken is tender and cooked through, about 30 minutes. Remove the chicken, and when cool enough to handle, shred.

2. Add the carrots, parsnip, garlic, scallions, ¼ cup of the dill, and salt to the pot and cook, stirring occasionally, until the vegetables are tender, about 10 minutes.

3. Add the egg noodles and cook until the noodles are tender but not falling apart, about 7 minutes. At serving time, return the broth to a simmer, add the chicken and the remaining dill, and cook just until heated through.

Per 2-cup serving: 303 calories • 27g protein • 5g fat (1g saturated) • 5.5g fiber 62mg calcium • 15mg vitamin C • 35g carbohydrate • 453mg sodium

Roasted Pepper Soup with Basil Meatballs

Hands-On Time: 30 minutes • **Total Time:** 55 minutes • **Makes:** 6 servings

The beauty of this soup is that it can be done in stages. The onions and peppers can be broiled (and peeled) ahead; or you can make the entire soup base (through step 5) ahead. The meatballs can be made ahead and even frozen. Refrigerate everything until ready to cook (bring the meatballs back to room temperature before cooking in the soup so the cooking times will still be correct). To have this during the Fade Away phase, make the meatballs without the bread crumbs.

Fat Releasers
Onions, bell peppers, tomatoes, vinegar, garlic, lean pork, multigrain bread, black pepper, basil, Parmesan cheese

2 sweet onions (1 pound total), thickly sliced

2½ pounds yellow bell peppers (4 large or 5 medium)

2 pounds plum tomatoes, cut into chunks

3 cups low-sodium chicken broth

1 tablespoon balsamic vinegar

2 cloves garlic, minced

¾ teaspoon salt

¾ pound ground pork

1 slice (1 ounce) multigrain bread, processed into fine crumbs

¼ teaspoon ground black pepper

¾ cup chopped fresh basil

2 tablespoons grated Parmesan cheese

1. Preheat the broiler to high. Line a baking sheet with foil. Place the onion slices on the baking sheet and lightly coat with cooking spray (preferably olive oil). Broil 4 inches from the heat until browned and lightly charred, about 11 minutes. Transfer the onions to a food processor and set aside.

2. Meanwhile, cut the bell peppers vertically into flat panels. Cut off the bottoms of the peppers and any other scraps of pepper left on the core, coarsely chop, and set aside. Discard the cores and any seeds.

3. Place the flat bell pepper panels, skin-side up, on the baking pan the onions were on and broil 4 inches from the heat until the skin is charred all over, about 12 minutes.

4. Remove from the oven, flip the pepper pieces over on the pan and let sit until cool enough to handle, then peel and add to the onions in the food processor. Puree the onions and peppers and transfer to a large saucepan. Add the tomatoes to the same processor bowl (no need to clean) and puree. Add to the pureed onions and peppers.

5. Stir in the reserved chopped bell peppers, the broth, vinegar, garlic, and salt. Bring to a low boil over medium-high heat. Reduce to a simmer and cook for 5 minutes to blend the flavors.

6. Meanwhile, in a medium bowl, thoroughly blend the ground pork, bread crumbs, black pepper, and ¼ cup of the basil. Shape the mixture into ¾-inch balls. (You should be able to make 48 meatballs.)

7. Drop the meatballs into the simmering soup and cook until they are cooked through, about 5 minutes. Stir in the remaining ½ cup basil. Serve topped with the Parmesan cheese.

COOKING FOR ONE: Make the soup base and freeze in 1½-cup portions. Spread the meatballs out on a tray to freeze; when frozen solid, divide them into equal portions (8 meatballs each) and store in individual storage bags. When ready to serve, reheat the soup base in a small saucepan and bring to a simmer; add one portion of thawed meatballs and cook for 5 minutes.

Per 1½-cup serving: 275 calories • 15g protein • 13g fat (5g saturated) 4.5g fiber • 96mg calcium • 310mg vitamin C • 25g carbohydrate 413mg sodium

Sweet Potato & Tomato Soup

Hands-On Time: 15 minutes • **Total Time:** 35 minutes • **Makes:** 4 servings

Have a cup of this for lunch (chilled or reheated in the microwave) along with 3 ounces cold poached or broiled chicken breast and a multigrain sandwich thin split, toasted, and spread with a wedge of Laughing Cow light cheese. Or have it all by itself for a snack.

Fat Releasers
Tomato paste, sweet potatoes, onion, black pepper, cinnamon, tomatoes, yogurt

- 1½ **teaspoons ground cumin**
- 2 **cups water**
- 2 **tablespoons no-salt-added tomato paste**
- 3 **small sweet potatoes (about ¾ pound), peeled and cut into chunks**
- 1 **large red onion, cut into chunks**
- ½ **teaspoon salt**
- ¼ **teaspoon ground black pepper**
- ⅛ **teaspoon ground cinnamon**
- 1 **cup grape tomatoes, halved (or quartered if large)**
- ¼ **cup chopped cilantro or parsley**
- ¼ **cup plain fat-free yogurt**

1. In a medium saucepan, cook the cumin over medium heat, stirring and shaking the pan frequently, until fragrant and toasted, about 2 minutes; take care not to burn.

2. Add the water, tomato paste, sweet potatoes, onion, salt, pepper, and cinnamon. Cover and bring to a boil over high heat. Reduce to a simmer and cook until the sweet potatoes and onion are tender, 15 to 20 minutes.

3. Let cool slightly and transfer the soup to a food processor or blender and puree. Return the puree to the pan, add the tomatoes, and stir over medium heat until heated through, about 2 minutes.

4. Remove from the heat and stir in the cilantro or parsley. Top each serving with 1 tablespoon yogurt. Serve the soup hot, at room temperature, or chilled.

Per generous 1-cup serving: 108 calories • 3g protein • 0.5g fat (0g saturated) 4g fiber • 64mg calcium • 27mg vitamin C • 24g carbohydrate • 326mg sodium

Creamy Double-Mushroom Barley Soup

Hands-On Time: 10 minutes ● **Total Time:** 1 hour ● **Makes:** 8 cups

Fat Releasers
Garlic, olive oil, barley, tofu

Have 2 cups of soup for lunch by itself; or have a 1-cup portion and pair it with a serving of Warm Broccolini Salad with Cashew Pesto (page 203) or simply with 2 cups steamed broccoli florets tossed with 1 tablespoon Digest Diet Vinaigrette (page 50). And if you're wondering what to do with the leftover silken tofu: Add it to a smoothie. Or puree it with water and use in place of soy milk.

2 cups boiling water

½ ounce dried wild mushrooms

16 ounces baby bella (cremini) mushrooms, cut into ½-inch chunks

4 cloves garlic, coarsely chopped

1 tablespoon extra-virgin olive oil

¼ teaspoon salt

4 cups water

3 tablespoons reduced-sodium soy sauce

1 cup pearled barley

1 cup silken tofu (a little over half a 16-ounce package)

Chopped chives, for garnish (optional)

1. In a heatproof bowl, pour the boiling water over the dried mushrooms and set aside to soften, about 15 minutes. Reserving the soaking liquid, scoop out the mushrooms with a slotted spoon and coarsely chop.

2. Meanwhile, in a food processor, combine half the cremini mushroom chunks and the garlic and pulse until the texture of coarse crumbs.

3. In a 3-quart saucepan, heat the oil over medium heat. Add the mushroom-garlic mixture and the salt and cook, stirring, until the mushrooms give up their liquid and the liquid evaporates, 2 to 3 minutes.

4. Add the mushroom soaking liquid (leave any grit behind in the bowl), water, soy sauce, and barley. Bring to a simmer, cover, and cook until the barley is mostly tender, about 35 minutes.

5. Add the remaining cremini mushroom chunks and the chopped dried mushrooms and cook for 5 minutes to soften the cremini.

6. Meanwhile, puree the tofu in a blender and stir into the soup. Sprinkle with the chives, if using. Serve hot, at room temperature, or chilled.

Per 2-cup serving: 290 calories ● 13g protein ● 6g fat (1g saturated) ● 9g fiber 61mg calcium ● 1mg vitamin C ● 49g carbohydrate ● 593mg sodium

Per 1-cup serving: 145 calories ● 6g protein ● 3g fat (0.5g saturated) ● 4.5g fiber 30mg calcium ● 0mg vitamin C ● 25g carbohydrate ● 296mg sodium

Chapter
6

Main Dishes

Feast your eyes and feed your tummy with these hearty, flavorful entrées. No going hungry on this diet!

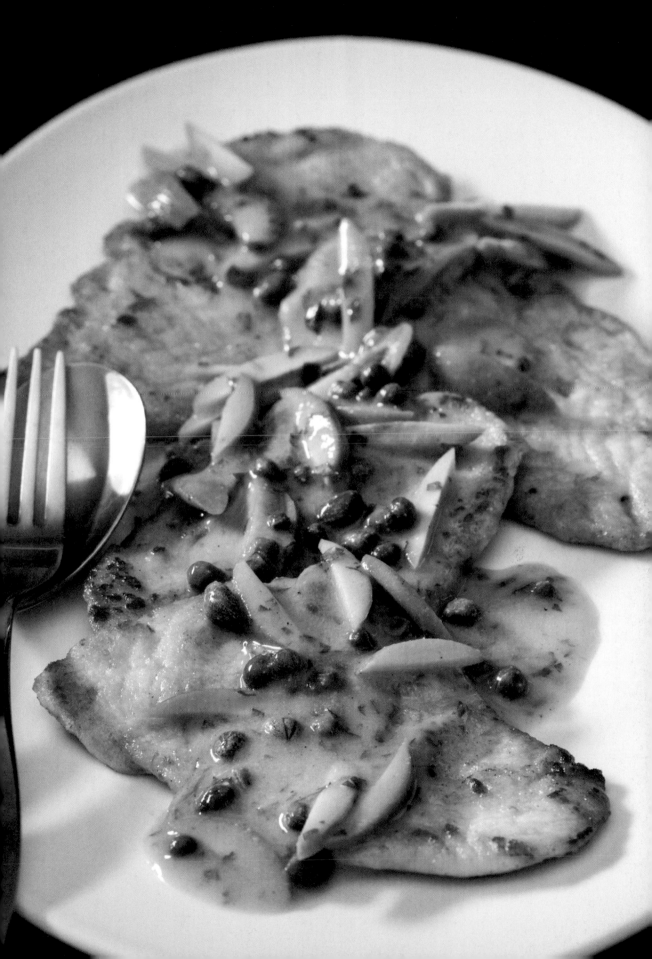

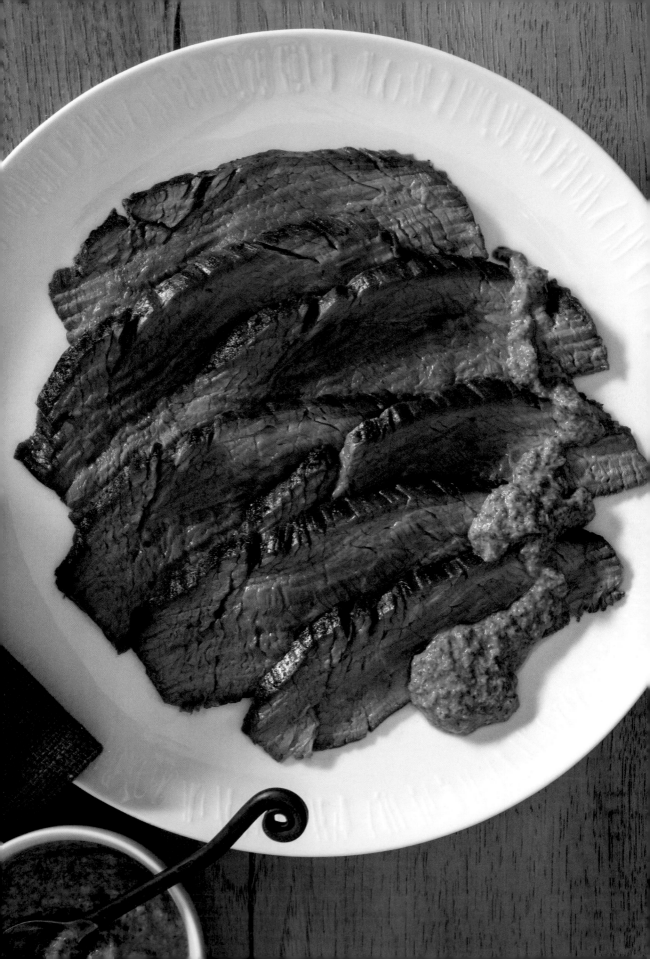

Flank Steak with Scallion Chimichurri

Hands-On Time: 25 minutes • **Total Time:** 30 minutes • **Makes:** 4 servings

Chimichurri, a specialty of Argentinean cuisine, is an herb condiment used to dress all manner of beef. It's generally made with parsley, oregano, garlic, onion, salt, and pepper and bathed in oil and vinegar. We've added some mustard and vinegar to the mix and some heat from a jalapeño. When the weather is nice, this is great on the grill.

Fat Releasers
Scallions, parsley, garlic, jalapeño, vinegar, olive oil, oregano, beef, black pepper

- 4 **scallions, sliced (¾ cup)**
- ⅔ **cup flat-leaf parsley leaves**
- 1 **clove garlic**
- 1 **pickled jalapeño pepper, seeds removed for less heat if desired**
- 1 **tablespoon red wine vinegar**
- 1 **tablespoon Dijon mustard**
- 4 **teaspoons extra-virgin olive oil**
- ¾ **teaspoon dried oregano**
- 2 **tablespoons water**
- 1 **pound flank steak**
- ½ **teaspoon salt**
- ¼ **teaspoon ground black pepper**

1. In a food processor, puree the scallions, parsley, garlic, pickled jalapeño, vinegar, mustard, oil, oregano, and 2 tablespoons water; set aside.

2. Preheat the broiler with the rack 4 inches from the heat source.

Sprinkle the flank steak with salt and pepper. Broil 5 minutes, then turn the steak over and broil 2 minutes longer for medium-rare. Let the meat stand for 5 minutes before slicing against the grain. Serve with the sauce.

COOKING FOR ONE: Swap in a 4-ounce sirloin steak or a 4-ounce chunk of flank steak for the larger steak. Serve with one-fourth of the chimichurri sauce and save the remainder for a snack (see below); it'll keep up to a couple of weeks in the fridge.

SAVE FOR A SNACK: Make a double or triple batch of the chimichurri and drizzle ⅓ cup over grilled winter or summer squash, bell peppers, or other vegetables for a snack.

Per serving: 209 calories • 25g protein • 11g fat (3g saturated) • 0.5g fiber 47mg calcium • 10mg vitamin C • 2g carbohydrate • 455mg sodium

Slow-Cooker Sunday Roast with Onion Gravy

Hands-On Time: 20 minutes • **Total Time:** 7 to 8 hours • **Makes:** 10 servings

Most gravies are thickened by flour; this one gets its heft from pureed onions (which are fat releasers). Serve the roast with Roasted Ratatouille (page 236) and a mixed green salad. If you aren't planning on having leftovers within the week after making the roast, slice or shred the beef, coat it with some leftover gravy, and freeze in 4-ounce (about ⅔ cup) portions.

Fat Releasers
Tomato paste, red wine, onions, garlic, ginger, black pepper, lean beef, olive oil

- 1 tablespoon tomato paste
- 2 cups red wine
- 2 large red onions, thinly sliced
- 3 cloves garlic, grated on a zester
- 1 inch fresh ginger, grated
- 2 teaspoons ground coriander
- ½ teaspoon salt
- ¼ teaspoon ground black pepper
- 3 pound rump roast (bottom round)
- 1 tablespoon plus 1 teaspoon extra-virgin olive oil

1. In a 6-quart slow cooker, stir the tomato paste into the red wine. Add the onions, garlic, ginger, coriander, salt, and pepper. Set to high and cook while you brown the meat.

2. Meanwhile, pat the meat dry. In a large nonstick skillet, heat the oil. Add the meat and brown on all sides, 8 to 10 minutes.

3. Add the meat to the hot liquid in the slow cooker, turn the heat to low, and cook for 4 hours. Turn the roast over, cover, and cook on low until the beef is tender and you can pull it apart with a fork, 3 to 4 hours. (Check at 3 hours; if it needs more time, turn the roast over again and cook for another hour.)

4. Let sit for 10 minutes before carving.

5. Meanwhile, reserving the cooking juices, strain the onions and transfer to a food processor. Process to a smooth puree. If the cooking juices have any fat on the surface, skim them a bit first, then add enough of the defatted juices to the onion puree to make a pourable gravy. (Save any remaining cooking juices for making soups, such as the Beef Soup opposite.)

Per serving: 265 calories • 30g protein • 9.5g fat (3g saturated) • 0.5g fiber 22mg calcium • 3mg vitamin C • 5g carbohydrate • 205mg sodium

❯ OPTIONS

This slow-cooker recipe was intentionally designed to produce way more than you would eat at a single meal to give you good leftovers for lunches—or even super-easy dinners. Here are some suggestions for using the leftovers.

Beef Salad (1 serving): Toss 4 ounces cut-up beef with ½ cup diced tomatoes, ¼ cup diced celery, and 1 cup baby arugula or spinach. Make a dressing of 1 teaspoon Dijon mustard, 2 teaspoons extra-virgin olive oil, and 2 teaspoons balsamic vinegar.

Per serving: 322 calories • 33g protein • 17g fat (4g saturated) • 2g fiber 74mg calcium • 17mg vitamin C • 8g carbohydrate • 196mg sodium

Beef Soup (4 servings): In a saucepan, combine 1 cup onion gravy (left over from the roast), 2 cups water, and 1 can (14.5 ounces) diced tomatoes with chiles. Stir in 12 ounces (2 cups) shredded beef and heat through. Stir in some chopped cilantro. Top each serving with 1 tablespoon of shredded reduced-fat cheese (your choice).

Per serving: 231 calories • 27g protein • 8g fat (3g saturated) • 1g fiber 91mg calcium • 14mg vitamin C • 6g carbohydrate • 168mg sodium

Beef Sandwich (1 serving): If you're in Finish Strong, moisten ⅓ to ½ cup shredded beef with a little onion gravy and roll it up in a whole-wheat tortilla with shredded lettuce, finely chopped red onion, and chopped grape tomatoes. Add a teaspoon or so of a piquant ingredient like small capers, minced pickled jalapeño, or minced dill pickle.

Per serving: 239 calories • 32g protein • 8.5g fat (2g saturated) 13g fiber • 69mg calcium • 4mg vitamin C • 20g carbohydrate 363mg sodium

Pan-Seared Sirloin with Red Wine Sauce

Hands-On Time: 15 minutes • **Total Time:** 15 minutes • **Makes:** 4 servings

Sirloin steaks are lean, reasonably priced, and cook quickly. If you're not a steak eater, this preparation works equally well with skinless, boneless chicken breast cutlets. In step 1, sauté the chicken for about 3 minutes instead of 5, then proceed with the recipe. Serve the steaks (or the chicken) with Baked Crispy Eggplant (page 233) and a big green salad. The almond butter in step 3 will thicken the sauce somewhat but will not make the sauce taste like almonds. If you don't mind a thinner sauce, you can leave it out.

Fat Releasers
Olive oil, beef, black pepper, onion, red wine, vinegar, thyme, almond butter

- 2 **teaspoons extra-virgin olive oil**
- 4 **sirloin steaks (4 ounces each)**
- ½ **teaspoon salt**
- ¼ **teaspoon ground black pepper**
- ¼ **cup minced red onion**
- ¾ **cup red wine**
- ⅓ **cup low-sodium chicken broth**
- 1 **tablespoon balsamic vinegar**
- ¼ **teaspoon dried thyme**
- 1 **tablespoon almond butter**

1. In a large nonstick skillet, heat the oil over medium heat. Season the steaks with ¼ teaspoon of the salt and the pepper. Cook the steaks until browned on both sides, about 5 minutes total for medium-rare. Transfer the steaks to a platter.

2. Add the onion to the skillet and cook, stirring, for 1 minute. Add the wine, broth, vinegar, thyme, and the remaining ¼ teaspoon salt and bring to a boil. Boil until reduced by half, about 5 minutes.

3. Whisk in the almond butter and cook until lightly thickened, about 1 minute. Serve the steaks with the sauce spooned on top.

Per serving: 251 calories • 21g protein • 12g fat (3.5g saturated) • 0.5g fiber 23mg calcium • 1mg vitamin C • 4g carbohydrate • 368mg sodium

Parmesan-Pecan Pork

Hands-On Time: 10 minutes • **Total Time:** 15 minutes • **Makes:** 4 servings

If your market carries only thinner pork chops (½ inch thick), reduce the cooking time by about 1 minute per side; but to be sure, cut into the meat toward the end of the cooking time. You want the pork to be juicy and just cooked through, with the faintest hint of pink in the center. The pork will continue to cook a bit after you take the pan off the heat and let the meat sit. The juices will also pull back into the meat to make the chop extra juicy.

Fat Releasers
Pecans, Parmesan cheese, black pepper, eggs, pork loin, olive oil

¼ **cup (1 ounce) pecans**

⅓ **cup grated Parmesan cheese**

Ground black pepper

2 **large egg whites**

4 **boneless pork loin chops (¾ inch thick, 4 ounces each)**

1 **tablespoon extra-virgin olive oil**

COOKING FOR ONE: Stir together 1 tablespoon finely chopped pecans, 4 teaspoons Parmesan cheese, and black pepper to taste. Dredge 1 pork chop in a beaten egg white and the pecan-Parm mixture. Coat a small nonstick skillet with olive oil cooking spray and cook the chop as directed.

1. In a mini food processor, grind the pecans and Parmesan cheese to the texture of fine bread crumbs. Place in a shallow bowl and season with pepper to taste. Put the egg whites in another shallow bowl and lightly beat.

2. Dip the pork in the egg whites (let the excess drip off) and then in the crumb mixture (pat the crumbs on thick). Place on a plate and let sit while you heat the oil.

3. In a large nonstick skillet, heat the oil over medium heat until shimmering. Add the pork and cook on the first side until the coating is golden, about 3 minutes. Carefully flip the pork and cook on the second side until the pork is mostly cooked through but with a hint of pink in the center, 3 to 4 minutes. Remove the pan from the heat and let the pork sit in the pan for 3 minutes. Serve hot.

Per serving: 259 calories • 24g protein • 17g fat (3.5g saturated) • 0.5g fiber 121mg calcium • 0mg vitamin C • 1g carbohydrate • 186mg sodium

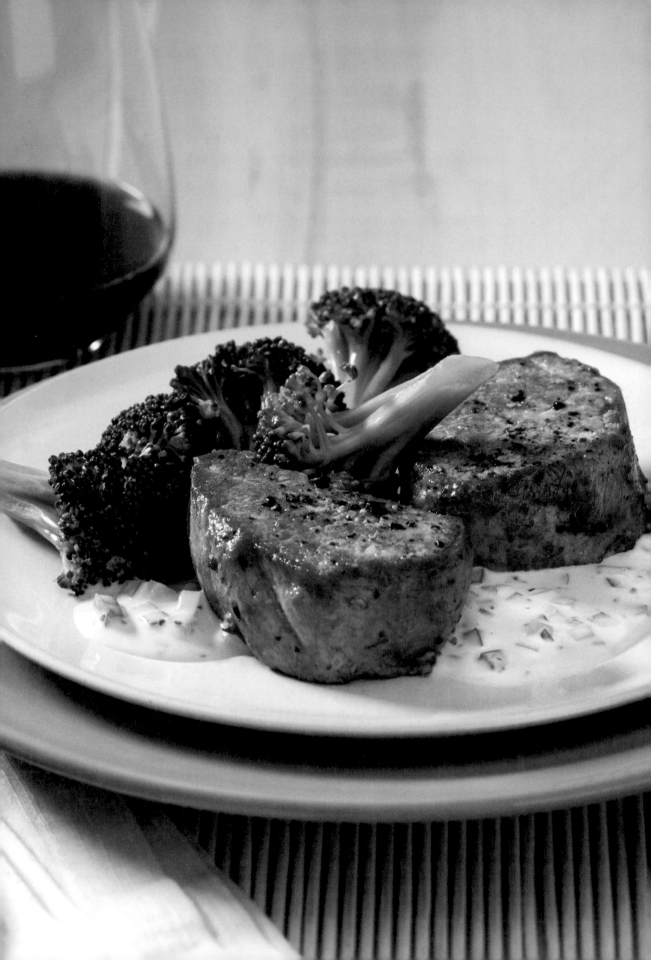

Pepper Loin Steaks

Hands-On Time: 25 minutes • **Total Time:** 35 minutes • **Makes:** 4 servings

Crushed black pepper gives this dish a kick, while the combo of broth and cream cheese makes for a creamy, soothing sauce. You can either crush peppercorns yourself for this dish or look for "butcher's grind" pepper in the supermarket. If you'd prefer, swap out the pork tenderloin for boneless pork loin chops or sirloin steaks. Serve the steaks with steamed broccoli or Lemon-Braised Fennel & Artichokes (page 228).

Fat Releasers
Pork, olive oil, black pepper, bell pepper, cream cheese, parsley

- 1 **pork tenderloin (1 pound)**
- 2 **teaspoons extra-virgin olive oil**
- ¼ **teaspoon kosher salt**
- 2 **teaspoons crushed black pepper**
- 1 **red bell pepper (or your favorite pepper), diced**
- 1 **cup low-sodium chicken broth**
- 3 **tablespoons ⅓-less-fat cream cheese**
- 2 **tablespoons minced parsley**

1. Cut the pork crosswise into 8 equal pieces (medallions).

2. In a large nonstick skillet, heat the oil over medium heat. Sprinkle the medallions with the salt and press the crushed black pepper into both sides. Brown the medallions on both sides and cook until cooked through but still juicy, 3 to 4 minutes per side. Transfer to a platter.

3. Add the bell pepper to the skillet and cook 2 minutes to soften slightly. Add the broth and bring to a boil. Boil to reduce to ⅔ cup, about 7 minutes. Whisk in the cream cheese and cook 1 minute, just until the cheese has melted. Stir in the parsley.

4. Return the medallions to the pan just to warm them. Spoon the sauce on dinner plates and top with the pork.

Per serving: 186 calories • 26g protein • 7g fat (2.5g saturated) • 1g fiber 25mg calcium • 41mg vitamin C • 3g carbohydrate • 356mg sodium

Roast Herb-Rubbed Turkey Breast

Hands-On Time: 10 minutes • **Total Time:** 50 minutes • **Makes:** 4 servings

Stuffing flavoring mixtures under the skin of the turkey ensures that the turkey flesh, not the skin, will pick up all of the flavor. Roasting with the skin on keeps the turkey juicy and also prevents the garlic-herb rub from burning. To make this a meal, serve with Red Quinoa Salad with Avocado (page 195) and Sauté of Peppers & Sugar Snap Peas (page 224). If you're on Finish Strong, try it with Barley Risotto with Collards (page 241) or Cajun Sweet Potato Fries (page 247) instead.

Fat Releasers
Garlic, rosemary, basil, olive oil, lemons, turkey

---

5 cloves garlic, coarsely chopped

¾ teaspoon kosher salt

1 tablespoon crumbled dried rosemary

2 teaspoons dried basil

1 tablespoon plus 1 teaspoon extra-virgin olive oil

1 tablespoon fresh lemon juice

1½-pound skin-on, boneless turkey breast half

1. Preheat the oven to 425°F. Place the garlic on a cutting board and sprinkle ¼ teaspoon of the salt over it. Chop it finely, and then with the flat side of your knife, mash it to a paste.

2. Transfer the mashed garlic to a bowl and add the rosemary, basil, oil, lemon juice, and remaining ½ teaspoon salt. Run your fingers under the skin of the turkey, being careful not to tear it, and lift it up but not off the turkey. Rub the garlic mixture all over the top side of the turkey and then fold the skin back in place.

3. Place in a small roasting pan and roast until the skin is browned and an instant-read thermometer inserted in the thickest part reads 160°F, about 30 minutes. Tent the turkey with foil and let rest 10 minutes before removing (and discarding) the skin and slicing the meat.

Per serving: 231 calories • 41g protein • 5.5g fat (1g saturated) • 0.5g fiber
43mg calcium • 3mg vitamin C • 2g carbohydrate • 431mg sodium

Yogurt Baked Chicken

Hands-On Time: 5 minutes • **Total Time:** 20 minutes + marinating time

Makes: 4 servings

Yogurt is a great tenderizer. Here it combines with hot sauce, black pepper, and some warm spices to make for chicken that is not only tender and juicy but spicy and incredibly flavorful. For Fade Away, serve with Red Quinoa Salad with Avocado (page 195) and steamed green beans or asparagus. If you're in Finish Strong, serve with Brown Basmati Risi e Bisi (page 244) and a cooling side salad of Belgian Endive & Grapes (page 221).

Fat Releasers
Yogurt, hot sauce, chili powder, ginger, black pepper, chicken

- ½ **cup 0% Greek yogurt**
- ¼ **cup hot sauce, such as Frank's RedHot**
- 2 **tablespoons reduced-sodium soy sauce**
- 1 **tablespoon water**
- ½ **teaspoon chili powder**
- ½ **teaspoon ground coriander**
- ½ **teaspoon ground ginger**
- ¼ **teaspoon ground black pepper**
- 4 **skinless, boneless chicken breast halves (6 ounces each)**

1. In a shallow baking dish with a cover, combine the yogurt, hot sauce, soy sauce, water, chili powder, coriander, ginger, and pepper. Add the chicken and spoon the yogurt mixture over the top. Cover and refrigerate for at least 6 hours or up to 24 hours.

2. Preheat the oven to 400°F. Line a rimmed baking sheet with parchment paper.

3. Lift the chicken from the marinade (discard the marinade). Place the chicken on the baking sheet and roast until the juices run clear and the chicken is cooked through but still moist, or until an instant-read thermometer registers 160°F, about 12 minutes.

Per serving: 185 calories • 35g protein • 4g fat (1g saturated) • 0g fiber 19mg calcium • 0mg vitamin C • 0g carbohydrate • 136mg sodium

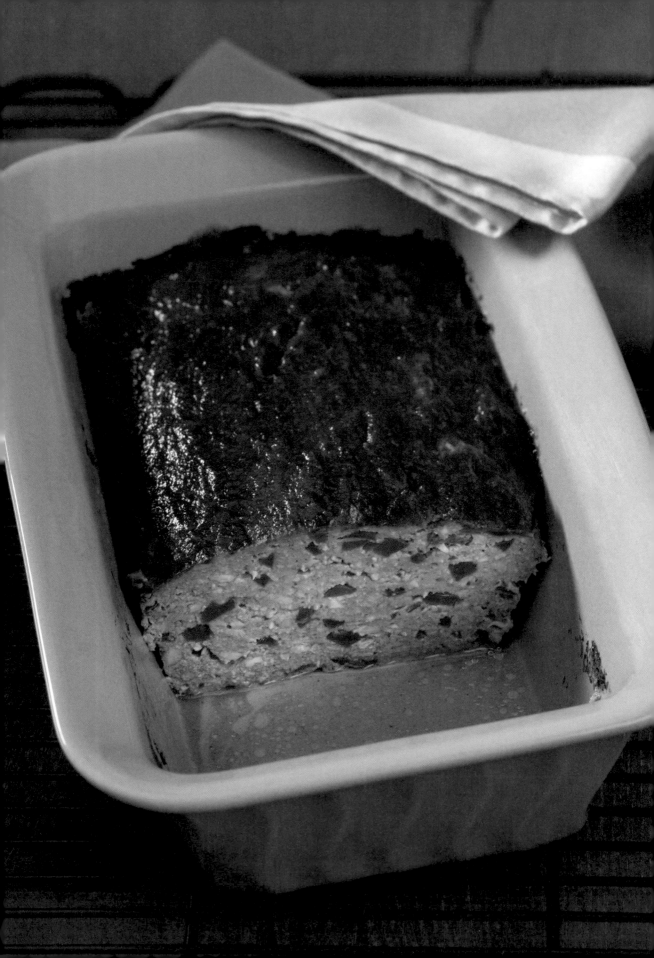

Confetti Meatloaf

Hands-On Time: 10 minutes • **Total Time:** 1 hour 25 minutes + standing time

Makes: 8 servings

When you make a meatloaf without bread or oats, the juices from the turkey and the other ingredients will naturally bubble up around the outside of the loaf. So, to give the juices time to absorb back into the loaf, you need to let the meatloaf sit for a while after baking. Or, if you are in the Finish Strong phase of the diet, you could add 2 slices of multigrain bread, finely crumbled, to the meatloaf mixture.

Fat Releasers
Edamame, bell pepper, turkey breast, tomato paste, olive oil, vinegar, eggs, garlic

- 1 cup (6 ounces) frozen shelled edamame, thawed
- 1 red bell pepper, diced (1 cup)
- 1¼ pounds ground turkey breast
- ½ pound ground turkey
- ¼ cup no-salt-added tomato paste
- 2 tablespoons extra-virgin olive oil
- 2 tablespoons balsamic vinegar
- 1 teaspoon salt
- 1 teaspoon smoked paprika
- 1 large egg
- 2 large egg whites
- 2 cloves garlic, grated on a zester

1. Preheat the oven to 350°F. Lightly coat a 9 x 5-inch loaf pan with cooking spray or use a nonstick pan.

2. In a food processor, pulse-chop the edamame until coarsely ground.

3. Transfer the edamame to a bowl and add the bell pepper and ground turkey.

4. In a small bowl, combine the tomato paste, oil, vinegar, salt, and paprika. Measure out 3 tablespoons and set aside to use as a glaze.

5. Add the remaining tomato paste mixture to the bowl with the turkey. Add the whole egg, egg whites, and garlic and use your hands to gently but thoroughly combine the mixture. Transfer the mixture to the loaf pan, making it higher at the center than at the edges.

6. Brush the reserved tomato glaze on top of the meatloaf and bake until cooked through and the juices run clear, 1 hour to 1 hour 15 minutes. Let stand for 10 minutes before serving.

Per serving: 204 calories • 28g protein • 8g fat (1.5g saturated) • 2g fiber
27mg calcium • 26mg vitamin C • 6g carbohydrate • 373mg sodium

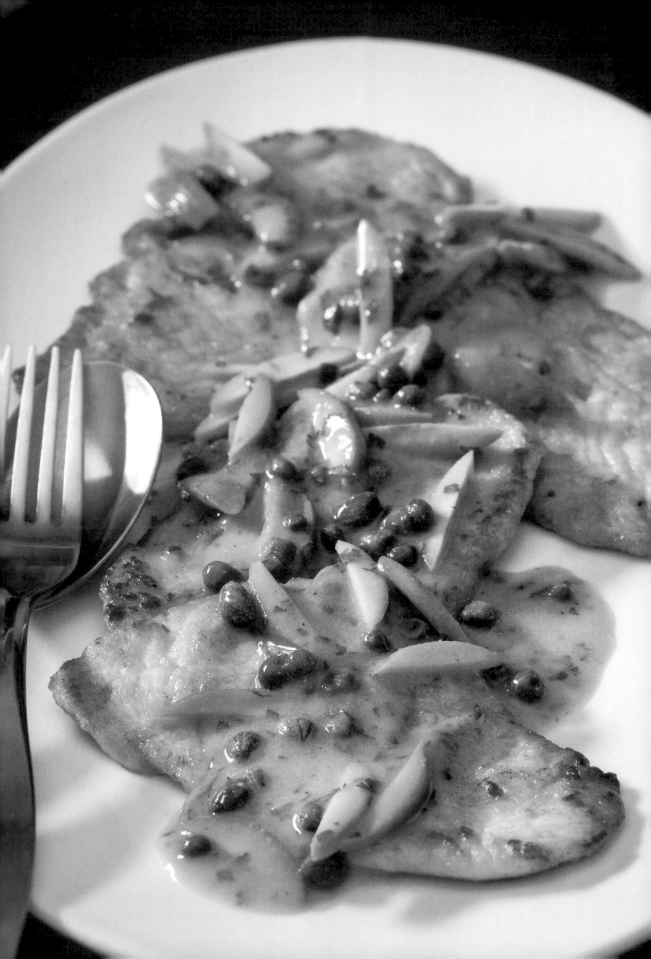

Chicken Piccata with Capers & Olives

Hands-On Time: 20 minutes • **Total Time:** 20 minutes • **Makes:** 4 servings

It's easy enough to make your own cutlets and less expensive, too. Here's how: Place skinless, boneless chicken breast halves in the freezer for 30 minutes to firm them up, then place them on a work surface and with a long-bladed knife or chef's knife, slice them horizontally to make ½-inch-thick cutlets.

Fat Releasers
Olive oil, chicken, chickpea flour, garlic, lemons, parsley

- 4 teaspoons extra-virgin olive oil
- 8 chicken cutlets (1 pound total)
- ¼ teaspoon salt
- ⅓ cup plus 2 tablespoons chickpea flour
- 2 cloves garlic, thinly sliced
- 1 cup low-sodium chicken broth
- ¼ cup fresh lemon juice
- 2 teaspoons nonpareil capers, rinsed
- ¼ cup green olives, pitted and coarsely chopped
- ½ cup coarsely chopped flat-leaf parsley

COOKING FOR ONE: Use 1 teaspoon olive oil, 2 chicken cutlets, ¼ teaspoon salt, 1 tablespoon chickpea flour, 1 clove garlic, ¼ cup broth, 1 tablespoon fresh lemon juice, ½ teaspoon capers, 1 tablespoon chopped olives, and 2 tablespoons chopped parsley. Omit the chickpea flour in the broth.

1. In a large nonstick skillet, heat 2 teaspoons of the oil over medium-high heat. Sprinkle the chicken with the salt, then dredge it in the ⅓ cup chickpea flour, shaking off the excess. Cook half the chicken until golden brown and cooked through, about 1 minute per side. Transfer to a platter. Repeat with the remaining chicken and oil.

2. Add the garlic to the skillet and cook until just beginning to color, about 1 minute. In a small bowl, stir 2 tablespoons broth into the remaining 2 tablespoons chickpea flour to make a smooth paste. Then stir in the remaining broth. Add the broth mixture to the skillet and bring to a boil. Cook until thickened, about 45 seconds. Off the heat, stir in the lemon juice, capers, olives, and parsley. Spoon the sauce over the chicken and serve.

Per serving: 220 calories • 26g protein • 8.5g fat (1.5g saturated) • 1.5g fiber 33mg calcium • 17mg vitamin C • 9g carbohydrate • 334mg sodium

Baked Pistachio-Lime Chicken Pockets

Hands-On Time: 15 minutes • **Total Time:** 45 minutes • **Makes:** 4 servings

Try different nut and citrus combinations in this simple stuffing for chicken: orange and pecan or lemon and walnut. Serve the chicken with steamed asparagus and Romaine with Guacamole Dressing (page 199).

Fat Releasers
Pistachios, garlic, ginger, limes, chicken breast, pistachio oil

- ¼ cup raw pistachios (1½ ounces)
- 1 small clove garlic, peeled and halved
- 1 teaspoon grated lime zest
- ½ teaspoon ground cumin
- ½ teaspoon ground ginger
- ⅓ teaspoon salt
- 2 tablespoons fresh lime juice
- 4 skinless, boneless chicken breast halves (6 ounces each)
- 2 teaspoons pistachio oil, peanut oil, or extra-virgin olive oil
- ½ teaspoon paprika

1. Preheat the oven to 400°F.

2. In a mini food processor, process the pistachios until coarsely ground. Add the garlic, lime zest, cumin, ginger, and salt and pulse until finely ground. Add 1 tablespoon of the lime juice and process until a thick paste forms.

3. With a sharp knife, make a horizontal cut into the flesh on the fat, smooth side of a chicken breast. Wiggle the knife around to make a pocket in the chicken.

Stuff the breast with one-fourth of the pistachio mixture (about 1 tablespoon). Repeat with the remaining breasts and pistachio stuffing.

4. In a small bowl, stir together the remaining 1 tablespoon lime juice, the oil, and paprika. Arrange the chicken on a rimmed baking sheet and brush or rub the lime-paprika mixture over the chicken.

5. Roast until the juices run clear and the chicken is cooked through but still moist, 20 to 25 minutes. Remove from the oven and let rest for 5 minutes before serving.

COOKING FOR ONE: Make up the whole amount of pistachio stuffing and use just 1 tablespoon to stuff a 6-ounce chicken breast. (Divide the remainder into 1-tablespoon portions and freeze for the next time you want to make this dish.) Brush the chicken with a mixture of 1½ teaspoons lime juice, ½ teaspoon oil, and a generous pinch of paprika. Bake as directed.

Per serving: 268 calories • 37g protein • 11g fat (2g saturated) • 1.5g fiber
33mg calcium • 3mg vitamin C • 4g carbohydrate • 156mg sodium

Herb-Crusted Salmon

Hands-On Time: 15 minutes • **Total Time:** 25 minutes • **Makes:** 4 servings

This mix of fresh herbs would also work well with other meaty fish such as tuna, cod, grouper, or swordfish. Because the salmon is oil-rich (and a great source of omega-3s), it should be paired with a very lean side dish, such as Lemon-Braised Fennel & Artichokes (page 228) or Sauté of Peppers & Sugar Snap Peas (page 224).

Fat Releasers
Salmon, lemons, black pepper, basil, parsley, scallions

- 4 **salmon fillets (6 ounces each)**
- 1 **tablespoon plus 1 teaspoon Dijon mustard**
- ¼ **cup fresh lemon juice**
- ¼ **teaspoon salt**
- ¼ **teaspoon ground black pepper**
- ¼ **cup chopped fresh basil**
- ¼ **cup flat-leaf parsley leaves, coarsely chopped**
- 2 **scallions, thinly sliced**
- **Lemon wedges, for serving**

1. Preheat the oven to 450°F.

2. Place the salmon on a rimmed baking sheet. In a small bowl, combine the mustard, lemon juice, salt, and pepper. Brush the mixture on the salmon. Sprinkle the salmon with the basil, parsley, and scallions, pressing to adhere.

3. Bake until the salmon is still slightly rare in the center, about 10 minutes. Serve with lemon wedges.

COOKING FOR ONE: Combine 1 teaspoon Dijon with 1 tablespoon lemon juice and a pinch each of salt and pepper. Brush the mixture onto 1 salmon fillet. Top the fillet with 1 tablespoon each chopped basil and parsley and 1 thinly sliced scallion. The baking time remains the same.

Per serving: 289 calories • 39g protein • 12g fat (2g saturated) • 0.5g fiber 40mg calcium • 13mg vitamin C • 3g carbohydrate • 354mg sodium

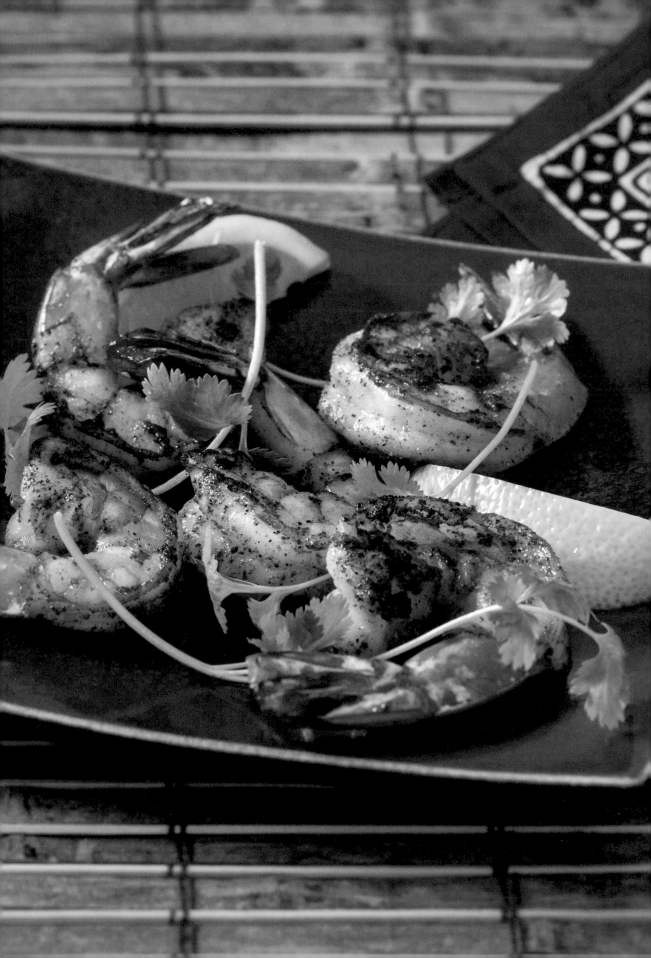

Indian-Spiced Shrimp

Hands-On Time: 20 minutes • **Total Time:** 20 minutes • **Makes:** 4 servings

Garam masala, common in Indian cooking, is a fragrant blend of both sweet and hot spices and can be found on supermarket shelves along with the other spices. It's great to have on hand and can be used in rubs for both meat and fish or stirred into soups and stews for a flavor boost. Cooking the shrimp on medium-low rather than over high heat keeps them tender. Leaving the tails on makes for a nice presentation but is not essential.

Fat Releasers
Shrimp, olive oil, lemons

2½ teaspoons garam masala

¼ teaspoon kosher salt

1½ pounds large shrimp (about 24), peeled and deveined, tails left on

4 teaspoons extra-virgin olive oil

½ cup chopped fresh cilantro

4 lemon wedges, for serving

1. In a medium bowl, stir together the garam masala and salt. Add the shrimp and toss well to coat.

2. In a large nonstick skillet, heat 2 teaspoons of the oil over medium-low heat. Add half the shrimp and cook, turning them until they turn pink, about 3 minutes. Repeat with the remaining shrimp and oil.

3. Transfer the shrimp to plates, sprinkle the cilantro over the shrimp, and serve with lemon wedges.

Per serving: 227 calories • 39g protein • 7g fat (1g saturated) • 0g fiber 112mg calcium • 7mg vitamin C • 1g carbohydrate • 566mg sodium

Sesame-Walnut Tofu Burgers

Hands-On Time: 25 minutes • **Total Time:** 25 minutes • **Makes:** 4 burgers

The combination of tofu and chickpea flour loads this vegetarian burger with protein; and the combination of flaxseed meal, walnuts, and sesame oil contributes huge amounts of good-for-you fats. The flavors and textures in these burgers are reminiscent of falafel (without the deep-fat frying, of course). You can form the patties ahead of time and freeze them for cooking later. Thaw them in the refrigerator. In Finish Strong, serve the burger with shredded lettuce in a small whole-wheat pita.

Fat Releasers
Tofu, egg, sesame oil, hot sauce, walnuts, scallions, flaxseed meal, chickpea flour, lemons

1 container (14 ounces) extra-firm tofu, well drained

1 large egg

1 teaspoon sesame oil

1 teaspoon hot sauce or vinegar (any type)

½ teaspoon ground cumin

½ teaspoon salt

⅓ cup walnut halves, toasted and finely chopped

2 scallions, very finely chopped

2 tablespoons flaxseed meal

6 tablespoons chickpea flour

Lemon wedges, for serving

1. In a large bowl, mash the tofu with a fork until it resembles ground meat. Then mash in the egg, sesame oil, hot sauce, cumin, and salt. Stir in the walnuts, scallions, flaxseed meal, and chickpea flour. Form into 4 patties about 4 inches in diameter.

2. Coat a large nonstick skillet with olive oil spray and heat over medium-high heat. Add the patties, reduce the heat to medium, and cook without turning for 4 minutes. Gently flip the patties and cook for 4 minutes on the second side. Cover the pan and cook until hot throughout, about 4 minutes. Serve with the lemon wedges.

Per burger: 240 calories • 16g protein • 16g fat (2g saturated) • 4g fiber 108mg calcium • 2mg vitamin C • 11g carbohydrate • 328mg sodium

Meatless Sloppy Joes

Hands-On Time: 25 minutes • **Total Time:** 25 minutes • **Makes:** 4 servings

Finely chopped cabbage and almonds give this vegetarian sloppy joe mixture a meaty texture. If you can find smoked portobellos, use them here in place of the regular. Pair the sloppy joes with Warm Goat Cheese on a Bed of Greens (page 198).

Fat Releasers
Cabbage, almonds, black beans, olive oil, scallions, garlic, tomato sauce, chili powder

- 1½ cups coleslaw mix or shredded cabbage
- ½ cup raw almonds
- 1 can (15 ounces) no-salt-added black beans, rinsed and drained
- 2 teaspoons extra-virgin olive oil
- 1 bunch scallions, chopped
- 2 cloves garlic, minced
- 1 can (8 ounces) no-salt-added tomato sauce
- 1 tablespoon Worcestershire sauce
- 1 teaspoon chili powder
- ½ teaspoon salt
- ½ cup water
- 4 portobello mushroom caps (the size of large hamburger buns)

1. In a mini food processor, pulse-chop the coleslaw mix to the texture of coarse crumbs. Transfer to a bowl. Add the almonds to the mini food processor and do the same thing. Add to the coleslaw mix. Add the beans to the mini food processor and carefully, in short bursts, pulse-chop the beans; you don't want them to turn into a paste. Toss the ingredients together.

2. In a large nonstick skillet, heat the oil over medium-high heat. Add the scallions and garlic and cook until softened, about 3 minutes.

3. Add the coleslaw-almond mixture, the tomato sauce, Worcestershire sauce, chili powder, salt, and water. Stir well, bring to a simmer, cover, and cook until the cabbage is tender and the flavors have blended, about 8 minutes. Check occasionally to make sure it isn't sticking. Uncover, and if the mixture is still very wet, stir until the mixture is sloppy but not soupy, 1 or 2 minutes.

4. Meanwhile, coat the mushrooms lightly with cooking spray. Cook the mushrooms in a sandwich press, hinged electric grill, or on a stovetop grill pan until tender but not shriveled, 8 to 10 minutes, depending on the thickness of the mushrooms.

5. To serve, place a portobello cap gill-side up on a plate and top with about ¾ cup of the sloppy joe mixture.

Per serving: 266 calories • 13g protein • 12g fat (1g saturated) • 10g fiber
132mg calcium • 16mg vitamin C • 31g carbohydrate • 395mg sodium

Jerk Steak

Hands-On Time: 10 minutes ● **Total Time:** 15 minutes + marinating time
Makes: 4 servings

Jerk, a style of cooking in Jamaica and the Caribbean, relies on either a dry rub or a wet marinade and is always spicy. This tamed-down version still has a bit of heat, but feel free to increase the amount of hot pepper sauce and black pepper; or, if you're so inclined, add some pickled jalapeño to the puree. Serve the steaks with Sweet & Sour Greens with Bacon (page 237) and Chickpea Salad with Carrot Dressing (page 220).

Fat Releasers
Scallions, garlic, lime juice, honey, hot sauce, cinnamon, black pepper, beef

- 3 **scallions, sliced**
- 3 **cloves garlic, peeled**
- 2 **tablespoons fresh lime juice**
- 1 **tablespoon reduced-sodium soy sauce**
- 2 **teaspoons honey**
- ½ **teaspoon hot pepper sauce, such as Frank's RedHot**
- ½ **teaspoon dried thyme**
- ¼ **teaspoon ground allspice**
- ¼ **teaspoon ground cinnamon**
- ¼ **teaspoon ground black pepper**
- ¼ **teaspoon salt**
- 4 **sirloin steaks (4 ounces each)**

1. In a food processor, puree the scallions, garlic, lime juice, soy sauce, honey, hot pepper sauce, thyme, allspice, cinnamon, pepper, and salt.

2. Place the steaks in a nonreactive pan or in a resealable plastic bag and pour the mixture over them. Refrigerate at least 1 hour, turning the steaks over once.

3. Preheat the broiler. Broil the steaks 4 inches from the heat about 3 minutes per side for medium rare.

Per serving: 179 calories ● 27g protein ● 5g fat (2g saturated) ● 0.5g fiber 36mg calcium ● 5mg vitamin C ● 6g carbohydrate ● 350mg sodium

North Carolina Barbecued Tenderloin

Hands-On Time: 5 minutes • **Total Time:** 1 hour 5 minutes • **Makes:** 4 servings

Low and slow is how barbecue is generally done. Here the pork cooks at a relatively low temperature until just done. The cooking juices are then cooked down to make a sauce. Serve the pork with Parmesan-Crumbed Roasted Root Vegetables (page 248) and a large tossed salad.

Fat Releasers
Vinegar, honey, tomato paste, hot sauce, pork

⅓ cup cider vinegar

2 tablespoons honey

2 tablespoons no-salt-added tomato paste

2½ teaspoons hot sauce, such as Frank's RedHot

1 teaspoon smoked paprika

½ teaspoon salt

1 pork tenderloin (about 1 pound), halved crosswise

1. Preheat the oven to 300°F.

2. In a small roasting pan, whisk together the vinegar, honey, tomato paste, hot sauce, paprika, and salt. Add the pork, turning to cover.

3. Cover the pan and bake the pork 15 minutes. Turn it over in the marinade, cover, and bake 15 minutes longer. Uncover and bake until cooked through and an instant-read thermometer registers 145°F, about 30 minutes.

4. Lift the pork from the pan to a carving board and pour the pan juices into a small skillet. Bring the juices to a boil over high heat and cook until lightly thickened and reduced to a generous ⅓ cup, 2 to 3 minutes.

5. Thinly slice the pork and serve topped with the sauce.

Per serving: 168 calories • 24g protein • 2.5g fat (1g saturated) • 0.5g fiber 13mg calcium • 2mg vitamin C • 11g carbohydrate • 376mg sodium

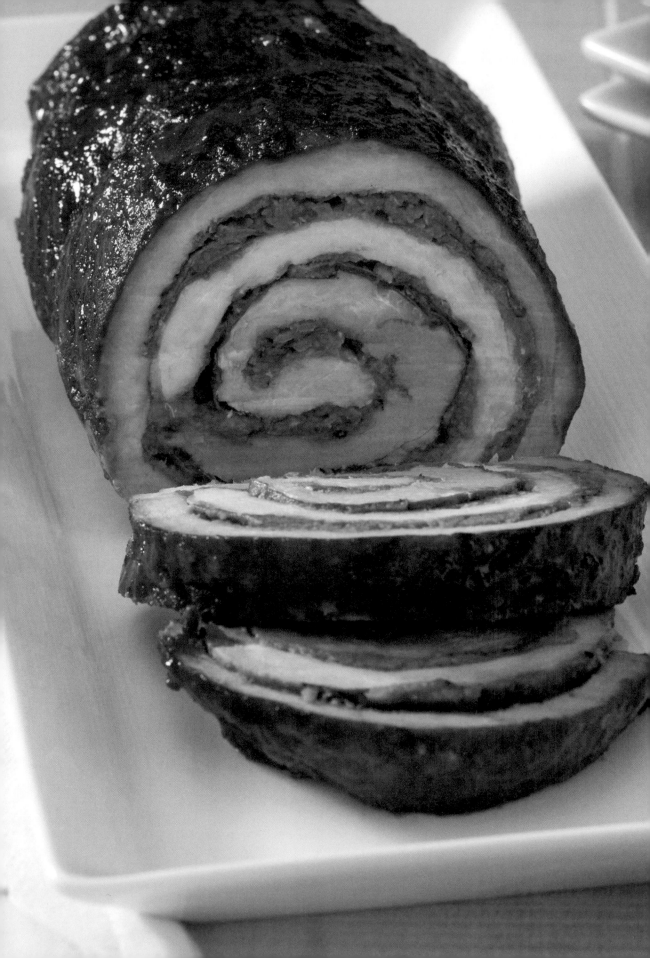

Tomato-Glazed Rolled Pork Roast

Hands-On Time: 15 minutes • **Total Time:** 1 hour 55 minutes + standing time

Makes: 10 servings

For dinner, pair this with Lemony Quinoa & Butternut Pilaf (page 239) and a simple side salad of mixed greens tossed with a little bit of Digest Diet Vinaigrette (page 50). You can use leftovers to make a week's worth of lunches: On one day, use 6 ounces of the leftover pork, cut up, in place of the chicken in Mexican Cobb Salad (page 193). The next day, top a multigrain sandwich thin with 2 ounces of leftover pork, sliced, 2 thin slices reduced-sodium Swiss cheese, red onion, and tomato. Then, add 3 ounces of the pork, cut up, to the Red Quinoa Salad with Avocado (page 195) to make it a main-dish salad.

Fat Releasers
Lentils, garlic, oranges, tomato paste, olive oil, lean pork, black pepper, spinach

¼ cup red lentils

2 cloves garlic, sliced

1 teaspoon smoked paprika

½ teaspoon salt

Grated zest and juice of
    ½ orange

6 tablespoons tomato paste

2 teaspoons extra-virgin
    olive oil

2½ pounds well-trimmed
    boneless center-cut pork
    loin

Ground black pepper

1 cup baby spinach

1. Preheat the oven to 450°F.

2. In a small saucepan of boiling water, simmer the lentils, garlic, ½ teaspoon of the smoked paprika, and the salt until the lentils are very tender, 7 to 8 minutes. Drain well and transfer to a mini food processor. Add the orange zest and 3 tablespoons of the tomato paste and process to a smooth puree.

3. Meanwhile, in a small bowl, combine the orange juice, remaining 3 tablespoons tomato paste, remaining ½ teaspoon smoked paprika, and the oil. Set the glaze aside.

4. Set the loin on a cutting board with a short end of the loin facing you (and if there's still any fat on the roast, set the loin fat-side up). Using a sharp knife, make a lengthwise, horizontal cut into the pork loin about ½ inch down from the top. Continue cutting into the pork, following the shape of the roast, as if you

continued on next page

continued from previous page

were unrolling a scroll. This will create a long piece of meat about 9 x 13 inches and ½ inch thick. With a meat pounder or small heavy skillet, pound any thick spots to even it out.

5. Sprinkle the pork lightly with pepper. Spread the lentil mixture over the pork, leaving a 1-inch border all around. Lay the spinach over the lentil mixture. Starting at a short end, roll up the roast. Tie in three places with kitchen string.

6. Place the roast seam-side down in a small roasting pan. Roast for 10 minutes. Brush with half the tomato glaze. Reduce the oven temperature to 325°F. Roast for 30 minutes. Brush with the remaining glaze and roast until the center of the pork reads 145°F on an instant-read thermometer, 40 to 50 minutes. Transfer to a cutting board and let sit for 15 minutes before slicing. (The internal temperature should rise to 150°F.)

Per serving: 253 calories • 25g protein • 14g fat (4.5g saturated) 1.5g fiber • 12mg calcium • 6mg vitamin C • 6g carbohydrate 168mg sodium

Pork Burgers with Chipotle Relish

Hands-On Time: 15 minutes • **Total Time:** 30 minutes • **Makes:** 4 servings

Serve the burger as is or on a whole-grain hamburger roll with lettuce. The relish that goes with these burgers can be used on all sorts of broiled or grilled meats or fish. It will keep in the refrigerator for at least 3 weeks.

Fat Releasers
Vinegar, chile powder, cauliflower, pork, kidney beans, scallions, yogurt, olive oil

RELISH
- ⅓ cup white wine vinegar
- ½ teaspoon chipotle chile powder
- 1½ cups small fresh or frozen cauliflower florets
- ¼ cup raisins

BURGERS
- 3 ounces low-sodium smoked ham or smoked pork, cut into cubes
- ⅔ cup canned no-salt-added kidney beans, rinsed and drained
- ¾ pound ground pork
- 4 scallions, chopped
- ¼ cup 0% Greek yogurt
- 1 tablespoon extra-virgin olive oil
- ¼ cup water

1. *To make the relish:* In a small saucepan, combine the vinegar and chipotle chile powder. Add the cauliflower and raisins and toss to coat. Cover and bring to a simmer. Cook until the cauliflower is tender but not soft, 3 to 5 minutes (slightly longer for fresh). Set the cauliflower aside to cool, drain it (reserving the vinegar) and transfer to a mini food processor. Pulse until it becomes the texture of hamburger relish adding a little of the vinegar if you want to wetter relish.

2. *To make the burgers:* In a mini food processor, pulse-chop the ham until finely ground. Transfer to a large bowl. Add the beans to the mini food processor and pulse-chop, but do not turn into a paste. Add it to the bowl. Add the ground pork, scallions, and yogurt and blend well. Form the mixture into 4 patties 3½ inches across.

3. In a large nonstick skillet, heat the oil over medium-high heat. Add the pork burgers and cook until nicely browned underneath, about 2 minutes. Flip the burgers and cook until they are browned on the second side, about 1 minute. Add the water to the pan, cover, and cook 2 minutes. Flip the burgers again, cover, and cook until cooked through but still juicy, 1 to 2 minutes.

4. Serve the burgers with the relish on top.

Per serving: 265 calories • 30g protein • 8.5g fat (2g saturated) • 5g fiber • 63mg calcium • 12mg vitamin C • 18g carbohydrate • 286mg sodium

Mexican Slow-Cooked Turkey Breast

Hands-On Time: 20 minutes • **Total Time:** 3 hours 15 minutes to 4 hours 15 minutes • **Makes:** 8 servings

Serve the turkey with ½ cup brown basmati rice per person and drizzle the turkey cooking juices over it. Have steamed broccoli rabe, broccolini, or broccoli as one side dish and Herb-Roasted Tomatoes (page 227) as another. Use leftovers in salads (such as Mexican Cobb Salad, page 193), soups (try Turkey, Black Bean & Winter Squash Soup, page 96), or sandwiches (like Smoked Turkey & Swiss Breakfast Sandwiches, page 86).

Fat Releasers
Oranges, sesame oil, garlic, oregano, cinnamon, black pepper, turkey, shallots, tomato paste

- 1 large orange
- 4 teaspoons sesame oil
- 6 cloves garlic, 1 grated on a zester and 5 sliced
- 2 teaspoons ground cumin
- 2 teaspoons dried oregano
- 1 teaspoon ground cinnamon
- 1 teaspoon hot paprika or cayenne pepper
- 1 teaspoon salt
- ½ teaspoon ground black pepper
- 5-to 6-pounds, skin-on, bone-in turkey breast
- 3 shallots or 1 small red onion, thickly sliced
- 3 tablespoons no-salt-added tomato paste

1. Grate the zest from ½ the orange and squeeze all of the juice.

2. In a small bowl, combine the orange zest, sesame oil, grated garlic, cumin, oregano, cinnamon, hot paprika, salt, and black pepper. Carefully separate the turkey skin from flesh with your fingers, then rub the spice paste all over the flesh. Replace the turkey skin (to help keep the turkey moist as it cooks).

3. Sprinkle the shallots and sliced garlic over the bottom of a 6-quart slow cooker. Stir the tomato paste into the orange juice and add enough water to come to 1½ cups liquid. Pour the mixture into the slow cooker, cover, and cook on low for 3 to 4 hours.

4. Transfer the turkey to a cutting board, cover, and let stand before removing (and discarding) the skin and carving.

5. Meanwhile, pour the cooking juices through a strainer, pressing on the solids to extract as much of the flavorful juices as possible. Skim the fat from the juices and serve alongside the turkey.

Per serving: 278 calories • 52g protein • 4g fat (1g saturated) • 1g fiber 40mg calcium • 8mg vitamin C • 7g carbohydrate • 384mg sodium

Pineapple Chicken

Hands-On Time: 10 minutes ● **Total Time:** 40 minutes ● **Makes:** 4 servings

Although this makes a great hot dish, it also makes a wonderful salad, which you can serve warm, at room temperature, or chilled. To make the salad, follow the recipe through step 4, but instead of spooning the sauce over the chicken, transfer the sauce to a medium bowl and whisk in 1 tablespoon extra-virgin olive oil. When the chicken is cool enough to handle, shred it and add it to the bowl along with the scallions, 3 cups shredded lettuce and 1 diced red bell pepper.

Fat Releasers
Pineapple juice, honey, ginger, garlic, chicken, scallions

⅔ cup unsweetened pineapple juice

1½ tablespoons honey

1½ tablespoons reduced-sodium soy sauce

¾ teaspoon ground ginger

3 cloves garlic, smashed

4 skinless, boneless chicken breast halves (about 6 ounces each)

2 scallions, thinly sliced

1. Preheat the oven to 375°F.

2. In a shallow baking dish just large enough to hold the chicken in a single layer, whisk together the pineapple juice, honey, soy sauce, ginger, and garlic. Add the chicken to the pan, spooning the juices over the top.

3. Bake the chicken until just cooked through, about 25 minutes. Lift the chicken from the pan and transfer the pan juices to a medium skillet; discard the garlic.

4. Bring the pan juices to a boil over medium heat and cook until syrupy, about 5 minutes. Serve with the sauce spooned over the chicken and the scallions scattered over the top.

COOKING FOR ONE: In a small baking dish, whisk together 3 tablespoons pineapple juice, 1 teaspoon each honey and soy sauce, ¼ teaspoon ground ginger, and 1 clove garlic. Bake 1 skinless, boneless chicken breast half in the marinade until cooked through, about 20 minutes. Garnish with 1 scallion.

Per serving: 254 calories ● 39g protein ● 4g fat (1g saturated) ● 0.5g fiber
33mg calcium ● 20mg vitamin C ● 14g carbohydrate ● 301mg sodium

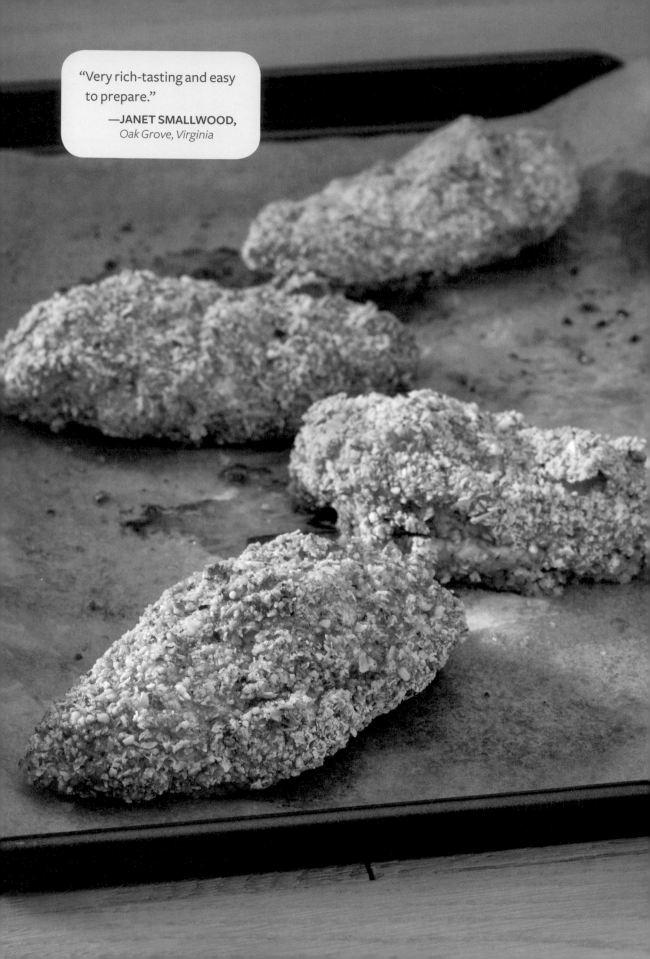

Oven-Fried Chicken

Hands-On Time: 10 minutes • **Total Time:** 40 minutes • **Makes:** 4 servings

Here's a little tip: Use a squeeze bottle (like those they use for mustard and ketchup) for "drizzling" oil over things like these coated chicken breasts. It gives you perfect control and you can drizzle evenly.

Fat Releasers
Eggs, garlic, oats, pecans, black pepper, chicken, olive oil

- 2 **egg whites**
- 2 **teaspoons Dijon mustard**
- 1 **clove garlic, grated on a zester**
- 6 **tablespoons quick-cooking oats**
- ¼ **cup pecans, coarsely chopped**
- ½ **teaspoon salt**
- ¼ **teaspoon ground black pepper**
- 4 **skinless, bone-in chicken breasts (7 ounces each) or 8 small skinless drumsticks (about 4 ounces each)**
- 1 **teaspoon extra-virgin olive oil**

COOKING FOR ONE: Beat together 1 egg white, 1 teaspoon Dijon, and ½ clove garlic. For the coating, mix 1½ tablespoons oats and 1 tablespoon chopped pecans. Season with a pinch each of salt and pepper. Coat a skinless, bone-in chicken breast or 2 small skinless drumsticks in the egg and oats, drizzle with ¼ teaspoon oil, and bake as directed.

1. Preheat the oven to 400°F. Line a baking sheet with parchment paper or a nonstick liner.

2. In a shallow bowl, whisk together the egg whites, mustard, and garlic.

3. In a mini food processor, pulse the oats until coarsely ground. Add the pecans, salt, and pepper and pulse to grind the pecans to the same texture as the oats. Transfer the mixture to a shallow bowl.

4. Dip the chicken first in the egg-mustard mixture, coating it all over. Then dip it into the oat mixture, pressing the mixture into the chicken to get even coverage.

5. Place the chicken on the baking sheet and drizzle each breast with ¼ teaspoon oil.

6. Bake until the chicken is cooked through but still juicy, 25 to 35 minutes.

Per serving (with breasts): 273 calories • 36g protein • 10g fat (1.5g saturated) 1.5g fiber • 30mg calcium • 0mg vitamin C • 7g carbohydrate • 456mg sodium

Per serving (drumsticks): 273 calories • 31g protein • 13g fat (2g saturated) 1.5g fiber • 28mg calcium • 0mg vitamin C • 7g carbohydrate • 515mg sodium

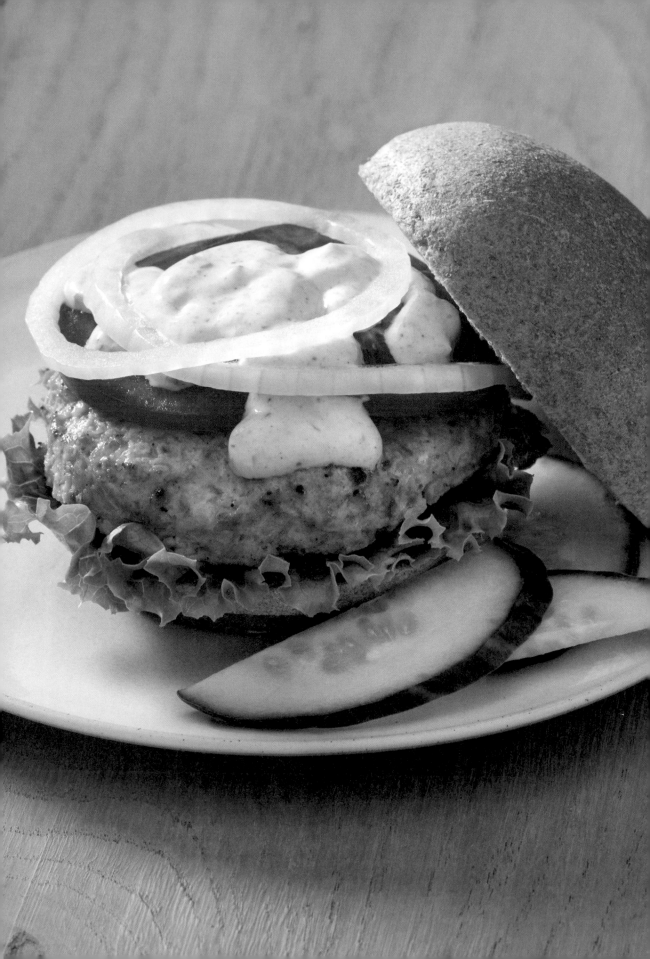

Chicken Burgers

Hands-On Time: 15 minutes • **Total Time:** 25 minutes • **Makes:** 4 servings

Chicken and apple are a classic combination. Here a sweet apple is grated and added along with grated onion to ground chicken. Choose lean ground chicken, not extra-lean: The burgers need a little bit of fat from dark-meat chicken to keep them moist. The burgers freeze nicely, also; just bring them to room temperature before cooking.

Fat Releasers
Yogurt, limes, chicken, multigrain bread, onion, rosemary, black pepper, lettuce, tomato

- ⅓ cup plus 3 tablespoons 0% Greek yogurt
- 2 teaspoons fresh lime juice
- 1 tablespoon minced cilantro
- Pinch of curry powder
- 1 pound lean ground chicken
- ½ slice multigrain sandwich bread, processed to fine crumbs
- 2 teaspoons Dijon mustard
- 2 tablespoons grated onion (1 small onion)
- 1 apple, such as Braeburn, peeled and grated
- ½ teaspoon salt
- ½ teaspoon crumbled dried rosemary
- ½ teaspoon ground black pepper
- 4 multigrain hamburger rolls (2 ounces each), split and toasted (optional)
- Toppings: lettuce, sliced tomato, sliced onion

1. In a small bowl, combine ⅓ cup of the yogurt, the lime juice, cilantro, and curry powder. Refrigerate the cilantro cream until ready to serve.

2. Preheat the broiler with the rack 4 inches from the heat source.

3. In a large bowl, combine the chicken, bread crumbs, remaining 3 tablespoons yogurt, the mustard, onion, apple, salt, rosemary, and pepper. Shape into 4 patties about 1 inch thick.

4. Broil the burgers until cooked through but still juicy, 6 to 8 minutes, turning the burgers over midway.

5. Serve the burgers (on buns, if using) with lettuce, tomato, and onion and a dollop of cilantro cream.

Per serving (without bun): 226 calories • 24g protein • 9.5g fat (2.5g saturated) 2g fiber • 53mg calcium • 8mg vitamin C • 12g carbohydrate • 422mg sodium

Per serving (with bun): 356 calories • 34g protein • 12g fat (2.5g saturated) 8g fiber • 133mg calcium • 8mg vitamin C • 26g carbohydrate • 682mg sodium

Apple-Brined Roast Chicken

Hands-On Time: 10 minutes • **Total Time:** 40 minutes + 8 hours brining
Makes: 6 servings

Brining makes for an incredibly juicy chicken. Before you start, make sure the container you're going to use will fit in your fridge. You can also brine chicken parts; just leave them in the brine for 4 hours for breast meat and up to 8 hours for bone-in thighs and drumsticks. Spatchcocking or butterflying a chicken (see step 3) makes it cook super fast, all in about 30 minutes. If you choose, you can skip that step and roast the chicken whole, for about 50 minutes. If you're using chicken parts instead, roast for about 25 minutes.

Fat Releasers
Rosemary, thyme, black pepper, garlic, chicken, lemons

1½ cups apple cider or juice
⅓ cup coarse salt
5 cups cold water
2 bay leaves
1 teaspoon dried rosemary
1 teaspoon dried thyme
½ teaspoon black peppercorns
5 cloves garlic, smashed
4 strips of lemon zest
1 whole chicken (3½ pounds)
1 large lemon, thinly sliced and seeded

1. In a container large enough to hold the chicken, stir together the apple cider and salt until the salt has melted. Add the cold water, bay leaves, rosemary, thyme, peppercorns, garlic, and lemon zest; stir to combine. Add the chicken and, if necessary, place a weight on top to keep it submerged. Refrigerate for 8 hours. (If you put the chicken in the fridge in the morning, you can make this for dinner.)

2. Preheat the oven to 475°F.

3. Lift the chicken out of the brine, rinse it, and pat it dry. Discard the brine. Using a pair of kitchen shears or a chef's knife, cut down the length of the chicken on either side of the backbone and remove it. Flip the chicken bone-side down and, with your hands, push down on the chicken to flatten it. (You should hear the rib bones crack.)

4. Place the chicken on a rimmed baking sheet. Carefully run your fingers under the skin of the chicken breast and thighs and place the sliced lemon underneath. Roast until cooked through, about 30 minutes. Remove the skin before eating.

Per serving: 237 calories • 39g protein • 4.5g fat (1.5g saturated) • 0g fiber
28mg calcium • 1mg vitamin C • 8g carbohydrate • 555mg sodium

Pomegranate-Glazed Salmon

Hands-On Time: 5 minutes • **Total Time:** 15 minutes • **Makes:** 4 servings

Because salmon is so rich, it marries well with the tangy flavor of pomegranate juice. Look for pomegranate juice, unsweetened, in the supermarket. Leaving the skin on as the salmon cooks makes it easy to lift it from the pan (leaving the skin behind). Use a thin-bladed spatula, place it between the fish and the skin, and lift the fish from the pan. This dish would go quite nicely with some steamed asparagus and Crispy Balsamic Potatoes (page 251).

Fat Releasers
Salmon, orange juice, honey, rosemary, vinegar

- 4 **skin-on salmon fillets (5 ounces each)**
- ¼ **teaspoon salt**
- 1 **cup pomegranate juice**
- 3 **tablespoons fresh orange juice**
- 1 **tablespoon honey**
- ¼ **teaspoon crumbled dried rosemary**
- 1 **teaspoon cider vinegar**

1. Preheat the oven to 450°F. Place the salmon, skin-side down, on a rimmed baking sheet and sprinkle with the salt. Roast until just cooked through, about 10 minutes.

2. Meanwhile, in a small skillet, combine the pomegranate juice, orange juice, honey, and rosemary and bring to a boil over high heat. Boil until reduced to 3 tablespoons, about 10 minutes. Stir in the vinegar.

3. With a metal spatula, lift the salmon from the baking sheet, leaving the skin behind. Serve the salmon with the sauce spooned over it.

COOKING FOR ONE: Reduce the pomegranate juice to ¼ cup, the orange juice to 2 teaspoons, the honey and vinegar to ¾ teaspoon each and cook them in a small saucepan until reduced to about 1 tablespoon. (Watch carefully because it should reduce in a minute or two.) Use 1 salmon fillet and a pinch of salt. The cooking time for the salmon will be the same, about 10 minutes.

Per serving: 286 calories • 32g protein • 10g fat (1.5g saturated) • 0g fiber
31mg calcium • 5mg vitamin C • 14g carbohydrate • 224mg sodium

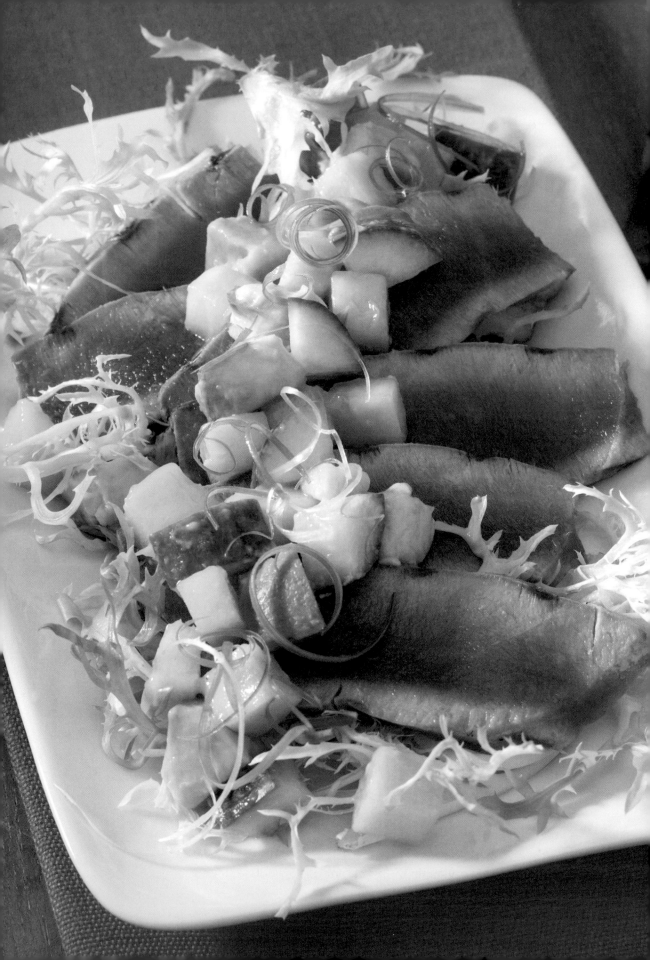

Jamaican Grilled Tuna with Avocado-Mango Relish

Hands-On Time: 15 minutes • **Total Time:** 20 minutes • **Makes:** 4 servings

Here are some good methods for cubing both mangoes and avocados: Halve and pit the avocado. Use a knife to cut the avocado flesh into cubes while it's still in the skin, then scoop the cubes out with a spoon. For the mango, hold it upright and cut downward along both sides of the pit. Place the halves cut-side up on a work surface, cut the flesh into cubes (still in the skin), turn the skin inside out to pop the cubes out, then cut them off. We've used kosher salt because it's coarser than regular table salt and distributes more evenly over the tuna.

Fat Releasers
Mango, avocado, scallions, limes, olive oil, tuna

- 1 **mango, cubed**
- 1 **Hass avocado, cubed**
- 1 **Kirby cucumber, quartered lengthwise and diced**
- 1 **scallion, thinly sliced**
- 2 **tablespoons fresh lime juice**
- 2 **teaspoons extra-virgin olive oil, plus a little for the grill**
- 4 **skinless tuna steaks (5 ounces each)**
- ½ **teaspoon kosher salt**

1. In a medium bowl, combine the mango, avocado, cucumber, scallion, and lime juice to make the relish.

2. Preheat the grill to medium and lightly oil the grates, or lightly brush a grill pan with oil. Brush the tuna with the oil and sprinkle with the salt. Grill 2 to 3 minutes per side for medium-rare. Serve the tuna with the relish spooned on top.

COOKING FOR ONE: Make the whole batch of relish (it makes about 2 cups) and save some for a snack (see below). Then simply cook 1 tuna steak and top with ½ cup relish.

SAVE FOR A SNACK: Make just the relish and have ½ cup as a snack. Serve with thin slices of crunchy jicama.

Per serving: 360 calories • 35g protein • 17g fat (3g saturated) • 4g fiber 35mg calcium • 38mg vitamin C • 18g carbohydrate • 300mg sodium

Pan-Fried Scallops with Citrus Dressing

Hands-On Time: 20 minutes • **Total Time:** 20 minutes • **Makes:** 4 servings

Don't be afraid to ask the fishmonger for a sniff before purchasing any seafood. Sea scallops, big and sweet, should smell briny, not fishy. Once you've gotten them home, keep them in the coldest part of the fridge and use them within a day. The orange juice becomes slightly syrupy when reduced, and the parsley and basil give heft and great flavor to the sauce. If you can't find sea scallops, look for large bay scallops or swap in thick chunks of firm, white-fleshed fish such as grouper or snapper.

Fat Releasers
Olive oil, scallops, whole-wheat flour, garlic, oranges, parsley, basil

- 5 **teaspoons extra-virgin olive oil**
- 1¼ **pounds sea scallops**
- ¼ **teaspoon kosher salt**
- ¼ **cup white whole-wheat flour**
- 3 **cloves garlic, finely chopped**
- ⅔ **cup fresh orange juice**
- ¼ **cup coarsely chopped parsley leaves**
- ¼ **cup coarsely chopped fresh basil leaves**

1. In a large nonstick skillet, heat 3 teaspoons of the oil over medium-high heat. Sprinkle the scallops with the salt and dredge them in the flour, shaking off the excess. Add half the scallops to the pan and cook until golden brown, about 3 minutes, turning them over midway. Transfer to a platter. Repeat with the remaining 2 teaspoons oil and scallops.

2. Add the garlic to the pan and cook until starting to color, about 1 minute. Add the orange juice and bring to a boil. Boil until reduced by half, about 3 minutes. Add the parsley and basil and spoon the sauce over the scallops.

Per serving: 184 calories • 18g protein • 6.5g fat (1g saturated) • 1g fiber 29mg calcium • 24mg vitamin C • 12g carbohydrate • 681mg sodium

Breaded Tofu Steaks

Hands-On Time: 20 minutes • **Total Time:** 30 minutes • **Makes:** 4 servings

Tofu is a flavor sponge, picking up the flavors of whatever it's coated with or tossed in. Here, a mix of sweet honey, spicy hot sauce, and herbs provides great taste while the bread crumb coating makes the tofu crisp on the outside and creamy within. To make this a meal, serve the tofu on a bed of arugula tossed with halved grape tomatoes and thinly sliced red onion. Serve toasted multigrain baguette slices on the side (2 ounces per person).

Fat Releasers
Tofu, whole-wheat bread, honey, hot sauce, marjoram, cinnamon, olive oil

- 1 container (14 ounces) firm tofu, drained
- 2 slices (1 ounce each) whole-wheat bread, toasted and torn into bite-size pieces
- 1 tablespoon honey
- ½ teaspoon hot sauce such as Frank's RedHot
- ½ teaspoon dried marjoram or oregano
- ¼ teaspoon ground cinnamon
- ½ teaspoon kosher salt
- 1 tablespoon plus 2 teaspoons extra-virgin olive oil

1. Halve the block of tofu lengthwise, then cut each piece crosswise into 4 "steaks," for a total of 8.

2. In a food processor, pulse the bread until coarse crumbs form. In a small bowl, stir together the honey, hot sauce, marjoram, and cinnamon. Brush the tofu with the honey mixture, sprinkle with the salt, and dredge in the bread crumbs, pressing to adhere.

3. In a large nonstick or cast-iron skillet, heat 1 tablespoon of the oil over medium-low heat. Add half the tofu and cook until crisp on both sides, turning the tofu over midway, 4 to 5 minutes total.

4. Repeat with the remaining tofu and 2 teaspoons oil.

Per 2-steak serving: 189 calories • 10g protein • 11g fat (1.5g saturated) • 2g fiber 132mg calcium • 0mg vitamin C • 14g carbohydrate • 297mg sodium

Chapter
7

One-Dish Mains

Minimize cleanup and maximize flavor and fat releasing with these scrumptious one-dish meals.

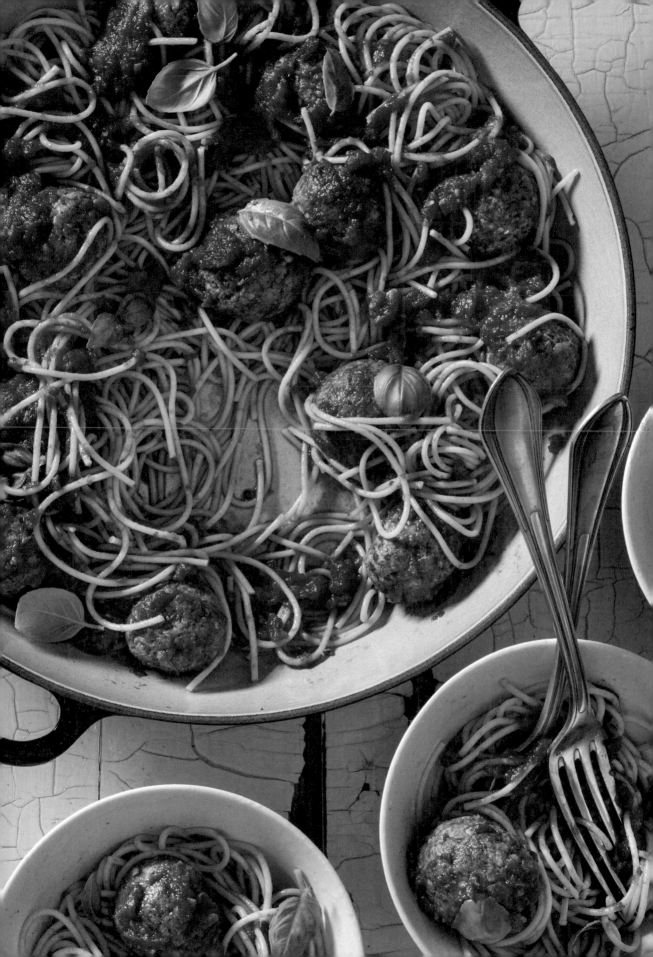

Quinoa Pasta with Peruvian Beef

Hands-On Time: 25 minutes • **Total Time:** 30 minutes • **Makes:** 4 servings

Quinoa—the ancient grain known for its complete protein—comes from Peru, as do the flavors in this beef sauce for quinoa pasta. The sauce is loosely based on a dish called *lomo saltado,* which is a Peruvian stir-fry of beef, onions, vinegar, soy, and tomatoes. If you can't find quinoa pasta, then you can turn this into a Finish Strong dish and make it with any whole-wheat or multigrain pasta.

Fat Releasers
Olive oil, garlic, chile pepper, sirloin, quinoa pasta, onion, bell peppers, vinegar, tomatoes, parsley

- 2 teaspoons extra-virgin olive oil
- 2 cloves garlic, minced
- 1 serrano chile pepper, seeded and minced (optional)
- 8 ounces well-trimmed sirloin, very thinly sliced
- 8 ounces quinoa rotelle pasta
- 1 small red onion, slivered
- 2 large red bell peppers, very thinly sliced
- 1 tablespoon reduced-sodium soy sauce
- 1 tablespoon red wine vinegar
- 2 plum tomatoes, slivered
- ½ cup chopped parsley

1. Bring a large pot of water to a boil.

2. In a large nonstick skillet, heat the oil over medium-high heat. Add the garlic and chile and cook for 1 minute. Add the beef and cook until browned on all sides, 1 to 2 minutes. Transfer the beef to a plate and set aside.

3. Add the pasta to the boiling water and cook according to package directions. Drain well and return to the pot.

4. Meanwhile, add the onion to the skillet and cook until softened, 2 to 3 minutes. Add the bell peppers, soy sauce, and vinegar. Cover and cook until softened, 2 to 3 more minutes. Add the tomatoes, cover, and cook until they start to break down, about 2 minutes.

5. Return the beef to the skillet and cook to heat through. Toss the beef sauce and the parsley with the cooked pasta.

Per 2-cup serving: 318 calories • 19g protein • 7g fat (1g saturated) • 5g fiber 49mg calcium • 121mg vitamin C • 44g carbohydrate • 191mg sodium

Stir-Fried Peanut Beef with Crisp Vegetables

Hands-On Time: 35 minutes • **Total Time:** 35 minutes • **Makes:** 4 servings

Frozen shelled edamame (green soybeans) can be found in most supermarkets along with the other frozen vegetables. Take what you need from the bag, then seal and freeze the remainder. And, if you haven't tried cooked radishes, you'll be surprised by how tasty they can be; they cook up crunchy with a slight bite.

Fat Releasers
Olive oil, edamame, radishes, garlic, ginger, beef, peanut butter, vinegar

- 4 teaspoons extra-virgin olive oil
- ½ pound green beans
- ¾ cup frozen shelled edamame, thawed
- 5 radishes, thinly sliced
- 3 cloves garlic, thinly sliced
- 2-inch piece fresh ginger, thinly sliced and cut into thin matchsticks
- 1 pound flank steak, thinly sliced against the grain
- 1½ tablespoons creamy natural peanut butter
- 1½ teaspoons rice vinegar or cider vinegar
- ½ teaspoon salt
- 2 tablespoons water

1. In a large nonstick skillet, heat 1½ teaspoons of the oil over medium-high heat. Add the green beans and edamame and cook until the green beans are starting to brown, about 4 minutes.

2. Add the radishes, garlic, and ginger and cook, stirring constantly, until the garlic and ginger are tender, about 1 minute. Transfer to a bowl.

3. Add the remaining 2½ teaspoons oil to the skillet. Working in batches, add half the steak and cook, stirring, until lightly browned, about 2 minutes; transfer to the bowl with the vegetables. Repeat with the remaining beef.

4. In a small bowl, whisk together the peanut butter, vinegar, salt, and water. Pour the peanut butter mixture into the skillet, return the beef and vegetables to the skillet, and toss until coated and heated through, about 1 minute.

Per serving: 297 calories • 31g protein • 15g fat (3.5g saturated) • 3.5g fiber 67mg calcium • 8mg vitamin C • 9g carbohydrate • 361mg sodium

Chicken "Lo Mein"

Hands-On Time: 25 minutes • **Total Time:** 25 minutes • **Makes:** 4 servings

In this spin on a classic dish that is usually made with noodles, thin shreds of napa cabbage stand in for the pasta. Finely shred or chop your leftover cabbage and toss with Digest Diet Vinaigrette (page 50; 1 tablespoon for every 2 cups of cabbage). Or save it to make Napa Cabbage with Garlic-Ginger Sauce (page 229).

Fat Releasers
Eggs, sesame oil, chicken, chickpea flour, honey, peanut oil, scallions, napa cabbage

- 1 large egg white
- 2 teaspoons plus 1 tablespoon reduced-sodium soy sauce
- 1 teaspoon sesame oil
- 1 pound skinless, boneless chicken breasts, cut across the grain into very thin slices
- 1 cup low-sodium chicken broth
- 2 cups water
- 2 teaspoons chickpea flour
- 2 teaspoons honey
- 1 tablespoon peanut oil or olive oil
- 5 scallions, cut into 1½-inch lengths
- 8 ounces cremini mushrooms, thinly sliced
- 10 large leaves napa cabbage, cut lengthwise into long, thin slivers

1. In a medium bowl, beat together the egg white, 2 teaspoons of the soy sauce, and the sesame oil. Add the chicken and toss to coat. Let sit while the chicken broth comes to a boil (next step).

2. In a medium saucepan, combine the chicken broth and water and bring to a boil. Set a colander over a bowl. Add the chicken to the boiling broth, stir to separate, and cook until the chicken turns white, about 30 seconds. Reserving the broth, drain into a colander. Set the chicken aside.

3. In a small bowl, stir together the chickpea flour, remaining 1 tablespoon soy sauce, the honey, and ¼ cup of the reserved broth.

4. In a nonstick Dutch oven, heat the peanut oil over medium-high heat. Add the scallions and mushrooms and toss to coat with the oil. Add the napa cabbage and another ¼ cup of the reserved broth (discard the remaining broth or save for making soup). Cover and steam just until the napa cabbage begins to wilt, about 1 minute. Add the chickpea flour mixture, stir well, cover, and cook until all the vegetables are tender, about 1 minute.

5. Uncover, add the chicken, and stir for 30 seconds to combine and heat through.

Per 1¼-cup serving: 219 calories • 28g protein • 8g fat (1.5g saturated) 1.5g fiber • 42mg calcium • 10mg vitamin C • 9g carbohydrate • 413mg sodium

Roast Chicken with Jicama & Brussels Sprouts

Hands-On Time: 20 minutes • **Total Time:** 45 minutes • **Makes:** 4 servings

Leaving the skin on the chicken keeps it moist as it roasts, but in this recipe, because the chicken and vegetables roast together, the chicken is cooked on a sheet of foil so the drippings don't cook into the vegetables. Jicama is a bulbous root vegetable with a texture similar to that of a potato. If you prefer, substitute a white or yellow turnip.

Fat Releasers
Olive oil, lemon, rosemary, Brussels sprouts, garlic, chicken, black pepper

- 1 tablespoon plus 1 teaspoon extra-virgin olive oil
- ½ teaspoon grated lemon zest
- 3 tablespoons fresh lemon juice
- ½ teaspoon crumbled dried rosemary
- 10 ounces Brussels sprouts, halved
- ½ pound jicama, peeled and cut into ½-inch chunks (1½ cups)
- 3 cloves garlic
- 4 skin-on, bone-in chicken breast halves (12 ounces each)
- ½ teaspoon salt
- ¼ teaspoon ground black pepper

1. Preheat the oven to 400°F. In a large bowl, whisk together 1 tablespoon of the oil, the lemon zest, lemon juice, and rosemary. Add the Brussels sprouts, jicama, and garlic to the bowl and toss to coat. Transfer to a rimmed baking sheet and push to one side (to make room for the chicken.)

2. With your fingers, carefully loosen the skin of the chicken and rub the remaining 1 teaspoon oil, the salt, and pepper under the skin, pulling the skin back over the chicken. Place the chicken on a sheet of foil. Fold the edges up to make a rim and place it on the baking sheet with the vegetables.

3. Roast, tossing the vegetables once or twice, until the vegetables are tender and the chicken is cooked through, about 25 minutes. Remove the chicken skin before serving.

Per serving: 355 calories • 52g protein • 10g fat (2.5g saturated) • 5g fiber 64mg calcium • 70mg vitamin C • 12g carbohydrate • 427mg sodium

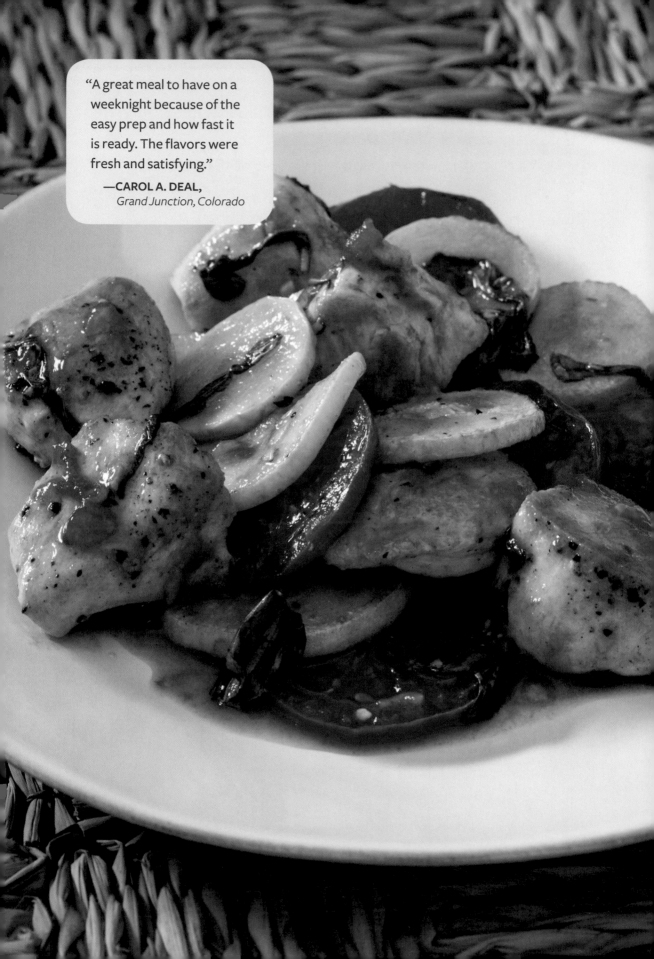

"A great meal to have on a weeknight because of the easy prep and how fast it is ready. The flavors were fresh and satisfying."

—CAROL A. DEAL,
Grand Junction, Colorado

Summer Sauté of Chicken & Yellow Squash

Hands-On Time: 25 minutes • **Total Time:** 25 minutes • **Makes:** 4 servings

Although this fresh-tasting sauté of chicken is at its best fresh out of the pan, it actually makes pretty nice leftovers. If you choose to have the leftovers for lunch (chilled or at room temperature), stir in a little lemon juice (to taste) and add some fresh basil to perk up the basil flavors.

Fat Releasers
Sesame oil, olive oil, chicken, summer squash, black pepper, tomatoes, basil

- 1 teaspoon sesame oil
- 3 teaspoons extra-virgin olive oil
- 1¼ pounds skinless, boneless chicken breasts, cut into ¾-inch chunks
- 4 small yellow summer squash (about 1 pound total), thinly sliced crosswise
- ½ teaspoon salt
- ¼ cup water
- ¼ teaspoon ground black pepper
- 4 plum tomatoes, thinly sliced
- ½ cup shredded fresh basil

1. In a large nonstick skillet or wok, heat the sesame oil and 1 teaspoon of the olive oil over medium-high heat. Add the chicken and stir-fry until opaque all over, 2 to 3 minutes. With a slotted spoon, transfer the chicken to a plate.

2. Add the remaining 2 teaspoons olive oil, the squash, ¼ teaspoon of the salt, and the water. Reduce the heat to medium, cover, and cook for 4 minutes to soften the squash a bit.

3. Stir in the tomatoes, cover, and cook until the tomatoes begin to collapse, about 3 minutes.

4. Return the chicken to the pan, sprinkle with the remaining ¼ teaspoon salt and the pepper, and stir to combine. Cook until the chicken is cooked through, about 3 minutes. Stir in the basil.

Per 1½-cup serving: 241 calories • 34g protein • 8g fat (1.5g saturated) • 3g fiber 54mg calcium • 30mg vitamin C • 7g carbohydrate • 363mg sodium

Vietnamese Pho with Chicken & Spaghetti Squash

Hands-On Time: 25 minutes • **Total Time:** 30 minutes • **Makes:** 4 servings

This classic Vietnamese meal in a bowl (called *pho*) is usually made with noodles, but in this lightened version, spaghetti squash stands in for them. You can easily prep this recipe in stages: Cook the spaghetti squash first; it can sit for an hour or so at room temp. You can also make the frizzled shallots (step 3) ahead of time.

Fat Releasers
Limes, spaghetti squash, olive oil, shallots, serrano chile, bell pepper, chicken

- 1 **lime**
- 1 **spaghetti squash (3½ pounds)**
- 1 **tablespoon plus 1 teaspoon extra-virgin olive oil**
- 4 **large shallots, thinly sliced**
- 4 **cups low-sodium chicken broth**
- ½ **teaspoon salt**
- 1 **serrano chile, seeded and minced**
- 1 **green bell pepper, finely slivered**
- 1 **pound skinless, boneless chicken breast, cut against the grain into very thin slices**
- 3 **tablespoons chopped cilantro**
- 3 **tablespoons chopped fresh mint**

1. Grate the zest of ½ lime into a large bowl. Squeeze in the juice of the whole lime.

2. Pierce the spaghetti squash in several places with a knife or kitchen fork. Microwave on high for 12 minutes, or until the squash is firm-tender (but not too soft). Holding the squash with a potholder, halve it lengthwise. When cool enough to handle, scoop out and discard the seeds, then use a fork to pull the squash flesh into strands. Gently toss the squash with the lime juice and set aside.

3. Meanwhile, in a large nonstick skillet, heat the oil over medium-high heat. Add the shallots and cook until very nicely browned, 5 to 7 minutes. Scrape onto a plate and set aside.

4. In a medium saucepan, combine the broth, salt, chile, and bell pepper and bring to a boil. Working in batches, place the chicken slices in a strainer and lower into the boiling broth to cook, just 45 seconds to 1 minute per batch. Set aside on a plate.

5. To serve, divide the hot broth and bell pepper among 4 large soup bowls. Place a portion of the "noodles" in the center. Top with the cooked chicken, fresh herbs, and fried shallots.

Per serving: 290 calories • 29g protein • 8.5g fat (1.5g saturated) • 5g fiber 79mg calcium • 40mg vitamin C • 26g carbohydrate • 547mg sodium

Wine-Braised Chicken & Leeks

Hands-On Time: 15 minutes • **Total Time:** 35 minutes • **Makes:** 4 servings

To wash leeks, fill a large bowl or the sink with lukewarm water. Slice the leeks, put them in the water, and swish them around. The sand will fall to the bottom and the leeks will float on top. Use a small strainer or a slotted spoon to scoop the leeks out. If you're in Finish Strong, serve this over ½ cup cooked brown rice.

Fat Releasers

Olive oil, chicken, rosemary, black pepper, leeks, zucchini, red wine, tomato paste

- 6 **ounces portobello mushroom caps, preferably smoked portobellos**
- 1 **tablespoon plus 1 teaspoon extra-virgin olive oil**
- 4 **skinless, boneless chicken breast halves (5 ounces each), cut crosswise into thirds**
- ½ **teaspoon crumbled dried rosemary**
- ¼ **teaspoon salt**
- ¼ **teaspoon ground black pepper**
- 4 **medium leeks, halved lengthwise and cut crosswise into ¾-inch pieces**
- 1 **cup low-sodium chicken broth**
- ¾ **pound zucchini, cut into ¾-inch chunks**
- 1 **cup dry red wine**
- 3 **tablespoons no-salt-added tomato paste**
- 3 **ounces low-sodium smoked ham, diced**

1. With a small spoon, scrape out the mushrooms' black gills. Cut the mushrooms into ¾-inch chunks.
2. In a large Dutch oven, heat 1 tablespoon of the oil over medium heat. Add the chicken and cook until golden brown on all sides, 3 to 4 minutes. Transfer the chicken to a plate.
3. Add the remaining 1 teaspoon oil and the mushrooms and sprinkle with the rosemary, salt, and pepper. Cook, without stirring, for 2 minutes.
4. Add the leeks and ¾ cup of the broth. Bring to a boil, cover, and cook, stirring occasionally, until the leeks just begin to soften, about 3 minutes. Stir in the zucchini, cover, and cook for 5 minutes. Add the wine, cover, and cook until the leeks are tender, about 3 minutes.
5. Meanwhile, stir the remaining ¼ cup broth into the tomato paste.
6. Stir the tomato paste mixture and ham into the pan. Return the chicken to the pan, nestling it down into the vegetables. Bring to a boil, reduce to a simmer, cover, and cook until the chicken is cooked through, 6 to 8 minutes.

Per serving: 378 calories • 40g protein • 10g fat (2g saturated) • 3.5g fiber • 95mg calcium • 29mg vitamin C • 21g carbohydrate • 476mg sodium

Spicy Chicken with Green Beans & Baby Bellas

Hands-On Time: 25 minutes • **Total Time:** 35 minutes • **Makes:** 4 servings

Smoked paprika and ancho chile powder used to be specialty items, but now all of the big-brand spice companies are carrying them. The paprika is both sweet and smoky, while the ancho chile powder gives a slight amount of heat. If you prefer, you can substitute regular paprika and your favorite chili powder.

Fat Releasers
Chile powder, chicken, olive oil, onion, garlic, ginger

- 1 teaspoon smoked paprika
- ¾ teaspoon ancho chile powder
- ¼ teaspoon kosher salt
- 1 pound skinless, boneless chicken breast, cut into 1-inch chunks
- 1 tablespoon plus 1 teaspoon extra-virgin olive oil
- ½ pound green beans, trimmed and cut into 2-inch lengths
- 6 ounces baby bella (cremini) mushrooms, quartered
- 1 small red onion, halved and thickly sliced
- ¾ cup low-sodium chicken broth
- 2 cloves garlic, thinly sliced
- 2 tablespoons minced fresh ginger

1. In a medium bowl, combine the paprika, ancho chile powder, and salt. Add the chicken and toss to coat.

2. In a large nonstick skillet, heat the oil over medium heat. Add the green beans, mushrooms, and onion and cook, stirring frequently, until the green beans are starting to brown, about 5 minutes. Add ¼ cup of the broth to the skillet and cook until the beans are crisp-tender, about 4 minutes.

3. Add the chicken, garlic, and ginger and toss to combine. Add the remaining ½ cup broth to the pan and cook until the chicken is just cooked through, about 5 minutes.

Per serving: 213 calories • 27g protein • 8g fat (1.5g saturated) • 2.5g fiber 43mg calcium • 10mg vitamin C • 9g carbohydrate • 273mg sodium

Poached Chicken & Vegetables with Lemon Sauce

Hands-On Time: 20 minutes • **Total Time:** 40 minutes • **Makes:** 4 servings

You'll end up with 2 to 3 cups of very flavorful broth. Freeze it for when you want to make soup.

Fat Releasers
Leeks, garlic, black pepper, zucchini, chicken, lemons, egg

- 2 **large leeks**
- 3 **cups low-sodium chicken broth**
- 2 **cloves garlic, smashed**
- 1 **bay leaf**
- **Ground black pepper**
- 2 **"jumbo" carrots (see page 171)**
- 2 **white turnips**
- 1 **small celeriac (celery root) or 3 ribs celery**
- 1 **zucchini**
- **Salt**
- 4 **small skinless, bone-in chicken thighs (4 ounces each)**
- 2 **skinless, boneless chicken breast halves (5 ounces each)**
- 2 **tablespoons fresh lemon juice**
- 1 **large egg**

1. Cut the leeks at the spot where the pale green turns dark. Thinly sliver enough dark greens to get ½ cup. Trim the roots from the white portion, and wash thoroughly. Then cut the leeks crosswise into 1-inch lengths.

2. In a large Dutch oven, combine the broth, slivered leek greens, garlic, bay leaf, and ¼ teaspoon pepper. Bring to a low simmer.

3. Quarter the carrots lengthwise and then cut crosswise into 1½-inch lengths. Cut the turnips, celeriac (or celery), and zucchini into similar largish pieces.

4. Add all the vegetables but the zucchini to the Dutch oven and sprinkle with ½ teaspoon salt. Bring the broth to a boil over high heat. Reduce to a high simmer, partially cover, and cook until the carrots are just tender, about 5 minutes.

5. Stir in the zucchini. Nestle the chicken well down into the vegetables and return to a boil. Reduce to a high simmer, cover, and cook until the thighs are cooked through, 10 to 15 minutes.

6. Meanwhile, in a small saucepan, whisk the lemon juice and ⅛ teaspoon salt into the egg, until well combined. Whisking constantly, add ½ cup of the hot broth from the chicken. Place the saucepan over medium-low heat and whisk until the sauce thickens slightly, 1 to 2 minutes.

7. Transfer the vegetables to shallow bowls. Halve the chicken breasts and serve each person 1 breast piece and 1 thigh. Spoon lemon sauce (2 generous tablespoons) over each serving and top with a pinch of pepper.

Per serving: 411 calories • 50g protein • 12g fat (3g saturated) • 6g fiber • 136mg calcium 45mg vitamin C • 26g carbohydrate • 678mg sodium

Turkey "Sausage" & Peppers

Hands-On Time: 25 minutes • **Total Time:** 25 minutes • **Makes:** 4 servings

The combination of flavors in this dish is similar to what you might find in a sausage and pepper hero. Store-bought Italian sausages (both pork- and turkey-based) tend to be very high in sodium, so we've made our own Italian-style sausage mixture. For a delicious pasta-like dish, toss the mixture with baked spaghetti squash. If you're on Finish Strong, add 1 large peeled and finely diced sweet potato to the pan in step 2 and toss in ¼ cup dried cranberries at the end or serve over whole-wheat pasta.

Fat Releasers
Turkey, oregano, black pepper, olive oil, onion, garlic, bell peppers, cheese

1¼ **pounds lean ground turkey**

2 **teaspoons paprika**

1 **teaspoon ground fennel**

½ **teaspoon dried oregano**

½ **teaspoon salt**

½ **teaspoon ground black pepper**

1 **tablespoon plus 1 teaspoon extra-virgin olive oil**

1 **large onion, halved and thinly sliced**

2 **ribs celery, thinly sliced**

2 **cloves garlic, thinly sliced**

2 **red bell peppers, thinly sliced**

10 **ounces baby bella (cremini) mushrooms, thinly sliced**

½ **cup shredded reduced-fat Italian cheese blend**

1. In a large bowl, mix together the turkey, paprika, fennel, oregano, salt, and pepper.

2. In a large nonstick skillet, heat the oil over medium heat. Break off tablespoonsful of the "sausage" mixture and add to the skillet along with the onion, celery, and garlic. Cook, stirring frequently, until the onion starts to soften, about 5 minutes.

3. Add the bell peppers and mushrooms and cook, stirring frequently, until the sausage is cooked through and the vegetables are tender, about 10 minutes.

4. Serve topped with the cheese.

Per serving: 343 calories • 35g protein • 17g fat (5.5g saturated) • 3.5g fiber 148mg calcium • 80mg vitamin C • 13g carbohydrate • 389mg sodium

Moroccan Chickpea Stew

Hands-On Time: 45 minutes • **Total Time:** 1 hour • **Makes:** 4 servings

Chock-full of vegetables and nutty-tasting chickpeas, this is perfect to make in the summer, when the freshest zucchini and eggplant are in season. This can be made a day or two ahead (save the cheese for when you're ready to serve) and refrigerated, or it can be frozen up to 3 months.

Fat Releasers
Olive oil, onion, garlic, zucchini, bell pepper, tomatoes, chickpeas, cheese, pumpkin seeds

- 1 tablespoon plus 1 teaspoon extra-virgin olive oil
- 1 medium onion, coarsely chopped (¾ cup)
- 3 cloves garlic, thinly sliced
- 1 zucchini, halved lengthwise and thickly sliced
- 1 red bell pepper, cut into ½-inch chunks
- 1 eggplant (10 ounces), cut into 1-inch chunks (3 cups)
- 1½ teaspoons smoked paprika
- ½ teaspoon salt
- ½ cup water
- 1 can (14.5 ounces) no-salt-added diced tomatoes
- 1 can (15 ounces) no-salt-added chickpeas, rinsed and drained
- ½ cup chopped cilantro
- ⅓ cup crumbled reduced-fat feta cheese
- ¼ cup hulled pumpkin seeds

1. In a large nonstick saucepan or Dutch oven, heat the oil over medium-low heat. Add the onion and garlic and cook, stirring frequently, until starting to soften, about 5 minutes. Add the zucchini and cook, stirring frequently, until it becomes translucent, about 10 minutes.

2. Add the bell pepper, eggplant, paprika, and salt and stir to coat. Add the water, cover, and cook until the eggplant has softened, about 5 minutes.

3. Stir in the tomatoes, chickpeas, and cilantro and bring to a boil. Reduce to a simmer, cover, and cook for 10 minutes to blend the flavors and thicken the stew. Serve sprinkled with feta and pumpkin seeds.

Per serving: 304 calories • 14g protein • 11g fat (2.5g saturated) • 12g fiber 138mg calcium • 94mg vitamin C • 39g carbohydrate • 524mg sodium

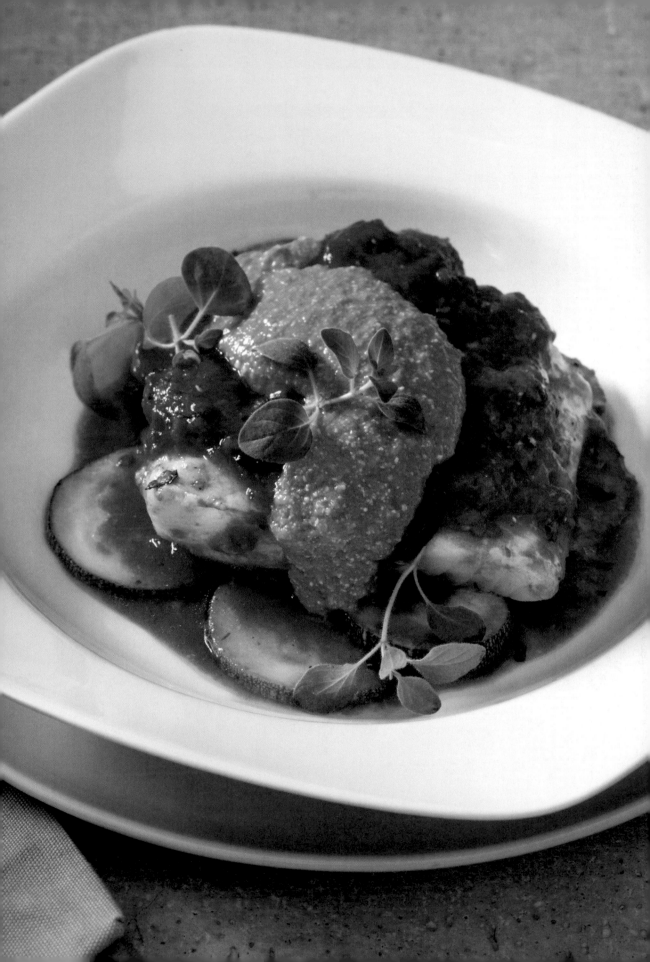

Cod, Roasted Red Pepper & Feta Bake

Hands-On Time: 30 minutes • **Total Time:** 50 minutes • **Makes:** 4 servings

With red peppers, zucchini, mint, feta, and tomato, this dish has a definite Mediterranean feel. While we've used cod, feel free to swap in grouper, hake, or shrimp.

Fat Releasers
Bell pepper, cheese, olive oil, zucchini, tomatoes, oranges, oregano, black pepper, cod

- 1 **red bell pepper, cut vertically into 4 flat panels**
- 3 **ounces reduced-fat feta cheese**
- 2 **teaspoons extra-virgin olive oil**
- 1 **zucchini (6 ounces), thinly sliced**
- 1 **can (15 ounces) no-salt-added crushed tomatoes**
- ⅔ **cup fresh mint leaves, coarsely chopped**
- 2 **strips orange zest plus 2 tablespoons juice**
- ½ **teaspoon dried oregano**
- ¼ **teaspoon salt**
- ⅛ **teaspoon ground black pepper**
- 1¼ **pounds skinless cod fillet, cut into large chunks**
- **Small sprigs fresh oregano, for garnish (optional)**

1. Preheat the broiler. Place the flat bell pepper panels, skin-side up, on the broiler pan and broil 4 inches from the heat until the skin is charred, about 10 minutes. Flip the pepper pieces over on the pan and let cool. Peel and transfer to a food processor, add the feta, and puree until smooth.

2. Preheat the oven to 375°F.

3. Meanwhile, in a large ovenproof nonstick skillet, heat the oil over medium heat. Add the zucchini and cook, stirring frequently, until tender, about 7 minutes. Transfer to a plate. Add the tomatoes, mint, orange zest and juice, oregano, salt, and black pepper to the skillet and bring to a boil. Reduce the heat slightly and boil gently for 5 minutes to lightly thicken and blend the flavors.

4. Add the cod to the skillet and spoon the tomato sauce on top. Transfer to the oven and bake until the cod is cooked through, about 25 minutes.

5. Remove the cod to a plate. To serve, divide the zucchini among 4 plates. Top each with a portion of baked cod and dollop with the pepper-feta sauce. Garnish with oregano sprigs, if desired.

Per serving: 228 calories • 30g protein • 6g fat (2.5g saturated) • 4g fiber
153mg calcium • 68mg vitamin C • 11g carbohydrate • 525mg sodium

Stir-Fried Shrimp with Yellow Grape Tomatoes

Hands-On Time: 30 minutes • **Total Time:** 30 minutes • **Makes:** 4 servings

You don't need any fancy tools to peel and devein shrimp, just use a pair of thin-bladed scissors to cut through the rounded top of the shell and into the flesh of the shrimp to reveal the vein. Now, pull off the shell and the vein will come with it. Rinse before cooking. If you prefer, you can buy frozen peeled and deveined shrimp—thaw and drain before using. For Finish Strong, serve over ½ cup cooked brown rice.

Fat Releasers
Olive oil, shrimp, sugar snap peas, tomatoes, garlic, basil

- 4 teaspoons extra-virgin olive oil
- 1½ pounds large shrimp, peeled and deveined
- 4 ounces sugar snap peas, trimmed
- 1 cup yellow or red grape tomatoes, halved
- ½ small jicama (4 ounces), peeled and cut into matchsticks
- 3 cloves garlic, thinly sliced
- ¼ teaspoon salt
- ½ cup fresh basil leaves, thinly sliced

1. In a large nonstick skillet, heat 2 teaspoons of the oil over medium heat. Add half the shrimp and cook, turning the shrimp as they color, until opaque, about 4 minutes. Transfer to a bowl. Add the remaining shrimp to the skillet and cook until opaque throughout. Add to the bowl.

2. Add the remaining 2 teaspoons oil to the skillet along with the sugar snaps, tomatoes, jicama, garlic, and salt and cook, tossing frequently, until the sugar snaps are crisp-tender and the tomatoes begin to soften and collapse, about 5 minutes.

3. Return the shrimp to the pan, add the basil, and toss until heated through, about 30 seconds.

Per serving: 263 calories • 41g protein • 7.5g fat (0.5g saturated) • 2.5g fiber 136mg calcium • 40mg vitamin C • 7g carbohydrate • 593mg sodium

Tofu Lasagna

Hands-On Time: 20 minutes • **Total Time:** 45 minutes • **Makes:** 4 servings

Firm tofu stands in for lasagna noodles in this dish. A little bit of ⅓-less-fat cream cheese makes the cottage cheese creamy, and egg whites help the dish set up. Frozen spinach is great to have on hand, but if you prefer, you can substitute another vegetable, such as zucchini. (Use about 2; thinly slice and add to the pan when you would have added the spinach.)

Fat Releasers
Cottage cheese, cream cheese, eggs, olive oil, garlic, spinach, tomatoes, oregano, tofu, Parmesan cheese

1 cup 1% cottage cheese

3 tablespoons (1½ ounces) ⅓-less-fat cream cheese

3 large egg whites

2 teaspoons extra-virgin olive oil

2 cloves garlic, thinly sliced

1 package (10 ounces) frozen chopped spinach, thawed and squeezed dry

1 can (15 ounces) no-salt-added crushed tomatoes

¼ teaspoon dried oregano

¼ teaspoon salt

1 package (14 ounces) firm tofu

⅓ cup grated Parmesan cheese

1. Preheat the oven to 375°F. In a food processor, combine the cottage cheese, cream cheese, and egg whites and puree until very smooth, about 2 minutes.

2. In a large nonstick skillet, heat the oil over medium-low heat. Add the garlic and cook until just tender, about 2 minutes. Add the spinach and cook, stirring frequently, until tender, about 5 minutes.

3. Add the tomatoes, oregano, and salt and cook, stirring frequently, until lightly thickened, about 5 minutes.

4. Cut the block of tofu crosswise into 8 slices. Arrange half the tofu in a single layer in the bottom of a baking dish that is ideally 6 inches square, but 6 x 8 inches and 8 x 8 inches can also work. Top with the spinach-tomato mixture and the remaining tofu. Pour the cottage cheese mixture on top and sprinkle with the Parmesan cheese.

5. Bake until the filling is set and the sauce is bubbling, 25 to 30 minutes. Let stand 10 minutes before cutting.

Per serving: 270 calories • 26g protein • 12g fat (3.5g saturated) • 4.5g fiber 376mg calcium • 20mg vitamin C • 13g carbohydrate • 609mg sodium

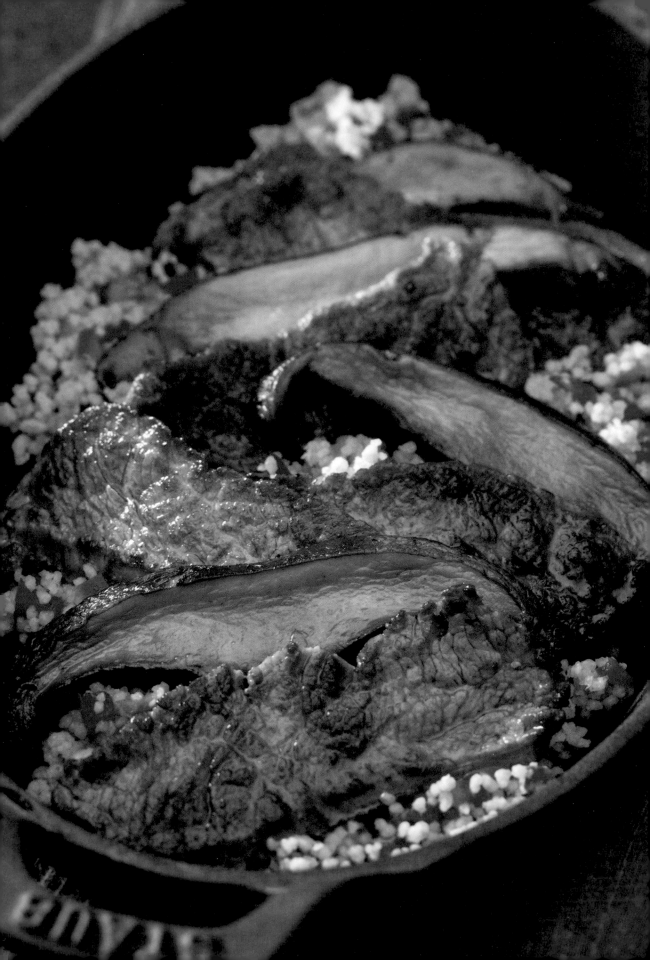

Beef & Portobello Sauté

Hands-On Time: 15 minutes • **Total Time:** 20 minutes • **Makes:** 4 servings

The thinner you can cut the beef, the more tender and flavorful this sauté will be. Put the steak in the freezer for about 20 minutes before you cut it to make it easier to get really thin pieces.

Fat releasers
Lean beef, garlic, bell peppers, black pepper, whole-wheat couscous, olive oil

¾ pound well-trimmed flank steak

12 ounces portobello mushroom caps

1 cup plus 2 tablespoons water

1 clove garlic, grated

1 small green bell pepper, finely diced

1 small red bell pepper, finely diced

Salt

Ground black pepper

¾ cup whole-wheat couscous

2 teaspoons extra-virgin olive oil

1. Cut the flank steak with the grain into 2-inch-wide strips. Cut each strip against the grain (and with the knife at an angle to the cutting board) into very thin slices.

2. Using a teaspoon, scrape the black gills out of the mushroom caps. Cut the caps crosswise into ½-inch-wide strips.

3. In a small saucepan, combine 1 cup water, garlic, bell peppers, ¼ teaspoon salt, and a large pinch of black pepper. Bring to a boil, add the couscous, and stir well. Remove from the heat, cover, and let stand for 5 minutes. Fluff with a fork and cover to keep warm.

4. Meanwhile, in a large nonstick skillet, heat 1 teaspoon of the oil over medium-high heat. Add half the beef and a pinch of salt and stir, using tongs or a fork to pull the beef apart, until lightly browned but still pinkish, 1 to 2 minutes. With a slotted spoon, transfer to a plate. Repeat with the remaining oil and beef.

5. Add the mushrooms to the skillet and let cook without turning for 2 minutes. Sprinkle with a pinch of salt, add 2 tablespoons water, and return the beef (and any juices from the plate) to the pan. Stir to combine with the mushrooms, cover, and cook for 3 minutes to develop juices.

6. Serve over the couscous.

Per serving: 339 calories • 31g protein • 10g fat (3.5g saturated) • 6.5g fiber
39mg calcium • 39mg vitamin C • 33g carbohydrate • 275mg sodium

Beef & Tomatillo Chili

Hands-On Time: 20 minutes • **Total Time:** 55 minutes • **Makes:** 4 servings

Fresh tomatillos—similar to, but with a slightly sweeter taste than, green tomatoes—can be found in the produce section of many supermarkets. (You could also use canned tomatillos, but the canned version is exceptionally high in sodium, so fresh is best if you can find them.) Decidedly Mexican in flavor, you can doll this chili up, if you'd like, by serving it with whole-grain tortillas and topping the chili with Greek yogurt, chopped tomato, and an additional sprinkling of fresh cilantro.

Fat Releasers
Tomatillos, onion, garlic, almonds, olive oil, beef, bell pepper, sweet potato, chili powder

- ¾ **pound fresh tomatillos, husked, rinsed, and quartered (2 cups)**
- 1 **cup cilantro, leaves and stems**
- ½ **medium red onion, cut into chunks**
- 3 **cloves garlic**
- 2 **tablespoons raisins**
- 2 **tablespoons slivered almonds**
- 1 **tablespoon plus 1 teaspoon extra-virgin olive oil**
- ¾ **pound flank steak, cut into ½-inch chunks**
- 1 **large green bell pepper, cut into ½-inch chunks**
- ¾ **pound sweet potato, peeled and cut into ½-inch chunks**
- ¾ **teaspoon chili powder**
- ½ **teaspoon salt**
- ⅔ **cup water**

1. In a food processor, puree the tomatillos, cilantro, onion, garlic, raisins, and almonds.

2. In a large nonstick saucepan or Dutch oven, heat the oil over medium heat. Add the steak and cook until browned, about 5 minutes. With a slotted spoon, transfer the steak to a plate.

3. Add the bell pepper and sweet potato to the pan and stir to coat. Add the tomatillo paste and cook for 5 minutes so it no longer tastes raw.

4. Return the meat to the pan along with the chili powder, salt, and water. Bring to a boil, reduce to a simmer, cover, and cook until the meat is tender, about 35 minutes.

Per 1¼-cup serving: 300 calories • 22g protein • 13g fat (2.5g saturated) 5.5g fiber • 74mg calcium • 54mg vitamin C • 27g carbohydrate • 368mg sodium

Chipotle Pork Stew

Hands-On Time: 15 minutes • **Total Time:** 30 minutes • **Makes:** 4 servings

The "jumbo" carrots called for here are not just big regular carrots but a variety of carrot. They are sweet and tasty and, because they're sold loose, you can buy only the amount you need. Of course you can substitute 1 pound of any carrot you want. Serve the stew with brown basmati rice or whole-wheat couscous.

Fat Releasers
Tomato paste, chile powder, whole-wheat flour, black pepper, pork, olive oil, garlic, bell peppers, green peas, lemons

- ½ cup plus 2 tablespoons water
- 3 tablespoons no-salt-added tomato paste
- ½ teaspoon chipotle chile powder
- ½ teaspoon ground cumin
- 2 teaspoons grated lemon zest
- ½ teaspoon salt
- 3 tablespoons white whole-wheat flour
- ¼ teaspoon ground black pepper
- ¾ pound boneless pork loin chops, cubed
- 4 teaspoons extra-virgin olive oil
- 2 cloves garlic, minced
- 1 pound "jumbo" carrots, halved lengthwise and thinly sliced on the diagonal
- 2 green bell peppers, cut into ½-inch squares
- 2½ cups low-sodium chicken broth
- 1 cup frozen green peas, thawed
- 1 tablespoon fresh lemon juice

1. In a small bowl, stir together ½ cup water, tomato paste, chipotle chile powder, cumin, lemon zest, and ¼ teaspoon of the salt. Set aside.

2. In a shallow bowl, mix together the flour, pepper, and remaining ¼ teaspoon salt. Add the pork and toss to coat. Shake off the excess. Reserve 1 tablespoon of the dredging mixture.

3. In a nonstick Dutch oven, heat 1 tablespoon of the oil over medium-high heat. Add the pork and cook until white all over, about 2 minutes. Transfer the pork to a plate.

4. Reduce the heat to medium-high and add the garlic and remaining 1 teaspoon oil. Cook until fragrant, about 30 seconds. Add the carrots, bell peppers, and 2 tablespoons water. Cover and cook until the peppers begin to soften, 4 to 5 minutes.

5. Sprinkle the vegetables evenly with the reserved dredging mixture and stir well. Add the broth and tomato paste mixture, stir well, and bring to a simmer. Cover and cook until the carrots are tender, about 8 minutes.

6. Add the peas, return the pork to the pan, return to a simmer, and cook for 3 minutes. Stir in the lemon juice.

Per 2-cup serving: 272 calories • 24g protein • 8.5g fat (2g saturated) • 7.5g fiber
71mg calcium • 64mg vitamin C • 27g carbohydrate • 407mg sodium

Pasta with Pork & Caramelized Onions

Hands-On Time: 35 minutes • **Total Time:** 40 minutes • **Makes:** 4 servings

Caramelized onions, golden brown from long cooking, are sweet and mellow. Green beans give a slight crunch, but feel free to swap in a cup of frozen peas if you'd like. Adding the Parmesan cheese to the pasta and sauce helps to thicken and coat.

Fat Releasers
Olive oil, pork, onions, garlic, whole-wheat pasta, Parmesan cheese

- 1 tablespoon plus 1 teaspoon extra-virgin olive oil
- ½ pound boneless center-cut pork loin chops, cut into thin strips (as for stir-fry)
- 2 large onions, halved and thinly sliced (4 cups)
- 1 large carrot, shredded (1 cup)
- 3 cloves garlic, thinly sliced
- ¼ pound green beans, cut into 1-inch lengths
- 2 cups low-sodium chicken broth
- ½ teaspoon salt
- 8 ounces whole-wheat linguine
- ⅓ cup grated Parmesan cheese

1. In a large nonstick skillet, heat 1 teaspoon of the oil over medium heat. Add the pork and cook until lightly browned, about 3 minutes. Transfer to a plate.
2. Add the remaining 1 tablespoon oil, the onions, carrot, and garlic to the pan and cook, stirring frequently, until the onions are golden brown and tender, about 20 minutes.
3. Add the green beans, broth, and salt and bring to a boil. Reduce to a simmer and cook, stirring occasionally, until the beans are tender, about 5 minutes. Return the pork to the pan and heat gently until warmed through, about 1 minute.
4. Meanwhile, in a large pot of boiling water, cook the pasta according to package directions. Drain and return the pasta to the pot.
5. Add the sauce and Parmesan cheese to the cooked pasta and toss to coat.

Per 2¼-cup serving: 400 calories • 24g protein • 11g fat (3g saturated) • 9.5g fiber 145mg calcium • 11mg vitamin C • 55g carbohydrate • 472mg sodium

Garlicky Chicken Stew with Artichokes

Hands-On Time: 20 minutes • **Total Time:** 45 minutes • **Makes:** 4 servings

If you purchase fennel with its frilly green fronds attached, reserve them and use them as a garnish. They're quite flavorful and pretty, too.

Fat Releasers
Olive oil, chicken, fennel, garlic, marjoram, artichokes, peas

- 4 teaspoons extra-virgin olive oil
- 1 pound skinless, boneless chicken breasts, cut into large chunks
- 1 small bulb fennel, stalks discarded, bulb halved lengthwise and thinly sliced
- 5 cloves garlic, peeled
- ½ teaspoon dried marjoram
- ¼ teaspoon salt
- 8 ounces small potatoes, cut into ½-inch-thick slices
- 1 can (14 ounces) water-packed artichoke hearts, quartered lengthwise
- 1½ cups low-sodium chicken broth
- 1 cup frozen green peas, thawed

1. In a nonstick Dutch oven, heat 2 teaspoons of the oil over medium heat. Add half the chicken and cook until golden brown, about 1½ minutes per side. With a slotted spoon, transfer the chicken to a bowl. (It will cook more later.) Repeat with the remaining chicken and oil.

2. Add the fennel, garlic, marjoram, and salt to the pan and cook until the fennel is golden brown, about 5 minutes. Add the potatoes, artichoke hearts, and broth and bring to a simmer. Cover and cook until the potatoes are tender, about 15 minutes.

3. Return the chicken to the pan along with the peas and simmer until the chicken is cooked through, about 3 minutes.

Per 2-cup serving: 292 calories • 30g protein • 8g fat (1.5g saturated) • 6.5g fiber 58mg calcium • 20mg vitamin C • 26g carbohydrate • 679mg sodium

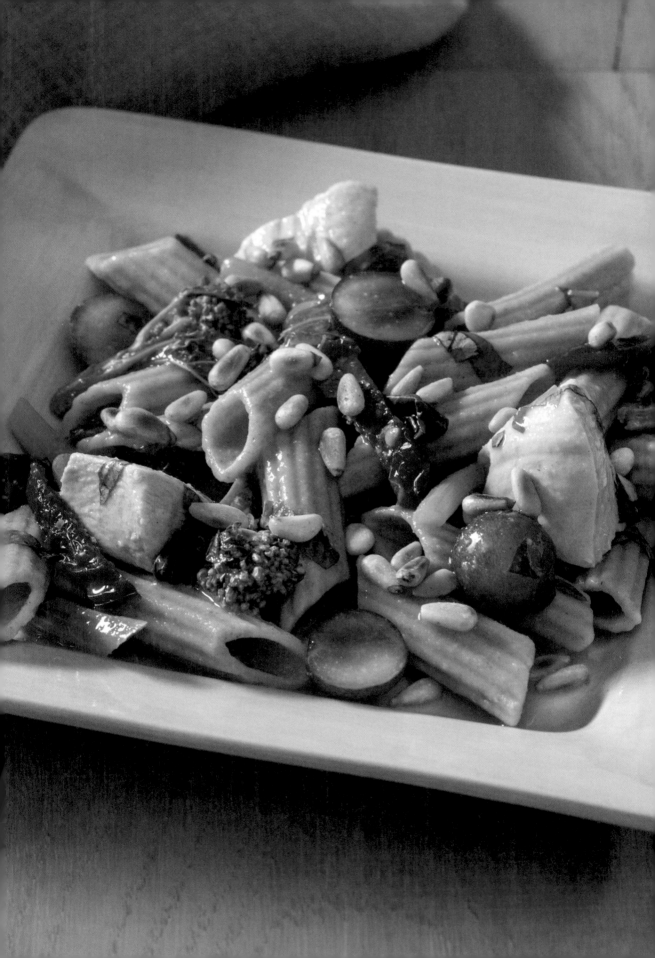

Pasta with Chicken, Broccoli Rabe & Sun-Dried Tomatoes

Hands-On Time: 15 minutes • **Total Time:** 25 minutes • **Makes:** 4 servings

Broccoli rabe has a slight bitterness, but when paired with sun-dried tomatoes and grapes, it mellows out. The flour that gets added to the mixture helps to thicken the sauce slightly so that it coats the pasta.

Fat Releasers
Whole-wheat penne, broccoli rabe, chicken, sun-dried tomatoes, basil, whole-wheat flour, red grapes, pine nuts

- 8 **ounces whole-wheat penne**
- 1½ **cups low-sodium chicken broth**
- ½ **teaspoon salt**
- 8 **ounces broccoli rabe, cut into 1-inch pieces (4 cups)**
- 10 **ounces skinless, boneless chicken breast, cut into 1-inch chunks**
- ⅓ **cup sun-dried tomatoes, thinly sliced**
- ⅓ **cup chopped fresh basil**
- 2½ **teaspoons whole-wheat flour blended with 1 tablespoon cold water**
- 1 **cup seedless red grapes, halved**
- 1 **tablespoon toasted pine nuts**

1. In a large pot of boiling water, cook the pasta according to package directions; drain. Return the pasta to the pot.

2. Meanwhile, in a large skillet, bring the broth and salt to a boil over medium heat. Add the broccoli rabe, chicken, sun-dried tomatoes, and basil and reduce to a simmer. Cook, uncovered, until the chicken is just cooked through and the broccoli rabe is tender, about 7 minutes. Whisk in the flour mixture and simmer until lightly thickened, about 1 minute.

3. Add to the pasta to the skillet along with the grapes and toss to combine. Divide among 4 bowls and top with the pine nuts.

Per 2-cup serving: 375 calories • 27g protein • 5g fat (0.5g saturated) • 6g fiber 64mg calcium • 55mg vitamin C • 56g carbohydrate • 390mg sodium

Country Captain

Hands-On Time: 15 minutes ● **Total Time:** 1 hour 10 minutes
Makes: 4 servings

Country Captain is a classic Southern dish, dating from the 18th century, when sea captains regularly brought spices to this country from the East Indies—hence, the curry spices used in the dish. This connection makes it all the more fitting that it be served with basmati rice, which also has its roots in India.

Fat Releasers
Chicken, black pepper, brown rice, olive oil, onions, garlic, thyme, bell pepper, tomatoes, almonds, parsley

1¼ **pounds skinless, boneless chicken breasts**

1 **bay leaf**

1¼ **teaspoons salt**

6 **black peppercorns**

⅔ **cup brown basmati rice**

4 **teaspoons extra-virgin olive oil**

4 **slices thin-cut turkey bacon, cut into pieces**

1 **Vidalia or other sweet onion (10 ounces), chopped**

1 **large clove garlic, minced**

2 **teaspoons curry powder**

½ **teaspoon dried thyme**

1 **green bell pepper, chopped**

3 **plum tomatoes (4 ounces each), diced**

¼ **teaspoon ground black pepper**

¼ **cup dried currants or chopped raisins**

¼ **cup slivered almonds, toasted**

Chopped parsley, for garnish

1. In a saucepan just big enough to hold the chicken side by side, place the chicken, bone-side up, and add the bay leaf, 1 teaspoon of the salt, the peppercorns, and water to just cover (about 4 cups). Cover, bring to a simmer, and cook (keeping it at a simmer) until the chicken is cooked through but still pink in the center, about 12 minutes. Transfer the chicken to a plate and set aside. Strain the broth and discard the solids. Measure out ½ cup broth to be used in step 4 and save the remainder for cooking the rice.

2. Cook the rice according to package directions, but use the remaining chicken broth (plus water if needed) in place of the water called for.

3. Meanwhile, in a large nonstick saucepan or Dutch oven, heat 2 teaspoons of the oil over medium-high heat. Add the bacon and cook until fragrant, about 1 minute. Add the

remaining 2 teaspoons oil, the onion, garlic, curry powder, and thyme, and cook until the onion begins to soften, about 2 minutes. Add the bell pepper and cook until the pepper is slightly softened, about 2 minutes.
4. Add the tomatoes, black pepper, remaining ¼ teaspoon salt, and the reserved ½ cup chicken broth. Bring to a boil, reduce to a simmer, and cook for 10 minutes.
5. Remove the chicken meat from the bone and coarsely chop. Add it to the pot along with the currants, cover, and simmer for 10 minutes.
6. To serve, mound ½ cup rice in each of 4 large soup bowls. Ladle some of the juices from the pan over the rice. Scoop 1¼ cups of the chicken mixture and place alongside each portion of rice. Sprinkle the almonds over the chicken and chopped parsley over the rice.

Per serving: 420 calories • 39g protein • 11g fat (2g saturated) • 6g fiber 80mg calcium • 41mg vitamin C • 43g carbohydrate • 414mg sodium

Penne & Turkey with Creamy Broccoli Pesto

Hands-On Time: 20 minutes • **Total Time:** 40 minutes • **Makes:** 4 servings

Cut the turkey as thinly as possible so that it will cook very quickly. To make it easier to cut thin strips of turkey, place the cutlets in the freezer for 20 to 30 minutes to firm them. You could use thawed frozen broccoli here; because it tends to be a little watery, you may not need to add as much liquid to the pesto when you puree it.

Fat Releasers

Broccoli, basil, Parmesan cheese, yogurt, sunflower seeds, garlic, olive oil, black pepper, whole-wheat penne, turkey, bell pepper

- ¾ **cup packed small broccoli florets**
- ¼ **cup coarsely chopped fresh basil**
- 3 **tablespoons grated Parmesan cheese**
- 3 **tablespoons 0% Greek yogurt**
- 3 **tablespoons hulled sunflower seeds, toasted**
- 1 **small clove garlic, peeled**
- 1 **tablespoon extra-virgin olive oil**
- **Salt**
- **Ground black pepper**
- 8 **ounces whole-wheat penne**
- ¾ **pound turkey breast cutlets, cut into thin strips**
- 1 **red bell pepper, slivered**

1. In a steamer, cook the broccoli until just tender but still bright green, 6 to 7 minutes. Rinse the broccoli under cold running water to cool it.

2. In a food processor or mini food processor, combine the broccoli, basil, Parmesan cheese, yogurt, sunflower seeds, garlic, oil, ¼ teaspoon salt, and a pinch of pepper. Pulse to combine, then add 2 or 3 tablespoons water (whatever you need to get the puree going), and process to as smooth a puree as you can get (don't worry if it's still a bit coarse).

3. When ready to make dinner, cook the pasta in a large pot of lightly salted boiling water according to package directions. Add the turkey and bell pepper for the last 1 minute of cooking time.

4. Scoop out some of the pasta cooking water and set aside. Drain the pasta and return to the pot. Add the pesto and toss. Add some of the reserved cooking water if the pesto seems too thick.

Per 1½-cup serving: 390 calories • 34g protein • 9g fat (1.5g saturated) • 6g fiber 97mg calcium • 66mg vitamin C • 47g carbohydrate • 409mg sodium

Southwestern Turkey Tacos

Hands-On Time: 20 minutes ● **Total Time:** 30 minutes ● **Makes:** 4 servings

If you'd like a little more heat, swap in a poblano chile pepper for the green bell pepper. Poblanos, available in many supermarkets, are dark green, thin skinned, about the size of a bell pepper, but usually longer and slightly tapered.

Fat Releasers
Olive oil, scallions, garlic, bell peppers, chili powder, turkey, tomatoes, peas, yogurt, whole-wheat tortillas

- 1 tablespoon plus 1 teaspoon extra-virgin olive oil
- 3 scallions, thinly sliced
- 3 cloves garlic, thinly sliced
- 1 small green bell pepper, diced
- 1 small red bell pepper, diced
- 1½ teaspoons mild to medium chili powder
- 1½ teaspoons ground coriander
- 1½ teaspoons ground cumin
- ½ teaspoon salt
- 1 pound ground turkey (93% lean) or chicken
- 1 can (14.5 ounces) no-salt-added crushed tomatoes
- 1 cup frozen peas, thawed
- ¼ cup 0% Greek yogurt
- 4 whole-wheat tortillas (taco size)

1. In a large saucepan or Dutch oven, heat the oil over medium heat. Add the scallions and garlic, and cook until the scallions are tender, about 2 minutes.

2. Stir in the bell peppers and cook, stirring occasionally, until tender, about 5 minutes. Stir in the chili powder, coriander, cumin, and salt and cook for 1 minute.

3. Add the turkey and cook, stirring to break up the meat, until no longer pink, about 5 minutes. Add the tomatoes and cook until lightly thickened, about 5 minutes. Stir in the peas and cook until just heated through, about 2 minutes.

4. Serve the taco mixture with a dollop of Greek yogurt and a tortilla for wrapping.

Per serving: 345 calories ● 33g protein ● 15g fat (3g saturated) ● 13g fiber 120mg calcium ● 60mg vitamin C ● 25g carbohydrate ● 638mg sodium

Tangy Shrimp and Vegetables with Linguine

Hands-On Time: 15 minutes • **Total Time:** 35 minutes • **Makes:** 4 servings

Carrot juice, tomato paste, and vinegar give this dish a sweet and sour tang, while a hefty amount of fresh ginger gives it some zing. This preparation works with other fish as well as with chicken or pork. Jicama is a root vegetable commonly used in Central and South American cuisines.

Fat Releasers
Tomato paste, vinegar, multigrain pasta, olive oil, garlic, ginger, shrimp, watercress

- ¾ **cup carrot juice**
- ¼ **cup no-salt-added tomato paste**
- ¼ **cup cider vinegar**
- 6 **ounces multigrain linguine or spaghetti**
- 1 **tablespoon extra-virgin olive oil**
- 1 **small jicama or large white turnip (about 8 ounces), halved and thinly sliced**
- 3 **cloves garlic, thinly sliced**
- 2-inch **piece fresh ginger, thinly sliced**
- 1½ **pounds peeled and deveined large shrimp**
- 1 **large bunch watercress, torn into bite-size pieces (4 cups)**

1. In a small bowl, stir together the carrot juice, tomato paste, and vinegar.

2. In a pot of boiling water, cook the pasta according to package directions; drain and return to the pot.

3. Meanwhile, in a large nonstick skillet, heat the oil over medium heat. Add the jicama, garlic, and ginger and cook, stirring frequently, until the jicama is crisp-tender, about 5 minutes.

4. Add the shrimp, tossing to combine. Add the carrot juice mixture and cook until the shrimp are just cooked through, about 5 minutes.

5. Transfer to the pasta pot along with the watercress and toss to combine.

Per 2½-cup serving: 428 calories • 48g protein • 7g fat (0.5g saturated) • 9g fiber 204mg calcium • 40mg vitamin C • 46g carbohydrate • 508mg sodium

Asparagus & Tuna Bake

Hands-On Time: 20 minutes • **Total Time:** 1 hour 5 minutes

Makes: 4 servings

Canned tuna that is packed in water retains more of its omega-3s than does oil-packed tuna. Make this casserole several hours ahead and serve at room temperature; or gently reheat it in a 250°F oven for 10 to 20 minutes. Leftovers store well and would make a nice lunch.

Fat Releasers
Olive oil, asparagus, onion, lemons, black pepper, tuna, spinach, chickpea flour, yogurt, eggs, cheese

---

- 3 teaspoons extra-virgin olive oil
- ½ pound red potatoes, cut into ½-inch cubes
- 1 pound asparagus, cut into 1-inch lengths
- 1 small red onion, slivered
- 2 teaspoons lemon juice
- ¼ teaspoon salt
- ¼ teaspoon ground black pepper
- 2 cans (5 ounces each) water-packed chunk white tuna, well drained
- 1½ cups loosely packed baby spinach or shredded spinach
- 2 tablespoons chickpea flour or whole-wheat flour
- 1⅓ cups 0% Greek yogurt
- 2 large eggs
- 2 teaspoons grated lemon zest
- ½ cup shredded reduced-fat Swiss cheese

1. Preheat the oven to 350°F. Coat the bottom and sides of a 7 x 11-inch glass baking dish with 1 teaspoon of the oil.

2. In a large pot of boiling water, cook the potatoes until just barely fork-tender, about 8 minutes. Add the asparagus for the last 1 minute of cooking. Drain well.

3. Meanwhile, in a medium nonstick skillet, heat the remaining 2 teaspoons oil over medium-high heat. Add the onion and cook until browned, 8 to 10 minutes.

4. Scrape the onion into a large bowl and stir in the lemon juice. Add the salt, pepper, potatoes, asparagus, tuna, and spinach, and toss to combine.

5. In a small bowl, blend the chickpea flour with ⅓ cup of the yogurt. Stir in the remaining 1 cup yogurt. Beat in the eggs. Beat in the lemon zest. Stir in the cheese.

6. Measure out 1 cup of the yogurt mixture and set aside. Add the remainder to the potato-tuna mixture and toss to coat. Scrape into the baking dish.

7. Spread the reserved yogurt mixture evenly over the top of the casserole. Bake for 45 minutes or until the top is nicely browned.

Per serving: 341 calories • 37g protein • 12g fat (4g saturated) • 4g fiber • 276mg calcium 17mg vitamin C • 22g carbohydrate • 362mg sodium

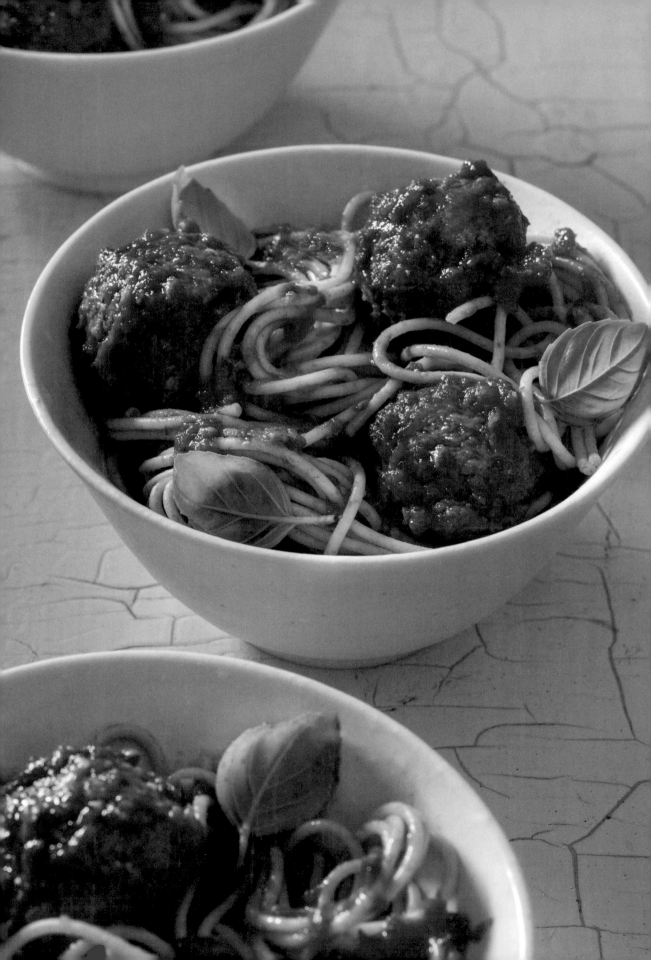

Eggplant "Meatballs" with Pasta

Hands-On Time: 20 minutes ● **Total Time:** 55 minutes ● **Makes:** 4 servings

When shopping for eggplants, look for firm, unblemished ones on the smaller side as they'll be less seedy than large eggplants. If you have a microwave, use it to steam the eggplant slices by placing them in a microwave-safe dish with a cover. For shaping the meatballs, a small ice cream or cookie scoop (if you have one) makes this chore a breeze. Otherwise, you can simply use a tablespoon to scoop them.

Fat Releasers
Parsley, Parmesan cheese, eggs, whole-wheat bread, black pepper, tomatoes, oranges, whole-wheat pasta

- 4 **medium eggplants (1¾ pounds total), peeled and cut into 1-inch-thick rounds**
- ½ **cup packed parsley leaves**
- ½ **cup grated Parmesan cheese (1 ounce)**
- 3 **large egg whites**
- ½ **cup fresh whole-wheat bread crumbs (from 1 slice bread)**
- ½ **teaspoon salt**
- ¼ **teaspoon ground black pepper**
- 1 **can (15 ounces) no-salt-added crushed tomatoes**
- 2 **strips orange zest**
- ¼ **cup fresh orange juice**
- 8 **ounces whole-wheat spaghetti**
- **Small basil leaves, for garnish (optional)**

1. Place the eggplant slices in a vegetable steamer and cook until tender, about 10 minutes.

2. Preheat the oven to 400°F. When the eggplant is cool enough to handle, squeeze the slices to get rid of excess moisture. Place the parsley in a food processor and pulse until coarsely chopped. Add the eggplant, Parmesan cheese, egg whites, bread crumbs, salt , and pepper and pulse until combined.

3. Shape the mixture into 16 "meatballs" (a generous tablespoon each) and place in a shallow baking dish. Bake 15 minutes, then add the tomatoes, orange zest, and juice and bake until the meatballs are firm, about 10 minutes more.

4. In a large pot of boiling water, cook the pasta according to package directions; drain. Transfer to a large bowl, add the sauce and meatballs, and gently toss. Serve the pasta and meatballs garnished with small basil leaves, if desired.

Per serving: 363 calories ● 20g protein ● 4.5g fat (2g saturated) ● 16g fiber 209mg calcium ● 37mg vitamin C ● 65g carbohydrate ● 531mg sodium

Vegetarian Posole

Hands-On Time: 10 minutes • **Total Time:** 50 minutes • **Makes:** 4 servings

Posole, a rich stew usually made with meat and always with hominy (large dried corn kernels), is often found on the menu in Mexican and Latin American restaurants. Look for canned hominy in supermarkets that carry Latin American products (it's usually in the aisle with the canned beans) or frozen hominy. If you can't find hominy, swap in 1½ cups of corn kernels (fresh, frozen, or canned) and add them 5 minutes before the dish is done. This vegetarian version is full of flavor from shiitake mushrooms, tomatoes, peppers, and sweet potato. Topped with cheese, we guarantee you won't miss the meat.

Fat Releasers
Olive oil, onion, bell pepper, jalapeño, garlic, sweet potatoes, tomatoes, oregano, cheese

1 tablespoon plus 1 teaspoon extra-virgin olive oil

1 large onion, coarsely chopped

1 green bell pepper, diced

1 jalapeño pepper, minced

3 cloves garlic, thinly sliced

6 ounces shiitake mushrooms, stems discarded, caps sliced

1 sweet potato (10 ounces), peeled, halved lengthwise, and cut into 1-inch chunks

1 can (14.5 ounces) no-salt-added diced tomatoes

½ teaspoon dried oregano

¼ teaspoon salt

1 can (15 ounces) hominy, rinsed and drained

1½ cups water

5 ounces shredded reduced-fat Mexican blend cheese

1. In a large saucepan, heat the oil over medium-low heat. Add the onion, bell pepper, jalapeño, and garlic, and cook, stirring occasionally, until the onion is tender, about 10 minutes. If necessary, add ¼ cup water to prevent sticking.

2. Add the mushrooms, sweet potato, tomatoes, oregano, and salt and stir to combine. Increase the heat to medium and bring to a boil.

3. Add the hominy and water and return to a boil. Cook until the hominy and sweet potatoes are tender, about 25 minutes. Serve sprinkled with the cheese.

Per 2½-cup serving: 303 calories • 15g protein • 13g fat (4.5g saturated) 6.5g fiber • 377mg calcium • 57mg vitamin C • 36g carbohydrate • 566mg sodium

Orzo Primavera

Hands-On Time: 25 minutes • **Total Time:** 35 minutes • **Makes:** 4 servings

A traditional pasta primavera uses heavy cream and high-fat pine nuts; we've swapped in reduced-fat cream cheese and almonds. And using whole-wheat orzo has two benefits: A smaller amount goes further because the pasta shape is small, and the whole wheat adds a nice amount of fiber. In fact, between the vegetables and the pasta, this dish has nearly half of the fiber you need in a day.

Fat Releasers
Olive oil, garlic, red pepper flakes, tomatoes, basil, whole-wheat pasta, zucchini, squash, asparagus, cream cheese, Parmesan cheese, peas, almonds

Salt

2 teaspoons olive oil

2 cloves garlic, minced

¼ teaspoon red pepper flakes

1 pint grape tomatoes, halved (or quartered if large)

½ cup shredded fresh basil, plus more for garnish

1½ cups whole-wheat orzo (9 ounces)

2 small zucchini (about ¾ pound total), cut into matchsticks

1 yellow summer squash (8 ounces), cut into matchsticks

½ bunch thinnish asparagus, cut on the diagonal into 1-inch pieces

3 tablespoons ⅓-less-fat cream cheese, cut into small pieces

⅓ cup grated Parmesan cheese

¾ cup frozen green peas, thawed

3 tablespoons slivered or sliced almonds, toasted

1. Bring a large pot of lightly salted water to a boil.

2. Meanwhile, in a large skillet, heat the oil over medium-high heat. Add the garlic and red pepper flakes and cook until fragrant, about 30 seconds. Add the tomatoes and a pinch of salt and cook until hot and beginning to collapse, 2 to 3 minutes. Stir in the basil and remove from the heat.

3. Add the orzo to the boiling water and cook according to package directions, adding the zucchini, squash, and asparagus for the last 4 minutes. Reserving ¼ cup of the cooking water, drain the orzo and return it to the pot.

4. Add the cream cheese, Parmesan cheese, a pinch of salt, and the reserved pasta cooking water to the hot pasta and stir to melt. Stir in the tomato mixture and peas.

5. Serve the pasta topped with the almonds and garnished with basil.

Per 2-cup serving: 398 calories • 17g protein • 11g fat (3g saturated) • 15g fiber 190mg calcium • 491mg vitamin C • 60g carbohydrate • 272mg sodium

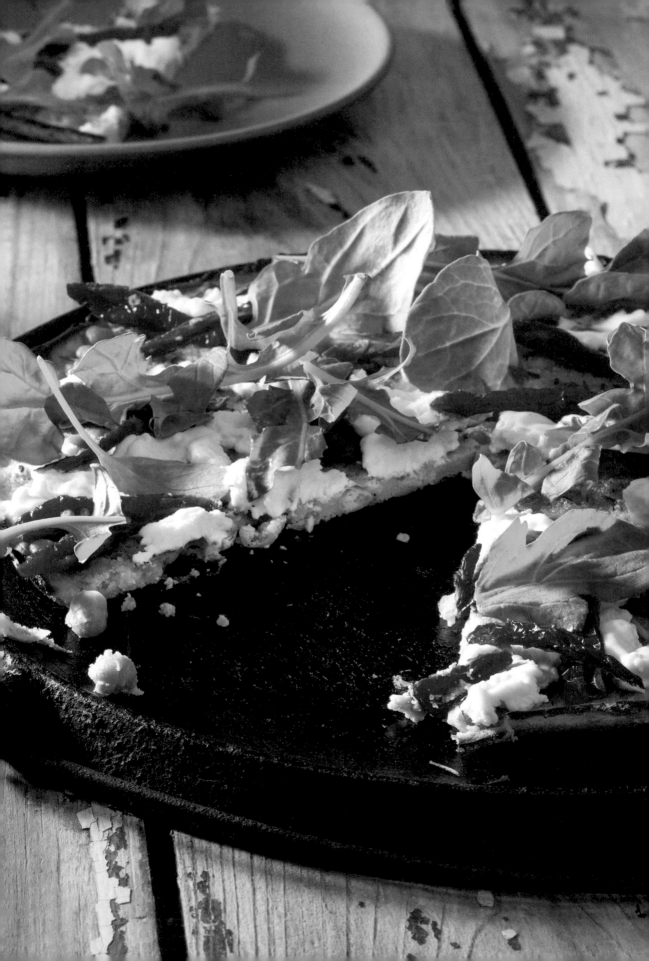

Chickpea & Arugula "Pizza"

Hands-On Time: 10 minutes • **Total Time:** 30 minutes + standing time

Makes: 4 servings

This dish, known as *socca* in France and *farinata* in Italy, is a cross between a pancake and a pizza. Chickpea flour (also called *besan* or *gram flour*) gives it a mildly nutty flavor. If you have a cast-iron skillet, use it here; it will produce an especially crispy crust.

Fat Releasers
Chickpea flour, rosemary, olive oil, chickpeas, sun-dried tomatoes, cheese

- ⅔ **cup chickpea flour**
- ½ **teaspoon salt**
- ½ **teaspoon crumbled dried rosemary**
- 1 **cup water, room temperature**
- 4 **teaspoons extra-virgin olive oil**
- 1 **cup no-salt-added canned chickpeas**
- ½ **cup sun-dried tomatoes, slivered**
- 4 **ounces reduced-fat goat cheese, crumbled**
- 1½ **cups (1½ ounces) baby arugula**

SAVE FOR A SNACK: This is great for a snack; simply cut into 6 portions. Or, if you have some left over, slices can be reheated in a 350°F oven for about 10 minutes or in a covered pan sprayed with nonstick cooking spray for 5 minutes on top of the stove.

1. In a large bowl, whisk together the chickpea flour, salt, and rosemary. Gradually whisk in the water until smooth. Stir in 2 teaspoons of the oil. Let stand 30 minutes or up to several hours at room temperature.

2. Preheat the oven to 450°F. Brush a large ovenproof skillet with the remaining 2 teaspoons oil and place in the oven for 5 minutes to heat up. Pour the chickpea flour mixture into the hot pan, scatter the chickpeas over the top, and bake until the top is set and starting to brown, 10 to 12 minutes.

3. Meanwhile, in a small pot of boiling water, cook the sun-dried tomatoes for 2 minutes to soften. Drain.

4. Scatter the cheese and sun-dried tomatoes on top of the pizza and bake until the cheese has melted somewhat, about 3 minutes. Remove from the oven and scatter the arugula over the top. Cut into wedges.

Per serving: 230 calories • 12g protein • 9.5g fat (2.5g saturated) • 5g fiber 104mg calcium • 4mg vitamin C • 26g carbohydrate • 436mg sodium

Chapter

8

Salads

Go way beyond iceberg lettuce with these versatile salads that can either complete a meal or be meals in themselves.

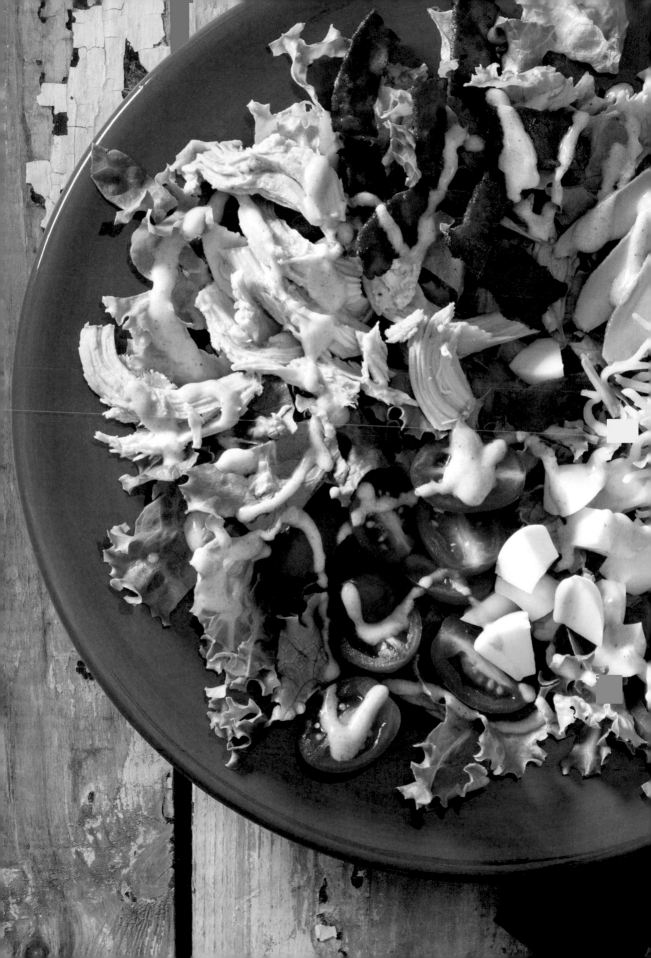

Thai Beef Salad

Hands-On Time: 25 minutes ● **Total Time:** 30 minutes ● **Makes:** 4 servings

A Thai beef salad would typically be served with egg noodles. In this light, refreshing version, zucchini are cut into thin noodle-like strands to take the place of the high-carb, high-calorie pasta.

Fat Releasers
Limes, olive oil, honey, red pepper flakes, bell pepper, zucchini, beef, scallions, cashews

1 teaspoon grated lime zest

¼ cup fresh lime juice

2 teaspoons extra-virgin olive oil

2 teaspoons honey

¼ teaspoon salt

Generous pinch of red pepper flakes

2 red bell peppers, cut into thin slivers

2 zucchini (8 ounces each), halved lengthwise and then crosswise, then cut into noodle-like strands

¾ pound sirloin steak

3 scallions, sliced

3 tablespoons chopped unsalted roasted cashews

Slivered fresh basil, mint, or cilantro (optional)

1. In a medium bowl, combine the lime zest, lime juice, oil, honey, salt, and red pepper flakes. Measure out 1 tablespoon and set aside. Add the bell pepper and zucchini to the dressing in the bowl and toss.

2. Preheat a grill or grill pan to medium-high heat. Cook the steak for 2 minutes, flip, and cook for 2 minutes. Repeat the process for medium-rare steak, a total of 8 minutes. Let the steak rest for 5 minutes before very thinly slicing against the grain.

3. Serve the sliced beef on a bed of the salad. Drizzle with the reserved 1 tablespoon dressing and top with the scallions, cashews, and fresh herb (if using).

Per serving: 248 calories ● 22g protein ● 12g fat (3.5g saturated) ● 3g fiber 50mg calcium ● 103mg vitamin C ● 14g carbohydrate ● 199mg sodium

Shrimp Cocktail Salad

Hands-On Time: 20 minutes • **Total Time:** 25 minutes • **Makes:** 4 servings

Choose a hot sauce that has heat but isn't too vinegary for this cocktail sauce. The salad can be eaten right after it's made, or you can refrigerate it until well chilled.

Fat Releasers
Tomato paste, vinegar, lemons, olive oil, hot sauce, black pepper, shrimp, lettuce, avocado

- ½ cup no-salt-added tomato paste
- 2 tablespoons cider vinegar
- 2 tablespoons fresh lemon juice, plus wedges for serving
- 2 tablespoons drained white horseradish
- 4 teaspoons extra-virgin olive oil
- 1 tablespoon water
- ½ teaspoon hot sauce, such as Frank's RedHot
- ½ teaspoon ground coriander
- ¼ teaspoon salt
- ¼ teaspoon ground black pepper
- 2 ribs celery, halved lengthwise and thinly sliced (1 cup)
- 1½ pounds medium or large shrimp, peeled and deveined
- 1 head buttercrunch lettuce (such as Bibb), separated into leaves
- 1 Hass avocado, sliced

1. In a large bowl, whisk together the tomato paste, vinegar, lemon juice, horseradish, 1½ teaspoons of the oil, the water, hot sauce, coriander, salt, and pepper. Add the celery and stir to combine.

2. In a large nonstick skillet, heat the remaining 2½ teaspoons oil over medium heat. Add half the shrimp and cook, turning them over as they color, until opaque throughout, about 4 minutes. Remove with a slotted spoon and repeat with the remaining shrimp.

3. Add the shrimp to the bowl of sauce and toss to combine. Serve at room temperature or chilled in lettuce leaves, with the avocado and lemon wedges on the side.

SAVE FOR A SNACK: Make a double batch of the cocktail sauce and have ½ cup as a dipper for vegetables.

Per serving: 292 calories • 35g protein • 12g fat (1.5g saturated) • 5g fiber 137mg calcium • 21mg vitamin C • 12g carbohydrate • 578mg sodium

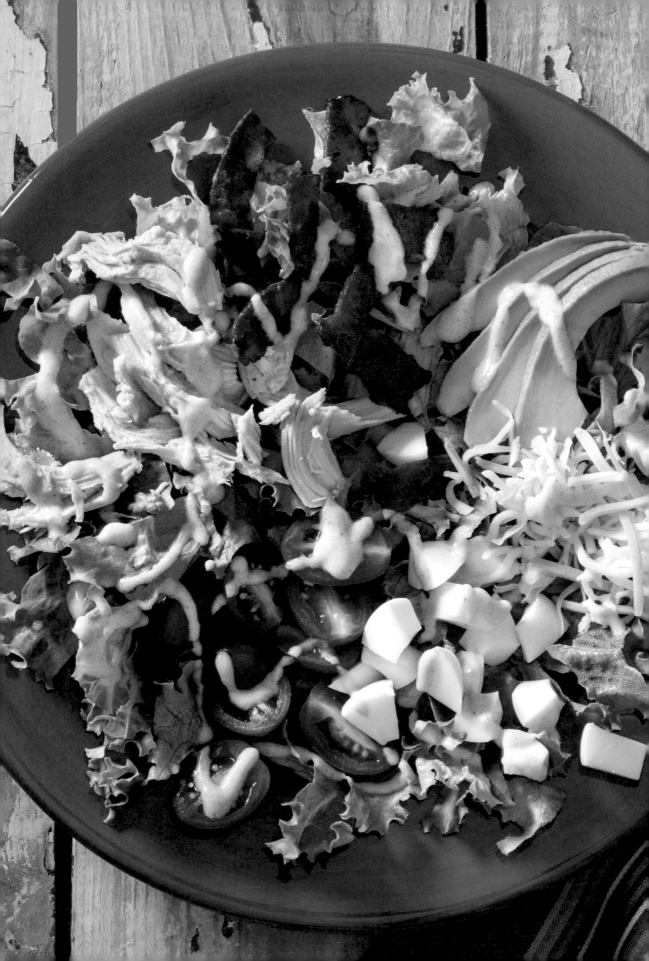

Mexican Cobb Salad

Hands-On Time: 15 minutes • **Total Time:** 30 minutes • **Makes:** 4 servings

You can make the dressing well ahead of time. (The longer it sits, the more garlicky it will get.) In fact, everything except the lettuce and avocado can be prepped ahead of time. If you have leftover chicken, use it for this recipe; you'll need about 1 cup shredded. Or if you're starting with raw chicken, follow the poaching directions in step 1 of Country Captain (page 176).

Fat Releasers
Yogurt, olive oil, limes, cayenne, garlic, lettuce, tomatoes, chicken, avocado, eggs, cheese

DRESSING

- ¼ cup fat-free yogurt
- 1 tablespoon extra-virgin olive oil
- 1 tablespoon fresh lime juice
- 1 teaspoon Worcestershire sauce (optional)
- ½ teaspoon ground cumin
- ¼ teaspoon salt
- Pinch of cayenne pepper
- 1 small clove garlic, minced
- 2 tablespoons water

SALAD

- 1 teaspoon olive oil
- 6 slices thin-cut turkey bacon, cut crosswise into ½-inch pieces
- 10 cups chopped or shredded crisp lettuce (such as iceberg, romaine, or leaf lettuce)
- 1 pint grape tomatoes, halved
- 1 large skinless, boneless chicken breast (8 ounces), cooked and shredded
- 1 Hass avocado, sliced
- 4 hard-boiled egg whites, cubed
- ¼ cup shredded reduced-fat Mexican blend cheese
- ½ cup minced cilantro

1. To *make the dressing:* In a screw-top jar, combine the yogurt, oil, lime juice, Worcestershire sauce, cumin, salt, pepper, garlic and the water. Cover and shake well.

2. *To make the salad:* In a medium nonstick skillet, heat the oil over medium-high heat. Add the bacon and cook until browned, 1 to 2 minutes. Drain on paper towels.

3. For each individual salad, make a bed of the lettuce on a large plate. Arrange the tomatoes, chicken, avocado, egg whites, bacon, and cheese in separate groups over the greens. Sprinkle with the cilantro.

4. Divide evenly, drizzling the dressing over the salads.

Per serving: 269 calories • 23g protein • 14g fat (3g saturated) • 5.5g fiber
154mg calcium • 30mg vitamin C • 14g carbohydrate • 438mg sodium

Fennel & Red Onion Salad with Blood Orange Vinaigrette

Hands-On Time: 15 minutes • **Total Time:** 15 minutes • **Makes:** 4 servings

Blood oranges have a deep ruby flesh and a juice that tastes faintly of raspberries. This is because blood oranges get their color from an antioxidant phytochemical called anthocyanin, the same compound that makes raspberries red. You can make the dressing and prep the vegetables for the salad ahead of time, but don't toss them together until shortly before serving. This would make a delicious accompaniment to Parmesan-Pecan Pork (page 117).

Fat Releasers
Oranges, fennel, onions, olive oil, black pepper

1 **blood orange or navel orange**

1 **large bulb fennel**

1 **red onion (6 ounces)**

1 **tablespoon extra-virgin olive oil**

2 **teaspoons Dijon mustard**

½ **teaspoon salt**

¼ **teaspoon ground black pepper**

1. Grate 2 teaspoons of zest from the orange into a salad bowl. Squeeze the orange juice into a screw-top jar.

2. Discard the fennel stalks but reserve a large handful of the fennel fronds. Quarter the fennel bulb through the core, cut out the core, and very thinly slice crosswise. (Use a mandoline-style cutter if you have one.) As you work, place the fennel in the salad bowl and toss with about 1 tablespoon of orange juice (from the screw-top jar) so it won't brown as it sits.

3. Mince the fennel fronds (to get about ¼ cup) and add to the sliced fennel. Halve the onion lengthwise, then thinly slice crosswise. Add to the other vegetables and toss.

4. Add the oil, mustard, salt, and pepper to the orange juice in the screw-top jar and shake to blend. Pour the dressing over the salad and toss.

Per 1¼-cup serving: 77 calories • 1g protein • 3.5g fat (0.5g saturated) 2.5g fiber • 41mg calcium • 19mg vitamin C • 11g carbohydrate • 383mg sodium

Red Quinoa Salad with Avocado

Hands-On Time: 15 minutes • **Total Time:** 25 minutes • **Makes:** 6 servings

Red quinoa is white quinoa's nutty-tasting cousin. It has all the same health benefits but a heartier flavor. It can be hard to find, though, so this salad would work just fine with regular quinoa. If you want to make the salad ahead of time, don't add the cucumber until you're ready to serve, because it tends to weep liquid as it sits and will make the salad watery.

Fat Releasers
Quinoa, yogurt, limes, olive oil, black pepper, avocado, sunflower seeds

1 **cup red quinoa**

¼ **teaspoon salt**

¼ **cup 0% Greek yogurt**

2 **tablespoons fresh lime juice**

2 **teaspoons extra-virgin olive oil**

¼ **teaspoon ground black pepper**

1 **Hass avocado**

½ **cup coarsely chopped cilantro**

1 **large cucumber, peeled, seeded, and cut into ¼-inch cubes**

2 **tablespoons hulled sunflower seeds, toasted**

1. In a pot of boiling water, cook the quinoa according to package directions, with the salt. Drain well and transfer to a salad bowl to cool slightly.

2. Meanwhile, in a small bowl, stir together the yogurt, 1 tablespoon of the lime juice, the oil, and pepper.

3. Cut the avocado into ¼-inch cubes and toss with the remaining 1 tablespoon lime juice.

4. Add the dressing, cilantro, and cucumber to the quinoa and toss gently. Add the avocado and toss very gently. Serve the salad sprinkled with the sunflower seeds.

MAKE IT A MAIN: Start with 1½ cups of the mixture and top it with 4 ounces roasted salmon or baked tofu for a one-dish dinner.

Per 1-cup serving: 189 calories • 6g protein • 8g fat (1g saturated) • 3.5g fiber • 34mg calcium • 5mg vitamin C • 25g carbohydrate • 110mg sodium

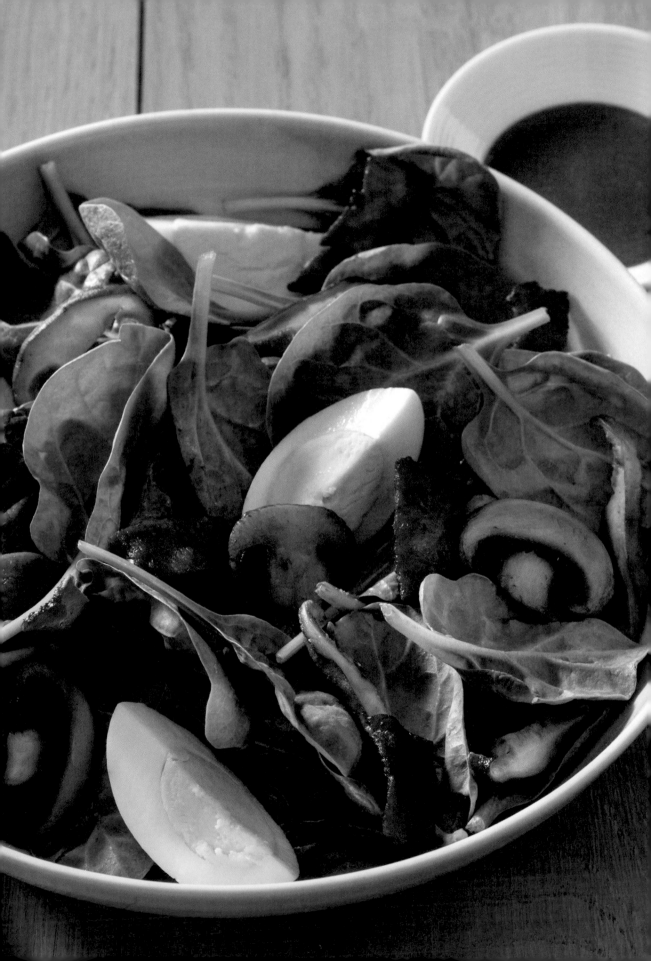

Old-School Spinach Salad

Hands-On Time: 25 minutes • **Total Time:** 25 minutes • **Makes:** 4 servings

A classic salad (from the '70s), updated with two types of mushrooms, turkey bacon, hard-boiled eggs, and baby spinach dressed in a light balsamic vinaigrette.

Fat Releasers
Eggs, vinegar, olive oil, spinach

4 large eggs

1 tablespoon Dijon mustard

2 tablespoons balsamic vinegar

1½ teaspoons extra-virgin olive oil

4 slices turkey bacon (1 ounce each), cut crosswise into ½-inch pieces

6 ounces shiitake mushrooms, stems discarded, caps thinly sliced

¼ cup water

8 ounces white mushrooms, thinly sliced

10 ounces (10 cups) baby spinach

1. Place the eggs in a small pot of cold water to cover. Bring to a boil over high heat. Remove from the heat, cover, and let stand 12 minutes. Drain, run under cold water, and peel. Cut lengthwise into quarters.

2. In a large bowl, whisk together the mustard, vinegar, and oil.

3. Meanwhile, in a large skillet, cook the bacon over medium heat until starting to color, about 1 minute. Add the shiitakes and water and cook until starting to soften, about 2 minutes. Add the white mushrooms and cook until tender, about 5 minutes.

4. Add the spinach to the bowl of dressing along with the bacon, mushrooms, and the eggs and toss to combine.

Per serving: 221 calories • 15g protein • 12g fat (3.5g saturated) • 5g fiber 94mg calcium • 13mg vitamin C • 15g carbohydrate • 585mg sodium

Warm Goat Cheese on a Bed of Greens

Hands-On Time: 10 minutes • **Total Time:** 20 minutes • **Makes:** 4 servings

This salad would make a nice starter course for a simple meal of Pepper Loin Steaks (page 119) and Green Beans with Basil & Toasted Walnuts (page 231)—a menu you could easily serve to dinner guests while still maintaining your diet.

Fat Releasers
Sesame seeds, cheese, olive oil, lemons, oregano, black pepper, watercress, greens

1½ tablespoons sesame seeds

4-ounce log of reduced-fat goat cheese, cut into 8 rounds

1 tablespoon plus 1 teaspoon extra-virgin olive oil

1 tablespoon lemon juice

2 teaspoons Dijon mustard

¼ teaspoon dried oregano

Large pinch of ground black pepper

1 bunch watercress, thick stems discarded, coarsely chopped

4 cups mixed field greens (about 4 ounces)

1. Preheat the oven to 300°F.

2. In a small ungreased skillet, stir the sesame seeds over medium heat until lightly browned and fragrant, about 3 minutes. Immediately pour into a shallow bowl or pie plate to stop the cooking and keep them from burning. Let them cool.

3. Dip both sides of the goat cheese rounds in the sesame seeds. Set on a small foil-lined baking pan in the fridge while you prep the rest of the salad ingredients.

4. In a large bowl, whisk together the oil, lemon juice, mustard, oregano, and pepper. Add the watercress and greens and toss.

5. Place the goat cheese in the oven to warm through but not melt, 5 to 7 minutes.

6. Divide the dressed greens among salad plates and top each salad with 2 warm goat cheese rounds.

Per serving: 120 calories • 6g protein • 9.5g fat (2.5g saturated) • 1.5g fiber 91mg calcium • 18mg vitamin C • 4g carbohydrate • 189mg sodium

Romaine with Guacamole Dressing

Hands-On Time: 10 minutes • **Total Time:** 10 minutes • **Makes:** 4 servings

The creamy dressing for this salad would also make an excellent dip. Prepare it as directed below, but don't add the water until you've processed everything else. Then add the water a tablespoon at a time until you get a dipping texture. Finish by stirring in the tomato. And if you want to take it in a guacamole direction, stir in a little chopped cilantro, too.

Fat Releasers
Avocado, limes, pepper sauce, tomato, lettuce, scallions

1 large Hass avocado
5 tablespoons fresh lime juice (2 to 3 limes)
¼ cup water
2 teaspoons cayenne pepper sauce
½ teaspoon salt
1 large plum tomato, finely chopped
8 cups shredded romaine lettuce
½ cup coarsely chopped cilantro
1 bunch scallions, thinly sliced

1. Scoop the avocado flesh into a mini chopper or blender. Add the lime juice, water, hot pepper sauce, and salt, and process until smooth.

2. Transfer the dressing to a large bowl and stir in the chopped tomato (and any tomato juices). Add the lettuce, cilantro, and scallions, tossing to coat.

MAKE IT A MAIN: Rub ¾ pound flank steak or chicken breast, or 1 pound peeled and deveined shrimp, with a little extra-virgin olive oil and cumin or chili powder. Broil or pan-grill. Slice the steak or chicken but leave the shrimp whole, and serve with lime wedges for squeezing over the meat or shrimp. Lightly coat slabs of zucchini and/or yellow squash with olive oil and grill to serve alongside.

COOKING FOR ONE: Make the whole amount of dressing (including the tomatoes) and store in the fridge; it should keep for about a week, well covered. To make a salad, toss 2 cups of salad greens with ½ cup of the dressing. (Be sure to stir before using, because the tomato will leak out liquid as the dressing sits.)

Per 2-cup serving: 88 calories • 3g protein • 5.5g fat (1g saturated) • 5g fiber 56mg calcium • 19mg vitamin C • 10g carbohydrate • 321mg sodium

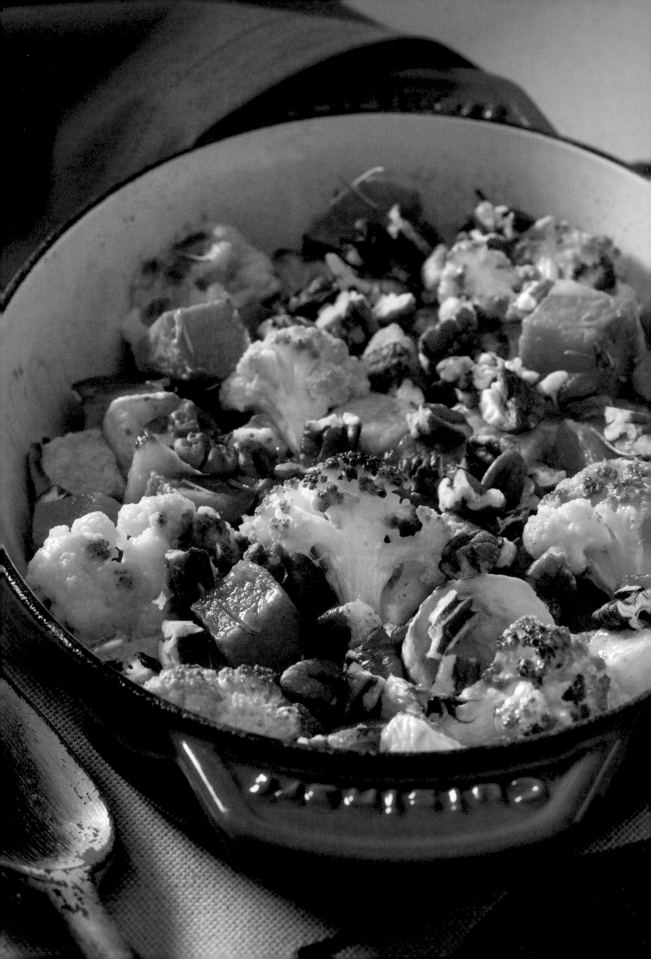

Roasted Winter Vegetable Salad

Hands-On Time: 20 minutes • **Total Time:** 1 hour 5 minutes • **Makes:** 4 servings

Hard vegetables like winter squash, cauliflower, jicama, and turnips take well to roasting, which brings out their natural sugars. Any combination of vegetables is good, so try them all to find your favorites! These are equally good hot, cold, or at room temperature.

Fat Releasers
Butternut squash, cauliflower, garlic, rosemary, olive oil, lemon, pecans

1 pound butternut squash, peeled and cut into 1-inch chunks

9 ounces cauliflower, cut into large florets

8 ounces jicama, peeled and cut into 1-inch chunks

5 ounces white turnips, cut into 1-inch chunks

3 cloves garlic, skin on

½ teaspoon crumbled dried rosemary

2 teaspoons plus 1 tablespoon extra-virgin olive oil

½ teaspoon salt

½ cup water

3 tablespoons fresh lemon juice

2 teaspoons Dijon mustard

¼ cup pecans, broken into bits

1. Preheat the oven to 425°F.

2. On a large rimmed baking sheet, toss together the squash, cauliflower, jicama, turnip, garlic, rosemary, 2 teaspoons of the oil, the salt, and the water. Roast, tossing occasionally, until the vegetables are lightly browned and tender, about 45 minutes.

3. Meanwhile, in a large bowl, whisk together the lemon juice, mustard, and the remaining 1 tablespoon oil.

4. Add the vegetables while still warm and toss to combine. Serve with the pecans sprinkled on top.

MAKE IT A MAIN: You can turn this into a vegetarian main dish by topping each portion with 1½ ounces of reduced-fat goat cheese. For a nonvegetarian main dish, toss each portion of the finished vegetables with 3 ounces of cooked chicken breast or pork tenderloin per person. Start the meal with Golden Gazpacho (page 99).

Per 1-cup serving: 185 calories • 4g protein • 11g fat (1.5g saturated) • 8g fiber 79mg calcium • 72mg vitamin C • 22g carbohydrate • 349mg sodium

Grilled Asparagus Salad with Balsamic Dressing

Hands-On Time: 5 minutes • **Total Time:** 15 minutes • **Makes:** 4 servings

When shopping for asparagus, look for stalks that have tightly closed tops and crisp stalks. Cooking the asparagus briefly in boiling water gives them a head start on grilling and ensures that they'll be cooked without scorching.

Fat Releasers
Vinegar, olive oil, asparagus, bell pepper, pumpkin seeds

½ cup balsamic vinegar

4 teaspoons extra-virgin olive oil

¼ teaspoon salt

2 pounds asparagus, preferably on the larger side, trimmed

1 red bell pepper, cut into thin strips

2 teaspoons hulled pumpkin seeds

1. In a small nonstick saucepan, combine the vinegar and 1 tablespoon of the oil and bring to a boil over medium-high heat. Boil until reduced to ¼ cup, 4 to 5 minutes. Transfer to a bowl and whisk in the salt.

2. Meanwhile, in a large pot of boiling water, cook the asparagus for 2 minutes to soften slightly. Drain well.

3. Lightly oil the grill grates or a grill pan with the remaining 1 teaspoon oil. Preheat the grill or pan to medium heat and cook the asparagus, turning them as they soften, to color and get grill marks, 3 to 5 minutes (depending on the thickness of the asparagus).

4. Halve the asparagus crosswise, place on a platter, drizzle the reduced vinegar dressing on top, and sprinkle with the bell pepper and pumpkin seeds. Serve warm or at room temperature.

Per serving: 99 calories • 4g protein • 4.5g fat (0.5g saturated) • 3g fiber 37mg calcium • 47mg vitamin C • 12g carbohydrate • 170mg sodium

Warm Broccolini Salad with Cashew Pesto

Hands-On Time: 10 minutes • **Total Time:** 25 minutes • **Makes:** 4 servings

Broccolini—also called broccolette, baby broccoli, and Asparation—is a cross between broccoli and Chinese broccoli. It is quite mild in flavor, and its main advantage is that the entire stalk is tender and edible. Broccolini's cousin, broccoli rabe, can be substituted in this recipe, if you're a fan of its slightly bitter flavor, because it is prepped and cooked the same way. Although this is served warm, it's quite tasty chilled, too.

Fat Releasers
Garlic, cashews, Parmesan cheese, basil, broccolini, lemons

3 cloves garlic, peeled

¼ cup unsalted roasted cashews

¼ cup grated Parmesan cheese

½ cup packed basil leaves

5 tablespoons water

Salt

2 bunches of broccolini (8 ounces each), cut into bite-size pieces

½ lemon

1. In a small saucepan of boiling water, cook the garlic for 2 minutes. Drain and transfer to a mini food processor.

2. Add the cashews to the food processor and pulse until coarsely ground. Add the Parmesan cheese, basil, and water and pulse to form a thick pesto-like sauce.

3. In a large pot of lightly salted boiling water, cook the broccolini until crisp-tender, about 5 minutes.

4. Drain the broccolini and transfer to a serving bowl and toss with the pesto. Squeeze the lemon over the broccolini and toss again. Let cool to warm.

Per 1-cup serving: 124 calories • 8g protein • 5.5g fat (1.5g saturated) • 2g fiber 153mg calcium • 109mg vitamin C • 12g carbohydrate • 228mg sodium

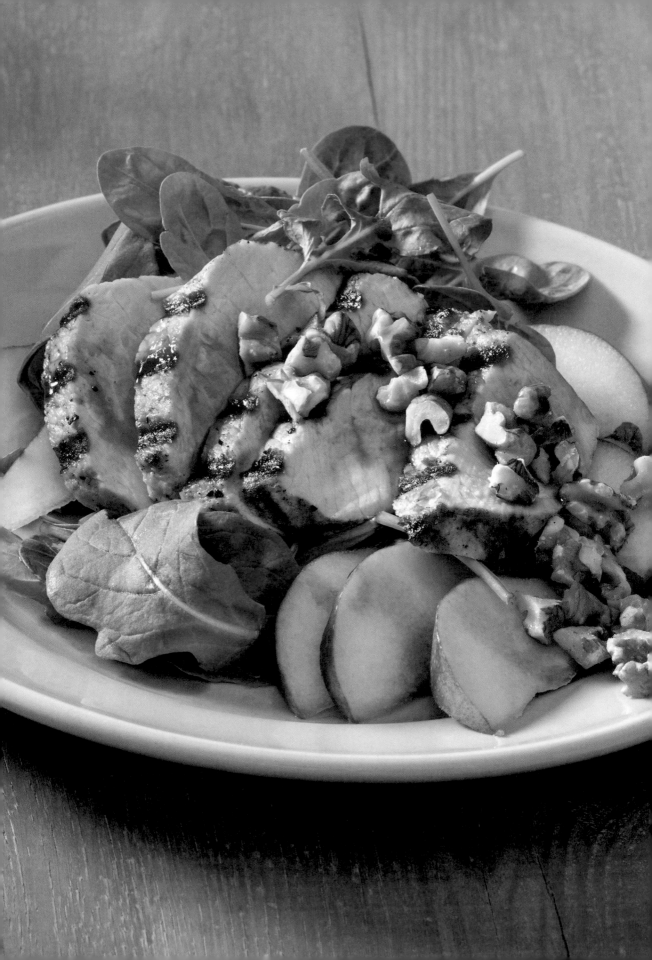

Grilled Pork & Pear Salad with Walnuts

Hands-On Time: 15 minutes • **Total Time:** 20 minutes • **Makes:** 4 servings

Bitter greens, such as arugula, are rich in an array of health-protective phytochemicals. Plus, their pungent flavor is a perfect counterpoint to the rich-tasting pork and the sweet pear.

Fat Releasers
Sesame oil, vinegar, pork loin, olive oil, black pepper, spinach, arugula, walnuts

DRESSING

- 2 teaspoons sesame oil
- 1 tablespoon reduced-sodium soy sauce
- 1 tablespoon sherry vinegar or cider vinegar

SALAD

- 4 well-trimmed boneless loin pork chops, ¾ inch thick (4 ounces each)
- 2 teaspoons extra-virgin olive oil
- Ground black pepper
- 4 cups baby spinach
- 4 cups baby arugula
- 2 pears, such as Bosc, thinly sliced lengthwise
- ¼ cup coarsely chopped toasted walnuts

1. *To make the dressing:* In a small bowl, whisk together the sesame oil, soy sauce, and vinegar. Measure out 2 teaspoons of the mixture and set aside in another small bowl.

2. *To make the salad:* Preheat a grill or a grill pan. Brush the pork chops with the olive oil and season with pepper. Grill until cooked through but still juicy, 2 to 3 minutes per side. Let sit for 5 minutes before slicing.

3. In a large bowl, toss the spinach and arugula with the dressing.

4. Pour the meat juices into the 2 teaspoons of reserved dressing. Serve the pork and pears on a bed of the greens. Drizzle with the dressing-juice mixture and top with the walnuts.

COOKING FOR ONE: Make the full amount of dressing and set aside 2 teaspoons for the salad that you're about to have. Save the remaining dressing to use on another night on a simple side dinner salad of mixed greens. Divide all the other ingredients by 4.

Per serving: 314 calories • 24g protein • 17g fat (3.5g saturated) • 5g fiber 100mg calcium • 12mg vitamin C • 19g carbohydrate • 238mg sodium

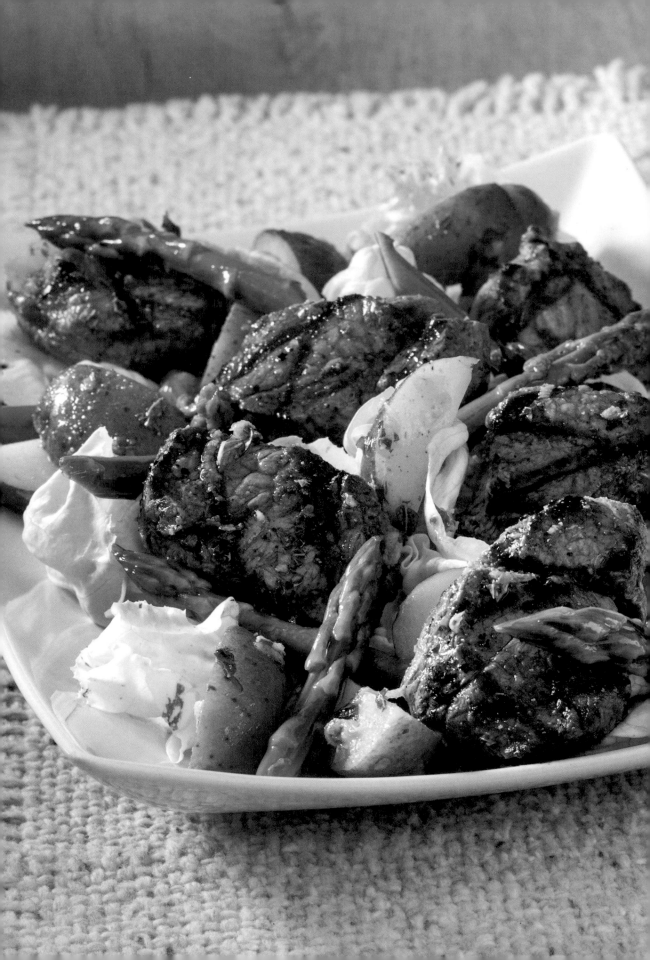

Grilled Lamb & Asparagus Salad

Hands-On Time: 20 minutes • **Total Time:** 35 minutes + marinating time
Makes: 4 servings

You can cook the potatoes and asparagus a couple of hours ahead of time if you so desire. The only last-minute cooking here is grilling the lamb (or beef). If you often like to marinate meat or other dishes, consider buying a vacuum-style marinator (such as the Vacu Vin Marinator). It takes only 5 minutes of marinating and you're good to go. If you're in Fade Away, substitute an equal amount of jicama or butternut squash for the potatoes. The squash will take a shorter amount of time to steam, so keep an eye on it.

Fat Releasers
Hot pepper sauce, olive oil, vinegar, garlic, asparagus, greens

- ½ **teaspoon hot pepper sauce**
- 3 **tablespoons extra-virgin olive oil**
- 3 **tablespoons cider vinegar**
- 3 **tablespoons finely chopped fresh mint**
- ½ **teaspoon salt**
- 2 **cloves garlic, grated on a zester**
- 2 **teaspoons ground cumin**
- 1 **pound well-trimmed leg of lamb or beef sirloin, cut into 1-inch cubes**
- 1 **pound small red potatoes, quartered (cut into eighths if larger than 2 inches)**
- 1 **pound asparagus, cut on the diagonal into 2-inch pieces**
- 6 **cups mixed baby greens**

1. In a large salad bowl, combine the hot pepper sauce, oil, vinegar, mint, and ¼ teaspoon of the salt. Measure out 3 tablespoons of the mixture for a marinade and transfer to a medium bowl.

2. Add the garlic, cumin, and lamb to the bowl with the marinade, tossing to coat. Let stand at room temperature for at least 15 minutes (or up to 2 hours in the fridge).

3. Meanwhile, in a vegetable steamer, cook the potatoes until firm-tender, 12 to 14 minutes. Add the asparagus for the last 6 minutes of cooking time. Drain well and transfer to the salad bowl with the dressing. Add the remaining ¼ teaspoon salt and toss to coat well.

4. Preheat the grill. Thread the lamb on skewers. (Discard any remaining

continued on next page

continued from previous page

marinade.) Grill the skewers covered, turning once, for 6 to 8 minutes, or until the lamb is medium-rare.

5. Add the lamb to the potatoes and asparagus, tossing to coat thoroughly. Serve the salad warm or at room temperature on a bed of the greens.

COOKING FOR ONE: Make the dressing/marinade mixture by combining 1 tablespoon each oil, vinegar, and mint, and 1/8 teaspoon salt. Measure out 1 tablespoon of the mixture to use as a salad dressing. Stir ½ clove grated garlic and ½ teaspoon cumin into the remaining marinade mixture and toss with the meat. Just divide the rest of the ingredients by 4. The cooking times will all be the same.

Per serving: 327 calories • 27g protein • 14g fat (4g saturated) • 5g fiber 47mg calcium • 15mg vitamin C • 25g carbohydrate • 348mg sodium

Marinated Grilled Chicken Salad

Hands-On Time: 25 minutes • **Total Time:** 40 minutes + marinating time
Makes: 4 servings

If you're making the salad ahead, don't stir in the apple, scallions, and cilantro until you are ready to serve. Leftover salad makes a great lunch sandwich: Using only ¾ cup of the salad, stuff it into a small whole-wheat pita or wrap it in a multigrain sandwich wrap, and add torn or shredded lettuce.

Fat Releasers
Vinegar, tomato paste, olive oil, ginger, garlic, red pepper flakes, chicken, scallions

¼ cup frozen apple juice concentrate

¼ cup cider vinegar

2 tablespoons no-salt-added tomato paste

1 tablespoon plus 1 teaspoon extra-virgin olive oil

1 teaspoon ground ginger

Salt

2 cloves garlic, minced

1 pinch plus ¼ teaspoon red pepper flakes

1¼ pounds skinless, boneless chicken breasts

1 pound carrots, shredded

1 apple, peeled and shredded

6 scallions, minced

⅓ cup coarsely chopped cilantro

1. In a large bowl, combine the apple juice concentrate, vinegar, tomato paste, oil, ginger, and ½ teaspoon salt. Measure out ⅓ cup for a marinade and place in a shallow container. To the mixture remaining in the large bowl, add ½ teaspoon of the garlic and a pinch of red pepper flakes. Set the dressing aside.

2. Add the ¼ teaspoon red pepper flakes and remaining garlic to the marinade. Add the chicken and turn to coat. Marinate for 45 minutes at room temperature up to 2 hours in the fridge.

3. Meanwhile, in a medium pot of lightly salted boiling water, cook the carrots until crisp-tender, about 3 minutes. Drain well and set aside to cool slightly, then add to the bowl of dressing.

4. Preheat a grill to medium-high. Grill the chicken, covered, until cooked through but still juicy, 9 to 12 minutes (depending on the thickness of the chicken), turning over and basting halfway through. When cool enough to handle, shred the chicken and add to the salad bowl (along with any chicken juices).

5. Add the apple, scallions, and cilantro, tossing to combine.

Per 1¾-cup serving: 351 calories • 46g protein • 8g fat (2g saturated) • 4.5g fiber 83mg calcium • 14mg vitamin C • 23g carbohydrate • 451mg sodium

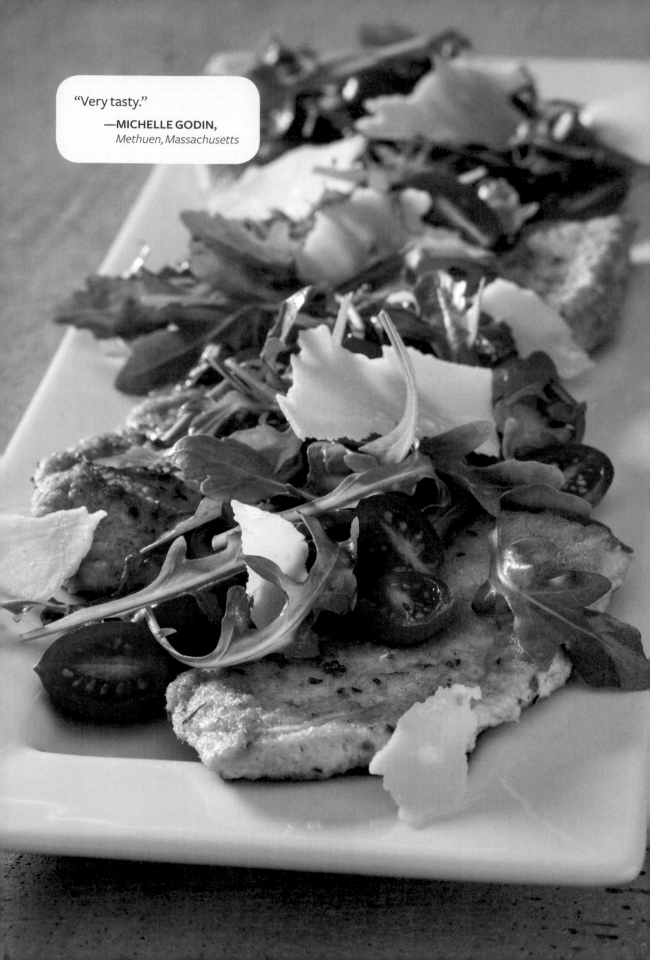

Turkey Milanese

Hands-On Time: 20 minutes • **Total Time:** 20 minutes • **Makes:** 4 servings

Hidden underneath the peppery-lemony arugula salad is a juicy turkey cutlet. The combo of warm cutlet and cool salad is especially pleasing. If you buy a chunk of Parmesan cheese, it's very easy to get thin shards by slicing them with a vegetable peeler. If you buy Parmesan cheese already grated, sprinkle 1½ teaspoons over each salad just before serving.

Fat Releasers
Turkey, oregano, whole-wheat flour, olive oil, lemons, tomatoes, arugula, Parmesan cheese

4 turkey cutlets (4 ounces each)
¾ teaspoon dried oregano
½ teaspoon salt
¼ cup whole-wheat flour
1 tablespoon plus 2 teaspoons extra-virgin olive oil
2 tablespoons fresh lemon juice
1⅓ cups grape tomatoes, halved
4 cups baby arugula
½ ounce Parmesan cheese, shaved with a vegetable peeler

1. Sprinkle the turkey cutlets with the oregano and salt and then dredge them in the flour, shaking off any excess.

2. In a large nonstick skillet, heat 1 tablespoon of the oil over medium heat. Add the turkey and cook, turning the turkey over midway, until golden brown and cooked through, about 2 minutes per side. Transfer to serving plates.

3. In a medium bowl, whisk together the remaining 2 teaspoons oil and the lemon juice. Add the tomatoes and arugula and toss to combine. Top the turkey with the salad and Parmesan cheese.

Per serving: 235 calories • 32g protein • 7.5g fat (1.5g saturated) • 2g fiber 91mg calcium • 21mg vitamin C • 10g carbohydrate • 453mg sodium

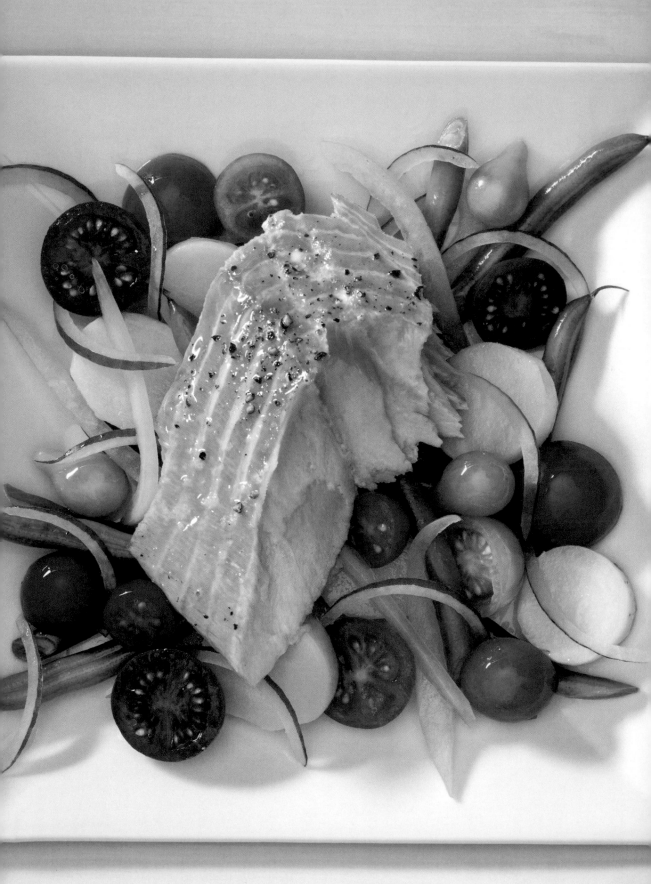

Salmon Niçoise

Hands-On Time: 15 minutes • **Total Time:** 30 minutes • **Makes:** 4 servings

Make this in the height of summer when the vegetables are at their most vibrant. Look in the farmers' market for baby heirloom tomatoes. (Don't buy them in the supermarket, though, because they'll be way too expensive.) If you like, add some capers to the salad for a briny bite.

Fat Releasers
Salmon, black pepper, green beans, lemons, olive oil, bell pepper, onion, tomatoes

- 4 **skin-on salmon fillets (6 ounces each)**
- ½ **teaspoon salt**
- ¼ **teaspoon ground black pepper**
- 1 **pound small potatoes**
- ½ **pound green beans, halved crosswise**
- 2 **tablespoons fresh lemon juice**
- 1 **tablespoon plus 1 teaspoon extra-virgin olive oil**
- ¾ **teaspoon Dijon mustard**
- 1 **yellow bell pepper, cut into strips**
- 1 **small red onion, halved and thinly sliced**
- 1½ **cups assorted small heirloom tomatoes or grape tomatoes, halved**

1. Preheat the oven to 450°F. Place the salmon skin-side down on a rimmed baking sheet. Sprinkle with ¼ teaspoon of the salt and the black pepper. Roast until just cooked through but still moist, about 10 minutes. With a metal spatula, lift the salmon from the baking sheet, leaving the skin behind.

2. Meanwhile, in a vegetable steamer, cook the potatoes until tender, about 15 minutes (depending on the size of the potatoes); add the green beans for the last 10 minutes of cooking. When cool enough to handle, peel the potatoes if you like, or leave the skins on, then thickly slice.

3. In a large bowl, whisk together the lemon juice, oil, mustard, and remaining ¼ teaspoon salt. Add the steamed vegetables along with the bell pepper, onion, and tomatoes and toss.

4. Divide the vegetables among 4 plates and top with the salmon.

Per serving: 450 calories • 43g protein • 17g fat (2.5g saturated) • 4.5g fiber 62mg calcium • 121mg vitamin C • 30g carbohydrate • 423mg sodium

Italian Tuna & Fennel Salad

Hands-On Time: 20 minutes • **Total Time:** 20 minutes • **Makes:** 4 servings

Fennel, sometimes called anise, has a crunch and texture similar to celery with a hint of licorice. The bulbous bottom of fennel is edible while the hollow stalks are not. To trim fennel, cut off and discard the stalks (or save for flavoring stock) and reserve the dark feathery fronds, if there are any, and use them as a garnish.

Fat Releasers
Oranges, lemons, olive oil, fennel, tomatoes, onion, nuts, tuna

2 tablespoons orange juice

1 tablespoon fresh lemon juice

1½ teaspoons Dijon mustard

1 tablespoon plus 1 teaspoon extra-virgin olive oil

1 bulb fennel (¾ pound), thinly sliced crosswise (1½ cups)

1 cup grape tomatoes, halved

1 small red onion, halved and thinly sliced (⅔ cup)

3 tablespoons raisins or dried currants

1 tablespoon pine nuts or slivered almonds

2 cans (5 ounces each) water-packed light tuna, drained

1. In a large bowl, whisk together the orange juice, lemon juice, and mustard until well combined. Whisk in the oil.

2. Add the fennel, tomatoes, onion, raisins, and pine nuts and toss. Add the tuna and toss gently.

Per serving: 203 calories • 20g protein • 6.5g fat (1g saturated) • 3g fiber 47mg calcium • 24mg vitamin C • 16g carbohydrate • 114mg sodium

Bulgur Salad with Tomatoes & Olives

Hands-On Time: 20 minutes • **Total Time:** 55 minutes • **Makes:** 4 servings

Tofu presents a wonderful blank canvas for other flavorful ingredients, but you need to get rid of some of the excess liquid first. Use the simple hands-off technique in step 1, and let the tofu drain while you prepare the ingredients in steps 2 and 3.

Fat Releasers
Tofu, tomatoes, olive oil, lemons, vinegar, garlic, basil, black pepper, walnuts

- 1 **container (14 ounces) extra-firm tofu, drained**
- 2 **large plum tomatoes**
- 1 **small cucumber**
- ¼ **cup pitted Kalamata olives**
- 1 **tablespoon plus 1 teaspoon extra-virgin olive oil**
- 2 **teaspoons lemon juice plus 2 teaspoons grated lemon zest**
- 3 **tablespoons balsamic vinegar**
- 2 **cloves garlic, 1 grated on a zester and 1 minced**
- 1 **teaspoon dried basil**
- ½ **teaspoon salt**
- 1½ **cups water**
- ¾ **cup bulgur (or cracked wheat)**
- **Ground black pepper**
- ⅓ **cup walnuts, toasted and chopped**

1. Slice the block of tofu in half horizontally. Place the tofu on a double layer of paper towels on a cutting board and top with another double layer of paper towels and a small baking pan with heavy weights in it (like canned goods). Let drain for at least 15 minutes.

2. Meanwhile, dice the tomatoes and place them in a salad bowl. Peel, seed, and dice the cucumber and add to the bowl. Chop the olives and add to the bowl. Add the olive oil and lemon juice and set aside.

3. Combine the vinegar, grated garlic, lemon zest, basil, and ¼ teaspoon of the salt in a shallow container big enough to hold all the tofu in a single layer.

4. Transfer the tofu to the container with the marinade. Use a knife to cut it into ½-inch cubes right in the container. Set aside to soak.

5. Meanwhile, in a small saucepan, combine the water, minced garlic, and the remaining ¼ teaspoon salt. Bring to a boil, add the bulgur, and stir. Remove from the heat, cover, and let stand until the liquid is absorbed, about 30 minutes.

6. Drain any liquid remaining in the bulgur and transfer into the bowl with the tomato mixture. Scrape the tofu and marinade onto the bulgur. Add lots of pepper and toss gently to combine. Serve sprinkled with walnuts.

Per 1½-cup serving: 328 calories • 16g protein • 17g fat (2g saturated) • 7.5g fiber 121mg calcium • 8mg vitamin C • 31g carbohydrate • 397mg sodium

Honey-Mustard Cabbage Slaw

Hands-On Time: 15 minutes • **Total Time:** 15 minutes + chilling time
Makes: 4 servings

To get the most flavor and nicest texture for this slaw, cut the cabbage into chunks and then pulse-chop in a food processor to finely chop. You can use bagged coleslaw mix in place of a head of red cabbage if you'd like, but even that should be very finely chopped.

Fat Releasers
Yogurt, vinegar, olive oil, honey, cabbage, scallions

- ⅓ cup 0% Greek yogurt
- 2 tablespoons cider vinegar
- 1 tablespoon Dijon mustard
- 1 tablespoon plus 1 teaspoon extra-virgin olive oil
- 1 tablespoon honey
- 1 teaspoon dried tarragon
- ½ teaspoon salt
- 5 cups very finely chopped red cabbage (½ small head, or 1 pound)
- 3 carrots, shredded
- 2 scallions, thinly sliced

1. In a large bowl, whisk together the yogurt, vinegar, mustard, oil, honey, tarragon, and salt.
2. Add the cabbage, carrots, and scallions, tossing to combine. Refrigerate for 1 hour or until chilled.

MAKE IT A MAIN: Brush a 1-pound pork tenderloin with a mixture of mustard and red wine and roast until cooked through but still juicy. Slice and serve on a bed of the cabbage slaw. Serve with Crispy Balsamic Potatoes (page 251) for a complete meal.

Per 1½-cup serving: 128 calories • 4g protein • 5g fat (0.5g saturated) • 4g fiber 87mg calcium • 69mg vitamin C • 19g carbohydrate • 452mg sodium

Lentil Salad with Feta

Hands-On Time: 10 minutes • **Total Time:** 35 minutes + cooling time
Makes: 6 servings

Lentils are an excellent source of fiber, especially heart-healthy soluble fiber. One serving of this has about a third of the dietary fiber you need for the whole day. This dish calls for regular supermarket lentils, but if you can find them, pardina lentils (often available in the Hispanic foods section of the supermarket) or French Puy lentils (in some supermarkets and gourmet food stores) would add a slightly peppery flavor and chewy texture to the salad.

Fat Releasers
Lentils, black pepper, limes, peanut oil, radishes, cheese

4 cups water

1 cup lentils

¾ teaspoon salt

¾ teaspoon ground black pepper

⅓ cup raisins, dried cranberries, or chopped dried cherries

3 tablespoons fresh lime juice

1 tablespoon plus 1 teaspoon peanut oil or extra-virgin olive oil

1¼ cups coarsely diced radishes (6 large; about ½ pound)

2 ounces reduced-fat feta cheese, crumbled

1. In a medium saucepan, bring the water to a boil. Add the lentils and ½ teaspoon each of the salt and pepper. Cook until tender, about 15 minutes. Remove from the heat and stir in the raisins; let sit for 1 minute. Drain.

2. Meanwhile, in a medium bowl, whisk together the lime juice, oil, and remaining ¼ teaspoon each salt and pepper.

3. Add the drained lentils to the dressing, toss and let cool to room temperature.

4. Add the radishes and feta, tossing to combine.

MAKE IT A MAIN: To make a one-dish meal, have the dish serve 4 instead of 6 and add 8 ounces grilled shrimp, chicken, or pork, cut into bite-size pieces. Swap diced sun-dried tomatoes for the raisins.

Per 1-cup serving: 195 calories • 11g protein • 4.5g fat (1.5g saturated) • 11g fiber 62mg calcium • 10mg vitamin C • 29g carbohydrate • 265mg sodium

Creamy Potato Salad

Hands-On Time: 15 minutes • **Total Time:** 40 minutes • **Makes:** 4 servings

Chunks of buttery Yukon Gold potatoes are roasted in their skins along with broccoli. Dressing the vegetables while they're still warm from the oven means the flavor will penetrate more readily. If you don't have buttermilk, you can use ⅔ cup plain 1% or 0% yogurt and thin it out with 1½ tablespoons water or milk. Or make your own buttermilk (see next page).

Fat Releasers
Broccoli, olive oil, garlic, buttermilk, sun-dried tomatoes

1 **head broccoli (10 ounces)**

1 **pound Yukon Gold potatoes, cut into ½-inch chunks**

4 **teaspoons extra-virgin olive oil**

3 **cloves garlic, unpeeled**

½ **teaspoon salt**

¾ **cup low-fat buttermilk**

¼ **cup sun-dried tomatoes, slivered**

1. Preheat the oven to 425°F. Separate the broccoli into florets and stalks. Cut the florets into bite-size pieces and peel and thinly slice the stalks.

2. In a 9 x 13-inch pan, toss the potatoes with 2 teaspoons of the oil. Roast 15 minutes. Add the broccoli and garlic, sprinkle with ¼ teaspoon of the salt, and roast 15 minutes longer until the potatoes are tender and the broccoli is lightly browned. Remove the garlic, peel it, and mash it.

3. Meanwhile, in a large bowl, whisk together the buttermilk, the remaining 2 teaspoons oil, and the remaining ¼ teaspoon salt. Add the mashed garlic, potatoes, broccoli, and sun-dried tomatoes and toss to combine. Serve warm or at room temperature.

MAKE IT A MAIN: For a one-dish meal, serve the potato salad on a bed of spinach and top each portion with 4 ounces cooked chicken or beef.

Per 1¼-cup serving: 174 calories • 6g protein • 5.5g fat (1g saturated) • 4.5g fiber 101mg calcium • 58mg vitamin C • 28g carbohydrate • 397mg sodium

Caesar Salad with Roasted Cauliflower & Pasta

Hands-On Time: 20 minutes • **Total Time:** 50 minutes • **Makes:** 4 servings

Roasting cauliflower makes it tender and sweet, and once you've tried it, chances are you'll always cook cauliflower this way. If you'd prefer, you can buy precut cauliflower florets from the produce section or the salad bar. Any leftover buttermilk can be frozen up to 3 months. Or, as an alternative, you can make your own buttermilk for this recipe by adding 1 tablespoon cider vinegar or distilled white vinegar to a measuring cup and enough 1% milk to make ¾ cup; let stand at room temperature for 30 minutes before using.

Fat Releasers
Cauliflower, olive oil, whole-wheat pasta, buttermilk, Parmesan cheese, hot sauce

- 5 **cups cauliflower florets (from 1 small or ½ medium head)**
- 2 **teaspoons extra-virgin olive oil**
- 2 **tablespoons water**
- 4 **ounces whole-wheat penne**
- ¾ **cup light (1.5%) buttermilk**
- 3 **tablespoons finely grated Parmesan cheese**
- 1 **teaspoon hot sauce, preferably Frank's RedHot**
- ¼ **teaspoon salt**
- 1 **rib celery, quartered lengthwise and thinly sliced**

1. Preheat the oven to 425°F. In a large bowl, toss the cauliflower with 1 teaspoon of the oil and the water. Transfer to a small rimmed baking sheet or pan and roast, tossing occasionally, until the cauliflower is tender and lightly browned, about 25 minutes.

2. Meanwhile, in a large pot of boiling water, cook the pasta according to package directions; drain.

3. In a large bowl, whisk together the buttermilk, Parmesan cheese, hot sauce, salt, and remaining 1 teaspoon oil. Add the pasta, cauliflower, and celery, and toss to combine.

MAKE IT A MAIN: Add either 12 ounces of cooked shrimp or sliced cooked chicken breast to the salad when tossing to combine.

Per 1½-cup serving: 203 calories • 11g protein • 6.5g fat (2g saturated) • 7g fiber 160mg calcium • 65mg vitamin C • 27g carbohydrate • 285mg sodium

Chickpea Salad with Carrot Dressing

Hands-On Time: 15 minutes • **Total Time:** 25 minutes • **Makes:** 4 servings

Pureeing a fresh carrot to use in this dressing not only adds a hefty amount of the antioxidant beta-carotene, it also adds fiber, a key nutrient for weight loss. You can vary this salad easily by switching out the type of beans and the type of nuts. Try one of these variations: black beans and pistachios (add ¼ teaspoon tarragon to the dressing), white beans and cashews (add a generous pinch of curry powder to the dressing), or pinto beans and pecans (add a generous pinch of chipotle powder or chili powder to the dressing).

Fat Releasers
Lemons, yogurt, honey, chickpeas, tomatoes, walnuts

½ small carrot (2 ounces), very thinly sliced

2 teaspoons grated lemon zest

1 tablespoon lemon juice

3 tablespoons 0% Greek yogurt

1 teaspoon honey

¼ teaspoon ground cumin

Large pinch of salt

1 can (15 ounces) no-salt-added chickpeas, rinsed and drained

1 pint grape tomatoes, halved (or quartered if large)

¼ cup walnut halves, toasted and chopped

1. In a small saucepan, combine the carrot, lemon zest, and lemon juice with water to just barely cover the carrot. Cover, bring to a boil, and cook until the carrot is very tender, 6 to 8 minutes.

2. Reserving the cooking liquid, drain the carrot and transfer to a mini food processor. Let cool slightly, then add the yogurt, honey, cumin, salt, and 1 tablespoon of the reserved cooking liquid. Puree to reach as smooth a texture as possible. Add more of the cooking liquid if the dressing seems too thick.

3. In a salad bowl, combine the chickpeas, tomatoes, dressing, and walnuts and toss to combine.

MAKE IT A MAIN: Add 12 ounces cubed roast turkey (or Mexican Slow-Cooked Turkey Breast, page 138), cut-up cooked shrimp, or baked tofu. Serve on a bed of shredded lettuce for a one-dish meal.

Per ¾-cup serving: 179 calories • 8g protein • 5g fat (0.5g saturated) • 5.5g fiber 57mg calcium • 23mg vitamin C • 26g carbohydrate • 89mg sodium

Belgian Endive & Grapes

Hands-On Time: 10 minutes • **Total Time:** 10 minutes • **Makes:** 4 servings

Belgian endive is sweet with a slight hint of bitterness. You'll find it in the market in boxes hidden under paper—this is to keep it from yellowing. Look for Belgian endive that is white with slightly yellow tips. While the contrast between the sweet dressing and the slightly bitter endive is nice, feel free to use your favorite type of green here.

Fat Releasers
Vinegar, honey, olive oil, arugula, red grapes

4 teaspoons cider vinegar

1 teaspoon honey

1 teaspoon Dijon mustard

¼ teaspoon salt

1 tablespoon extra-virgin olive oil

2 Belgian endives (4 ounces each), halved lengthwise and cut crosswise into ½-inch slices

2 cups baby arugula

1 cup seedless red grapes (6 ounces), halved

1. In a large bowl, whisk together the vinegar, honey, mustard, and salt. Whisk in the oil.

2. Add the endive, arugula, and grapes and toss to coat. Serve immediately.

MAKE IT A MAIN: Broil or grill 4 skinless, boneless chicken breast halves (6 ounces each) and serve atop the salad for a one-dish meal.

Per 1¼-cup serving: 79 calories • 1g protein • 3.5g fat (0.5g saturated) • 2g fiber 37mg calcium • 5mg vitamin C • 12g carbohydrate • 181mg sodium

Chapter

9

Side Dishes

Ever choose what to eat based on the side dish? You will with these mouthwatering recipes!

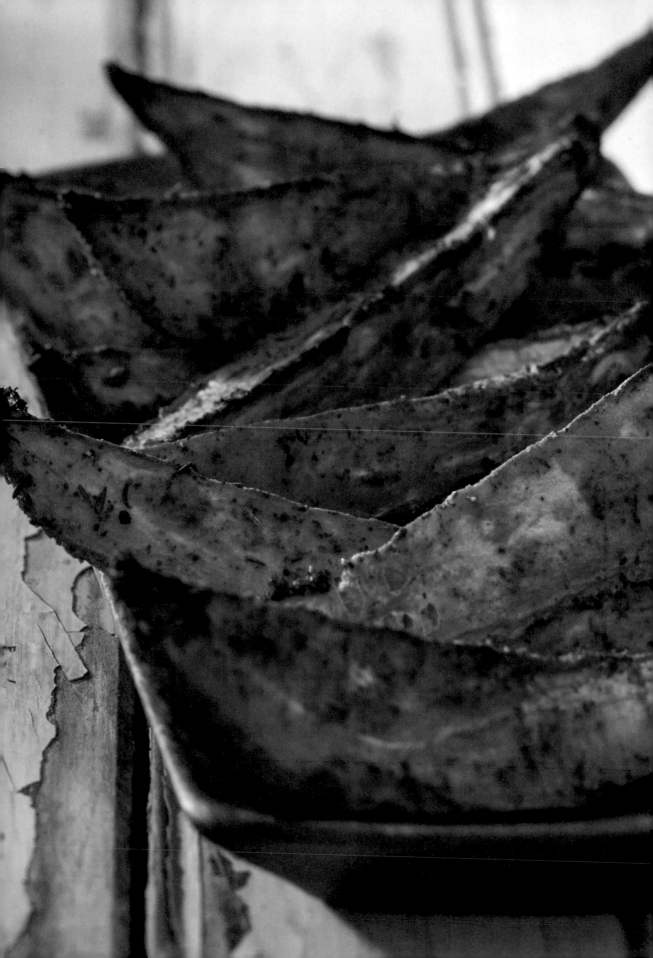

Sauté of Peppers & Sugar Snap Peas

Hands-On Time: 10 minutes • **Total Time:** 20 minutes • **Makes:** 4 servings

This is a super-quick side dish that makes a nice accompaniment to broiled or grilled meat or fish. Garam masala is an Indian blend of sweet and mildly hot spices found in the grocery aisle along with the other spices. If you prefer, you can swap ground coriander for the garam masala.

Fat Releasers
Olive oil, sugar snap peas, bell peppers, ginger

2 teaspoons extra-virgin olive oil

2 ribs celery, halved lengthwise and cut crosswise into 1-inch pieces

½ pound sugar snap peas, trimmed

1 red bell pepper, cut into thin strips

1 yellow bell pepper, cut into thin strips

¼ cup water

½ teaspoon salt

¼ teaspoon ground ginger

¼ teaspoon garam masala

1. In a large nonstick skillet, heat the oil over medium heat. Add the celery and cook until crisp-tender, about 3 minutes.

2. Add the sugar snaps and bell peppers and toss to combine. Add the water, salt, ginger, and garam masala and cook until the peppers and sugar snaps are crisp-tender, about 3 minutes.

Per serving: 67 calories • 2g protein • 2.5g fat (0.5g saturated) • 2.5g fiber 38mg calcium • 156mg vitamin C • 9g carbohydrate • 311mg sodium

Double-Sesame Bok Choy

Hands-On Time: 20 minutes • **Total Time:** 20 minutes • **Makes:** 4 servings

Bok choy is a type of Chinese cabbage. It is light, sweet, and crisp in texture and perfect for a quick stir-fry. The stalks take a little longer to cook than the leaves, so we've separated them and added them to the skillet at different times.

Fat Releasers
Olive oil, garlic, ginger, bok choy, scallions, sesame oil, sesame seeds

- 2 teaspoons extra-virgin olive oil
- 3 cloves garlic, thinly sliced
- 1-inch piece fresh ginger, thinly sliced
- 2 heads baby bok choy (12 ounces total), cut into 1-inch widths, stalks and leaves kept separate
- 3 scallions, thinly sliced
- ¼ teaspoon salt
- 1 teaspoon sesame oil
- 2 teaspoons sesame seeds

1. In a large nonstick skillet, heat the olive oil over low heat. Add the garlic and ginger and cook until the garlic is golden brown and the ginger is tender, 3 to 5 minutes.

2. Add the bok choy stalks and cook 3 minutes. Add the leaves, scallions, and salt, raise the heat to medium, and cook until the bok choy is crisp-tender, 3 to 5 minutes. Remove from the heat and sprinkle with the sesame oil and sesame seeds.

MAKE IT A MAIN: To make a one-dish meal, add 8 ounces of thinly sliced flank steak and cook until browned all over once the garlic and ginger have been sautéed. Remove the steak from the pan. Add another teaspoon of oil to the pan along with a thinly sliced bell pepper and cook it along with the bok choy stalks. Proceed with the recipe and return the steak to the pan in the last minute of cooking.

Per serving: 58 calories • 2g protein • 4.5g fat (0.5g saturated) • 1.5g fiber
14mg calcium • 3mg vitamin C • 4g carbohydrate • 184mg sodium

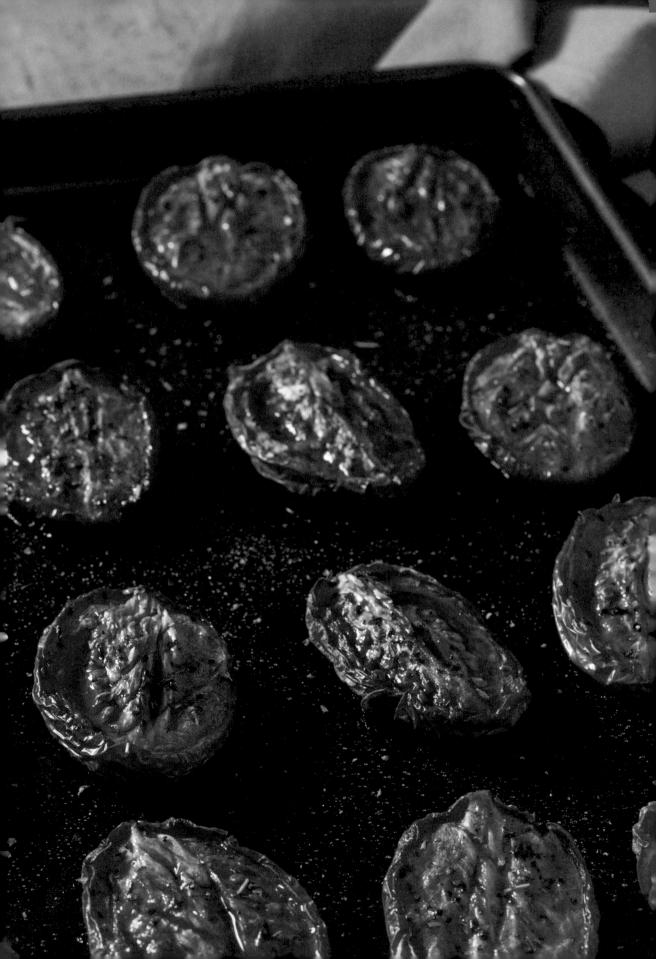

Herb-Roasted Tomatoes

Hands-On Time: 10 minutes • **Total Time:** 1 hour 40 minutes
Makes: 16 tomato halves

This is a recipe to make on a cool-weather weekend when you're lining up food for the week to come. You can serve these tomatoes hot, but they're great at room temperature and are a perfect addition to sandwiches or salads.

Fat Releasers
Tomatoes, olive oil, black pepper, Italian seasoning (contains oregano and basil)

8 **plum tomatoes (about 2 pounds)**
2 **teaspoons extra-virgin olive oil**
½ **teaspoon salt**
Ground black pepper
Italian seasoning

SAVE FOR A SNACK:
Have 3 tomato halves for a snack and top each with 2 teaspoons fat-free ricotta and a sprinkling of a fresh herb (whatever you have on hand: basil, dill, parsley, chives).

1. Preheat the oven to 375°F.
2. Halve the tomatoes lengthwise and place on a rimmed baking sheet. Brush the cut surfaces of the tomatoes with the oil. With a small, sharp knife, make a couple of cuts through the core (the hard flesh in the center of the tomato). Also cut through any flesh to either side of the core that might be covering the tomato seeds. (Exposing the juicy seeds makes it easier for the tomatoes to dry out as they roast.)
3. Sprinkle each tomato half with the salt. Then sprinkle with pepper and Italian seasoning to taste. Roast for 30 minutes.
4. Reduce the oven temperature to 300°F and bake until the tomatoes are collapsed, about 1 hour. Serve warm or at room temperature.

Per tomato half: 11 calories • 0g protein • 0.5g fat (0g saturated) • 0.5g fiber 3mg calcium • 4mg vitamin C • 1g carbohydrate • 74mg sodium

Lemon-Braised Fennel & Artichokes

Hands-On Time: 10 minutes • **Total Time:** 25 minutes • **Makes:** 4 servings

Braising vegetables in a mixture of olive oil, lemon juice, and herbs makes a tasty hot side dish. But you can also serve it chilled, more like a salad.

Fat Releasers
Olive oil, onion, garlic, lemons, oregano, fennel, artichokes, parsley, Parmesan cheese

- 1 tablespoon plus 1 teaspoon extra-virgin olive oil
- 1 small red onion (5 ounces), finely chopped
- 2 cloves garlic, minced
- 1 cup water
- 3 tablespoons fresh lemon juice
- 1 teaspoon dried oregano
- ½ teaspoon salt
- 1 large bulb fennel, cut into chunks the size of the artichokes
- 1 package (9 ounces) frozen artichoke hearts
- ¼ cup coarsely chopped flat-leaf parsley
- ¼ cup shredded Parmesan cheese

1. In a Dutch oven, heat the oil over medium heat. Add the onion and garlic, and cook, stirring often, until the onion begins to brown, 4 to 5 minutes.

2. Add the water, lemon juice, oregano, salt, fennel, and artichokes. Stir well to coat. Increase the heat to high, cover, and bring to a boil. Reduce to a simmer, cover, and cook until the fennel and artichokes are very tender, 10 to 15 minutes.

3. Stir in the parsley. Serve hot or at room temperature, topped with the Parmesan cheese.

MAKE IT A MAIN: Ten minutes before the fennel and artichokes are tender, top the vegetables with 4 pieces of halibut (6 ounces each), cod, or salmon, cover, and cook until the fish is cooked through. Transfer the fish to dinner plates, stir the parsley into the vegetables, and spoon onto the plate next to the fish. Top the vegetables with the Parmesan cheese. Serve with thick slices of beefsteak tomatoes sprinkled with grated lemon zest, black pepper, and balsamic vinegar.

SAVE FOR A SNACK: Have ¾ cup of the vegetables topped with 1 tablespoon Parmesan cheese.

Per 1-cup serving: 130 calories • 5g protein • 6.5g fat (1.5g saturated) • 6.5g fiber 143mg calcium • 24mg vitamin C • 15g carbohydrate • 452mg sodium

Napa Cabbage with Garlic-Ginger Sauce

Hands-On Time: 15 minutes • **Total Time:** 20 minutes • **Makes:** 4 servings

Napa cabbage is very mild compared with other cabbages, but it still contains the same important health-protective phytochemicals that its more pungent relatives have. All cabbages are cruciferous vegetables, a grouping known for its potential anticancer properties. Other members of this same group include broccoli, turnips, watercress, and radishes.

Fat Releasers
Garlic, ginger, bell peppers, napa cabbage, sesame oil

½ cup water

6 cloves garlic, grated on a zester

4 teaspoons grated fresh ginger

½ teaspoon salt

2 red bell peppers, finely slivered

5 cups shredded napa cabbage (1 small head or ½ large head)

1 teaspoon toasted (dark) sesame oil

1. In a medium saucepan, combine the water, garlic, ginger, and ¼ teaspoon of the salt. Bring to a simmer over medium-low heat, cover, and cook for 5 minutes to create a flavorful cooking liquid.

2. Add the bell peppers, cover, and cook until beginning to soften, 1 to 2 minutes.

3. Add the cabbage and toss until well coated. Sprinkle with the remaining ¼ teaspoon salt, cover, and cook until the cabbage is tender, about 3 minutes, stirring once halfway through.

4. Remove from the heat, drizzle with the sesame oil, and toss well.

Per 1-cup serving: 50 calories • 2g protein • 1.5g fat (0g saturated) • 3g fiber 43mg calcium • 92mg vitamin C • 8g carbohydrate • 303mg sodium

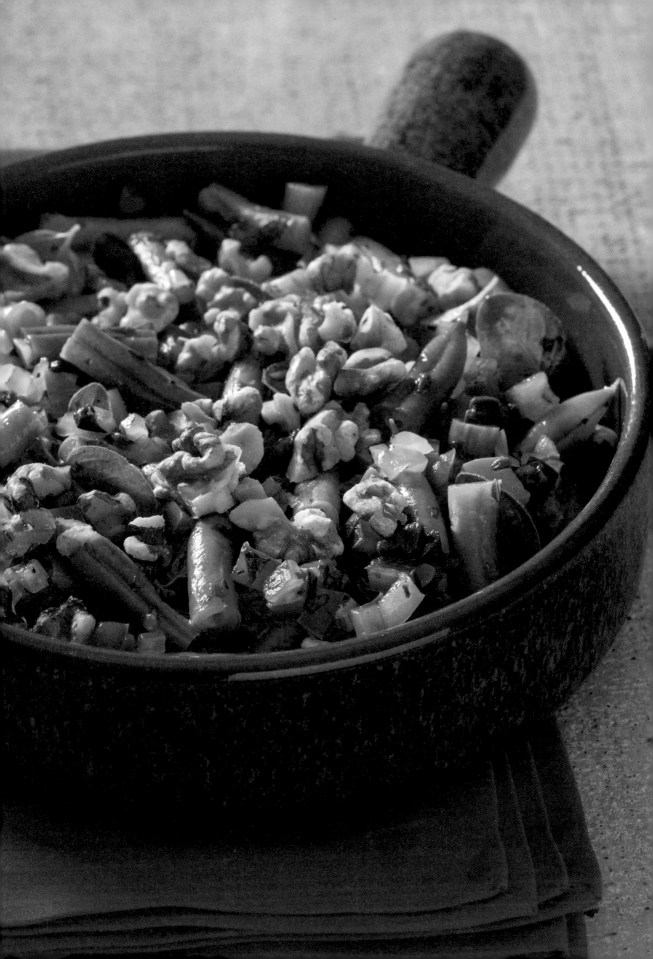

Green Beans with Basil & Toasted Walnuts

Hands-On Time: 25 minutes • **Total Time:** 40 minutes • **Makes:** 4 servings

The stir-steaming method here works with other vegetables, too. The idea is that you start with a combination of oil and water in a skillet and cover the pan to steam the vegetables. Then when you uncover the pan, you let any remaining liquid evaporate and the vegetables will sizzle a bit in the oil that's there. Try this with asparagus, carrots, sugar snaps, or broccoli. The cooking times will all be a bit different, depending on the density of the vegetables.

Fat Releasers
Olive oil, bell pepper, onion, black pepper, basil, oregano, walnuts, lemon

- 1 tablespoon extra-virgin olive oil
- 1 large green bell pepper, diced
- 1 small onion, finely chopped
- 1½ pounds green beans, cut into 1-inch pieces
- ¼ teaspoon salt
- ¼ teaspoon ground black pepper
- 3 tablespoons water
- ⅓ cup minced fresh basil
- 3 tablespoons minced Kalamata olives (6 or 7 olives)
- ½ teaspoon oregano
- 3 tablespoons chopped toasted walnuts
- 1 lemon, cut into wedges

1. In a large nonstick saucepan or Dutch oven, heat the oil over medium-high heat. Add the bell pepper, onion, green beans, salt, and black pepper, and stir for 1 minute. Add the water, cover, and cook, stirring occasionally, until the green beans are crisp-tender, 8 to 10 minutes.
2. Uncover, stir in the basil, olives, and oregano, and cook for a minute to evaporate some of the liquid.
3. Serve sprinkled with the walnuts. Pass lemon wedges for squeezing on the beans.

MAKE IT A MAIN: To make a one-dish meal, when the beans are still hot, squeeze the lemon juice over them and let them cool. Then toss in 1 cup quartered grape tomatoes, ⅓ cup crumbled reduced-fat feta cheese, and 2 cups diced cooked chicken breast. Add more shredded fresh basil or a little cilantro.

Per serving: 149 calories • 4g protein • 9g fat (1g saturated) • 5.5g fiber
78mg calcium • 58mg vitamin C • 16g carbohydrate • 264mg sodium

Cremini & Artichokes Arrabbiata

Hands-On Time: 20 minutes ● **Total Time:** 20 minutes ● **Makes:** 4 servings

In Italian, *arrabbiata* means angry, which is a way of describing the heat that the red pepper flakes bring to a dish. Serve this alongside Confetti Meatloaf (page 123) or Mexican Slow-Cooked Turkey Breast (page 138). Stick to frozen, rather than canned, artichoke hearts in this recipe; canned artichoke hearts are much higher in sodium.

Fat Releasers
Olive oil, onion, garlic, rosemary, red pepper flakes, tomatoes, artichokes

2   **teaspoons extra-virgin olive oil**

1   **red onion, finely chopped**

4   **cloves garlic, sliced**

12   **ounces cremini (baby bella) mushrooms, thinly sliced**

¾   **teaspoon crumbled dried rosemary**

½   **teaspoon salt**

¼ **to** ½ **teaspoon red pepper flakes**

1   **cup canned no-salt-added crushed tomatoes**

1   **package (9 ounces) frozen artichoke hearts, thawed**

1. In a large nonstick skillet, heat the oil over medium-high heat. Add the onion and garlic and cook for 3 minutes. Add the mushrooms, rosemary, salt, and red pepper flakes, and toss to combine. Cook, without stirring, for 2 minutes.

2. Add the tomatoes and artichokes and stir well. Return to a simmer and cook for 3 to 4 minutes to blend the flavors and heat through.

SAVE FOR A SNACK: Have 1 cup of the chilled mixture topped with 1 tablespoon 0% Greek yogurt.

Per 1-cup serving: 105 calories ● 5g protein ● 3g fat (0.5g saturated) ● 6g fiber 81mg calcium ● 17mg vitamin C ● 16g carbohydrate ● 339mg sodium

Baked Crispy Eggplant

Hands-On Time: 15 minutes • **Total Time:** 40 minutes • **Makes:** 4 servings

This dish is best straight out of the oven. However, if you do have leftovers, you can use them instead of slices of bread to make a hot mini-sandwich. Layer ½ ounce reduced-fat Swiss cheese and ½ ounce reduced-sodium smoked turkey on top of one leftover slice. Season with black pepper. Top with a second slice. Wrap in foil and reheat in a toaster oven until the eggplant is heated through and the cheese is melted; or wrap in a paper towel and reheat in a microwave.

Fat Releasers
Yogurt, tomato paste, lemons, cinnamon, black pepper, cashews, Parmesan cheese

- ½ cup 0% Greek yogurt
- 2 tablespoons no-salt-added tomato paste
- 2 teaspoons lemon juice plus 2 teaspoons grated lemon zest
- ¼ teaspoon ground cinnamon
- ¼ teaspoon salt
- ¼ teaspoon ground black pepper
- 2 ounces raw cashews or pecans (about ½ cup)
- ¼ cup grated Parmesan cheese
- 1 large eggplant (1¼ pounds), trimmed, peeled, and cut crosswise into ½-inch slices

1. Preheat the oven to 375°F. Line a baking sheet with parchment paper or a nonstick liner.
2. In a small bowl, whisk together the yogurt, tomato paste, lemon juice, cinnamon, salt, and pepper.
3. In a mini food processor, pulse-chop the cashews until they're the texture of coarse crumbs. Add the Parmesan cheese and process until the texture of fine crumbs. Pulse in the lemon zest and pour the mixture into a shallow bowl or pie plate.
4. Generously paint both sides of the eggplant slices with the yogurt mixture. Lightly dip one side into the nut mixture and place on the baking sheet nut-side down. When all the slices are in place, sprinkle the remaining nut mixture evenly over the tops of the slices.
5. Bake until the eggplant is tender and nicely browned on top, 24 to 26 minutes.

Per serving: 157 calories • 9g protein • 8g fat (2g saturated) • 5.5g fiber 98mg calcium • 6mg vitamin C • 16g carbohydrate • 242mg sodium

Slow-Cooker Vegetable Medley

Hands-On Time: 25 minutes • **Total Time:** 5½ to 6 hours • **Makes:** 12 cups

What a simple way to get an interesting mixture of vegetables for side dishes and snacks. This recipe makes 8 servings of 1½ cups each. Serve the vegetables as a hot or cold side dish with Oven-Fried Chicken (page 141), North Carolina Barbecued Tenderloin (page 133), Parmesan-Pecan Pork (page 117), or Herb-Crusted Salmon (page 127). You can also make a bunch of vegetable swaps: parsnips for carrots, rutabagas for turnips, broccoli for cauliflower, zucchini for squash. In Finish Strong, add ¾ pound red potatoes cut into small cubes.

Fat Releasers
Onions, cauliflower, tomatoes, bell peppers, squash, olive oil, garlic, thyme, lemons

1 large sweet onion, thinly sliced

½ head cauliflower (about 1 pound), cut into small florets

4 plum tomatoes, cut into chunks

3 carrots, thinly sliced

2 turnips (about 6 ounces each), cut into small cubes

1 red bell pepper, cut into squares

1 green bell pepper, cut into squares

1 yellow squash, cut into chunks

2 tablespoons extra-virgin olive oil

4 cloves garlic, grated on a zester

1½ cups water

2 teaspoons dried tarragon

1 teaspoon dried thyme

1 bay leaf

1¼ teaspoons salt

Grated zest and juice of 1 lemon

1. Place the onion, cauliflower, tomatoes, carrots, turnips, bell peppers, and squash in a 5- to 6-quart slow cooker.

2. In a small saucepan, heat the oil over medium heat. Add the garlic and stir until fragrant, about 30 seconds. Add the water, tarragon, thyme, bay leaf, and 1 teaspoon of the salt and bring to a boil. Pour the hot liquid (and herbs) over the vegetables. Cover and cook on high for 5 to 5½ hours until the hard vegetables like the cauliflower are tender.

3. Sprinkle the remaining ¼ teaspoon salt, lemon zest, and lemon juice over the vegetables and stir to combine. Serve hot, scooped out of the broth, or let cool in the broth to serve chilled.

Per 1½-cup serving: 98 calories • 3g protein • 4g fat (0.5g saturated) • 4g fiber 53mg calcium • 77mg vitamin C • 15g carbohydrate • 425mg sodium

▶ OPTIONS

This slow-cooker recipe was intentionally designed to produce much more than you would eat at a single meal. You'll have plenty of leftovers for lunches or super-easy side dishes. Here are some suggestions for using the leftovers.

Vegetable Salad (1 serving): Chill the vegetables in their broth. To serve, scoop out 1½ cups of the vegetables and toss with 1 tablespoon Digest Diet Vinaigrette (page 50) mixed with 1 tablespoon of the vegetable cooking broth.

Per serving: 140 calories • 3g protein • 8g fat (1g saturated) • 4g fiber
54mg calcium • 80mg vitamin C • 16g carbohydrate • 471mg sodium

Hot Vegetable Soup (1 serving): Scoop out 1½ cups vegetables and heat with 1 cup low-sodium chicken broth and some of the vegetable cooking broth (to taste). Add some ground black pepper or chili powder to taste. If you're on Finish Strong, stir in ¼ cup cooked brown rice or whole-wheat orzo.

Per serving (Fade Away): 113 calories • 5g protein • 4g fat (0.5g saturated)
4g fiber • 53mg calcium • 77mg vitamin C • 16g carbohydrate • 495mg sodium

Per serving (Finish Strong): 167 calories • 6g protein • 4g fat (0.5g saturated)
5g fiber • 57mg calcium • 77mg vitamin C • 27g carbohydrate • 498mg sodium

Gazpacho-Style Soup (1 serving): Scoop out 1½ cups vegetables and very coarsely chop with enough of the cooking broth to make a gazpacho-style soup. Serve chilled, sprinkled with 2 teaspoons toasted slivered almonds.

Per serving: 124 calories • 4g protein • 4g fat (0.5g saturated) • 4g fiber
65mg calcium • 77mg vitamin C • 15g carbohydrate • 425mg sodium

Vegetable Gratin (4 servings): Scoop out 3 cups vegetables and place in a shallow baking dish. Top with 2 tablespoons ground almonds (or flaxseed meal) mixed with 2 tablespoons grated Parmesan cheese. Place under a broiler preheated to high to brown the top.

Per serving: 80 calories • 3g protein • 4.5g fat (1g saturated) • 2.5g fiber
62mg calcium • 39mg vitamin C • 8g carbohydrate • 252mg sodium

Roasted Ratatouille

Hands-On Time: 20 minutes • **Total Time:** 1 hour • **Makes:** 4 servings

This is an easy recipe to double if you want to have extra on hand for snacks or for a cold side dish. (Ratatouille is actually perfectly designed to be served cold.) It also freezes nicely; pack it in 1-cup containers for perfect portions. Well sealed, it should last several months in the freezer.

Fat Releasers
Zucchini, tomatoes, olive oil, onion, garlic, marjoram, thyme, black pepper

- 4 Italian eggplants (4 ounces each)
- 4 small zucchini (5 ounces each)
- 6 plum tomatoes
- 1 tablespoon plus 1 teaspoon extra-virgin olive oil
- 1 red onion (½ pound), chopped
- 3 cloves garlic, minced
- 1 teaspoon dried marjoram or oregano
- ½ teaspoon dried thyme
- ½ teaspoon salt
- ¼ teaspoon black pepper

SAVE FOR A SNACK: This is so low in calories, you can have the whole 1¾ cups for a snack. Or have only 1 cup of the ratatouille and top it with 2 tablespoons of fat-free ricotta and a generous sprinkling of black pepper.

1. Preheat the oven to 375°F. Line a baking sheet with parchment paper or a nonstick liner.

2. Pierce the untrimmed eggplants, zucchini, and tomatoes in several places with the tip of a sharp knife. Place on the baking sheet and bake until the eggplant is tender, 35 to 40 minutes.

3. Meanwhile, in a medium nonstick saucepan, heat the oil over medium-high heat. Add the onion and garlic and cook, stirring occasionally, until the onion is softened, 5 to 7 minutes. Sprinkle in the marjoram and thyme and cook for 30 seconds. Remove from the heat and set aside until the vegetables are roasted.

4. When the vegetables are done and cool enough to handle, cut them into ¾-inch chunks. Add them to the saucepan with the onion and stir to combine. Sprinkle in the salt and pepper and stir over medium heat for 2 or 3 minutes to blend the flavors. Serve at room temperature or chilled.

Per 1¾-cup serving: 134 calories • 5g protein • 5.5g fat (1g saturated) • 7g fiber 60mg calcium • 46mg vitamin C • 21g carbohydrate • 312mg sodium

Sweet & Sour Greens with Bacon

Hands-On Time: 15 minutes • **Total Time:** 30 minutes • **Makes:** 4 servings

Shredding collards (or other sturdy greens) shortens their cooking time. Here they're briefly braised before being tossed with a little hot sauce, honey, and vinegar for a sweet and tangy finish to the dish. Feel free to swap in raisins for the prunes. And don't be put off by the amount of greens; they shrink substantially once cooked.

Fat Releasers
Olive oil, garlic, collard greens, vinegar, honey, hot sauce

- 1 tablespoon extra-virgin olive oil
- 3 slices turkey bacon, cut into thin strips
- 3 cloves garlic, thinly sliced
- 1 bag (16 ounces) cleaned collard greens, mustard greens, or turnip greens or a combination, shredded (24 loosely packed cups)
- ¼ cup water
- 3 small pitted prunes, diced (3 tablespoons)
- ¼ teaspoon salt
- 2 teaspoons red wine vinegar
- 1 teaspoon honey
- ¼ teaspoon (or more to taste) hot sauce, such as Frank's RedHot

1. In a Dutch oven, heat the oil over medium-low heat. Add the turkey bacon and cook until lightly crisped, about 5 minutes; remove with a slotted spoon. Add the garlic to the pan and cook until golden brown, about 3 minutes.

2. Add the collards and toss to coat. Add the water, prunes, and salt and cook, stirring occasionally, until soft and tender, about 5 minutes.

3. Return the bacon to the pan along with the vinegar, honey, and hot sauce and stir to combine. Serve hot.

Per 1-cup serving: 144 calories • 6g protein • 8g fat (1.5g saturated) • 4g fiber 200mg calcium • 25mg vitamin C • 14g carbohydrate • 427mg sodium

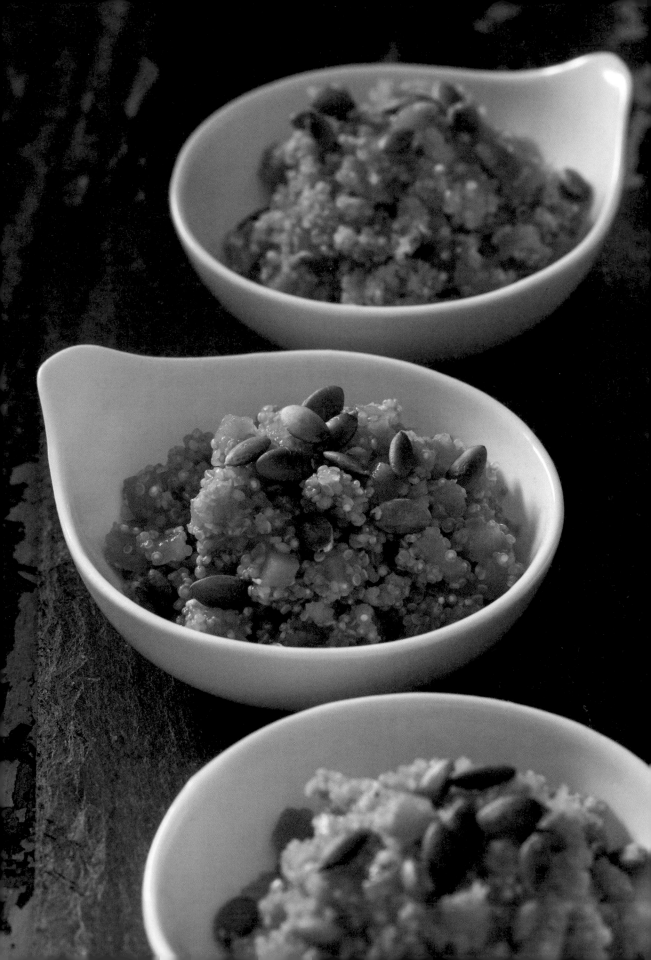

Lemony Quinoa & Butternut Pilaf

Hands-On Time: 20 minutes • **Total Time:** 40 minutes • **Makes:** 6 servings

Carrot juice—which you can find in the supermarket—gives this dish not only a natural sweetness but a spectacular amount of beta-carotene. Between the carrot juice and the butternut squash, one serving of the pilaf has almost 400% of your daily recommended allowance for this antioxidant.

Fat Releasers
Olive oil, onion, garlic, butternut squash, black pepper, quinoa, pumpkin seeds

- 1 tablespoon extra-virgin olive oil
- 1 medium onion, chopped
- 3 cloves garlic, minced
- 1½ cups finely diced butternut squash (about 8 ounces)
- 1 cup water
- ¾ cup carrot juice
- 2 teaspoons grated lemon zest
- ½ teaspoon salt
- ¼ teaspoon ground black pepper
- 1 cup quinoa
- 2 tablespoons hulled pumpkin seeds, toasted

1. In a medium nonstick saucepan, heat the oil over medium heat. Add the onion, garlic, and squash and cook until the onion is tender, about 7 minutes.

2. Meanwhile, in a small saucepan, combine the water, carrot juice, lemon zest, salt, and pepper and bring to a simmer.

3. Stir the quinoa into the sautéed vegetables and cook for 1 minute. Stir in the hot broth mixture. Bring to a boil, reduce to a simmer, cover tightly, and cook until tender and the liquid has been absorbed, 17 to 19 minutes.

4. Fluff with a fork. Serve sprinkled with pumpkin seeds.

MAKE IT A MAIN: Let the quinoa cool to room temperature and turn this into a one-dish meal. Stir in a little lemon juice and minced pickled jalapeño, both to taste. Add 8 ounces diced reduced-sodium smoked ham and a large green pepper, diced.

Per ¾-cup serving: 178 calories • 6g protein • 5.5g fat (1g saturated) • 3.5g fiber 48mg calcium • 13mg vitamin C • 28g carbohydrate • 217mg sodium

Hoppin' John

Hands-On Time: 15 minutes • **Total Time:** 1 hour • **Makes:** 8 servings

If you grew up in the South, then you know that Hoppin' John is the must-have dish for New Year's Day. Eating a bowl of it is said to guarantee good fortune for the upcoming year. So why not eat Hoppin' John all year long? The dish is traditionally on the soupy side (it's not like a pilaf), but if you'd prefer something with less liquid, omit 1 cup of the broth. The dish also freezes really well; just ladle it into 1-cup freezer containers.

Fat Releasers
Olive oil, garlic, black-eyed peas, brown rice, scallions, bell pepper

1 tablespoon olive oil

4 slices (1 ounce each) Canadian bacon, slivered

¼ cup water

2 cloves garlic, minced

5 cups low-sodium chicken broth

1 bay leaf

1⅓ cups (8 ounces) dried black-eyed peas

½ cup brown basmati rice

½ teaspoon salt

5 large scallions, sliced

1 small red bell pepper, diced

1. In a medium saucepan, heat the oil over medium heat. Add the Canadian bacon and stir-fry until beginning to crisp, about 3 minutes. With a slotted spatula, transfer to a plate and set aside.

2. Add the water and garlic to the pan and stir to get up the browned bits on the bottom of the pan. Add the chicken broth and bay leaf and bring to a boil. Add the black-eyed peas, brown rice, and salt. Reduce to a high simmer, cover, and cook until the rice and black-eyed peas are tender, about 45 minutes. About 10 minutes before the rice is done, stir in the scallions, bell pepper, and Canadian bacon. Discard the bay leaf before serving.

MAKE IT A MAIN: Double the portion size (to 1½ cups) and stir in 4 ounces shredded cooked turkey or chicken (per portion). Serve with a large tossed salad (per person) of 2 cups salad greens, 1 tablespoon Digest Diet Vinaigrette (page 50), and 2 teaspoons shredded reduced-fat cheese (your choice).

Per ¾-cup serving: 128 calories • 8g protein • 3.5g fat (0.5g saturated) • 3g fiber • 18mg calcium • 21mg vitamin C • 17g carbohydrate • 387mg sodium

Barley Risotto with Collards

Hands-On Time: 10 minutes • **Total Time:** 45 minutes • **Makes:** 4 servings

Swapping in barley for rice in this risotto adds a considerable amount of soluble fiber, which is important for heart health. Barley also adds a very satisfying chewiness to this flavorful side dish.

Fat Releasers
Olive oil, onion, barley, collard greens, Parmesan cheese, black pepper

- 1 teaspoon extra-virgin olive oil
- 1 small onion, finely chopped
- ⅔ cup pearled barley
- 2 cups water
- ½ teaspoon salt
- ¼ teaspoon turmeric (optional)
- 1 package (10 ounces) frozen chopped collard greens or spinach, thawed
- ¼ cup grated Parmesan cheese
- ¼ teaspoon ground black pepper

1. In a medium nonstick saucepan, heat the oil over medium-low heat. Add the onion and cook, stirring, until softened and beginning to brown, 5 to 7 minutes. Add the barley, stirring to coat.

2. Stir in the water, salt, and turmeric (if using). Increase the heat to high and bring to a boil. Reduce to a simmer, cover, and cook, stirring occasionally, until the barley is almost tender, about 25 minutes.

3. Stir in the collards and cook until the barley is fully tender, about 10 minutes. Remove from the heat and stir in the Parmesan cheese and pepper.

MAKE IT A MAIN: For each serving, rub a 4-ounce boneless pork loin chop with a mild chili powder and pan-grill. Serve the chop on a bed of the risotto (¾ cup). Toss 2 cups shredded romaine lettuce with 2 teaspoons lemon juice, 1 teaspoon olive oil, and 2 teaspoons grated Parmesan cheese and serve it alongside.

Per ¾-cup serving: 182 calories • 8g protein • 3g fat (1g saturated) • 7.5g fiber 219mg calcium • 20mg vitamin C • 33g carbohydrate • 406mg sodium

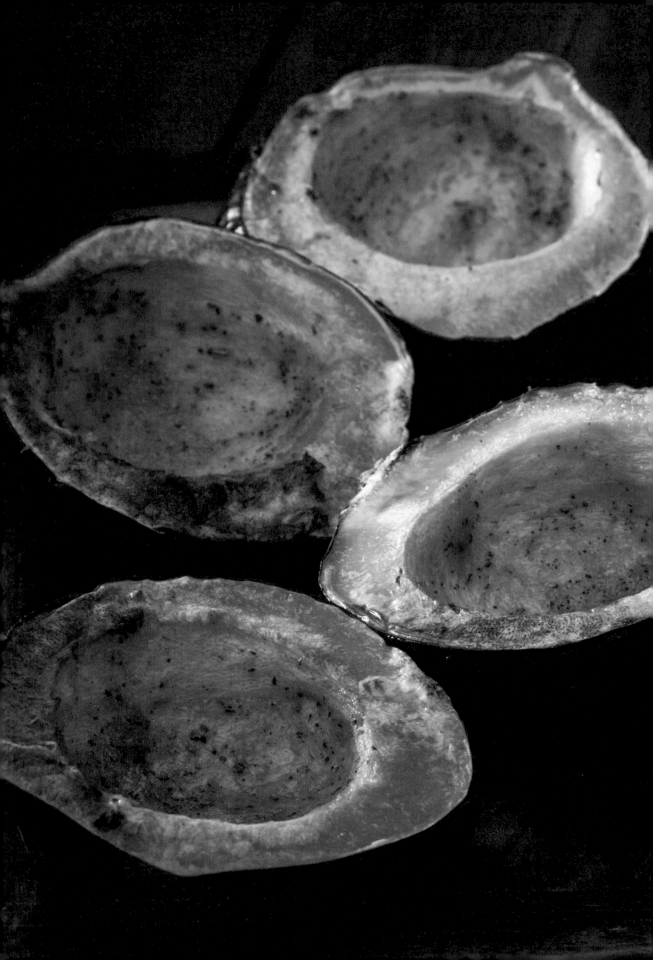

Honey-Roasted Acorn Squash

Hands-On Time: 10 minutes • **Total Time:** 1 hour 5 minutes
Makes: 4 servings

Acorn squash are the perfect size: Each one is enough for two and you can prepare as many as you want. And because, like all winter squash, they're naturally sweet, they don't need very much to make them shine. Pair with Pepper Loin Steaks (page 119) or Roast Herb-Rubbed Turkey Breast (page 120).

Fat Releasers
Acorn squash,
honey,
olive oil

- 2 **acorn squash (1 pound each), halved lengthwise, seeds removed**
- 1 **tablespoon honey**
- 1 **tablespoon extra-virgin olive oil**
- ¼ **teaspoon rubbed sage**
- ¼ **teaspoon salt**

1. Preheat the oven to 425°F. Place the squash halves cut-side down on a parchment-lined baking sheet (for easy cleanup) and bake 30minutes.

2. Meanwhile, in a small bowl, stir together the honey, oil, sage, and salt.

3. Turn the squash cut-side up and spoon the honey mixture into the cavity. Bake until the squash is tender and the filling is bubbling, about 25 minutes. Let stand 5 minutes before serving.

SAVE FOR A SNACK: Save a half for a snack, and top with 1 tablespoon reduced-fat goat or feta cheese.

COOKING FOR ONE: Divide the filling ingredients in half and roast just 1 squash; serve half one day and half another.

Per serving: 115 calories • 1g protein • 3.5g fat (0.5g saturated) • 2.5g fiber 58mg calcium • 19mg vitamin C • 22g carbohydrate • 151mg sodium

Brown Basmati Risi e Bisi

Hands-On Time: 5 minutes • **Total Time:** 55 minutes • **Makes:** 6 servings

Risi e bisi is a classic Italian dish of rice and peas, typically made with Arborio, a starchy short-grained rice. Here we're using brown basmati rice, which is low in starch and high in fiber.

Fat Releasers
Olive oil, onion, garlic, brown rice, thyme, black pepper, peas, parsley, lemons, Parmesan cheese

- 1 tablespoon extra-virgin olive oil
- 1 onion, coarsely chopped
- 2 cloves garlic, thinly sliced
- 1 cup brown basmati rice
- 2 cups low-sodium chicken broth
- ¼ teaspoon dried thyme
- ¼ teaspoon salt
- ¼ teaspoon ground black pepper
- 1 cup frozen peas, thawed
- ½ cup chopped flat-leaf parsley leaves
- 1 teaspoon grated lemon zest
- 1 tablespoon fresh lemon juice
- ⅓ cup grated Parmesan cheese

1. In a medium saucepan, heat the oil over medium heat. Add the onion and garlic and cook, stirring frequently, until the onion is lightly browned, about 8 minutes.

2. Add the rice to the pan and stir to coat. Add the broth, thyme, salt, and pepper and bring to a boil. Reduce to a simmer, cover, and cook until the rice is tender, about 40 minutes. Remove from the heat.

3. Stir in the peas, parsley, lemon zest, lemon juice, and the Parmesan cheese and cover until the peas are heated through, about 2 minutes.

MAKE IT A MAIN: Have the dish serve 4 instead of 6. Into the cooked rice and peas, stir 2 cups shredded cooked chicken breast or 8 ounces pork tenderloin, cooked, thinly sliced, and cut into strips. Serve with a salad of diced cucumber, minced red onion, and chopped cilantro dressed with store-bought yogurt-based salad dressing (1 tablespoon per person).

Per ½-cup serving: 178 calories • 6g protein • 4.5g fat (1.5g saturated) • 3g fiber 71mg calcium • 12mg vitamin C • 29g carbohydrate • 210mg sodium

Kasha & Orange Pilaf with Pecans

Hands-On Time: 15 minutes • **Total Time:** 20 minutes • **Makes:** 6 servings

Kasha is a term used to refer to the toasted seeds (called groats) of the buckwheat plant. In spite of the word *wheat* in its title, buckwheat is actually not a cereal grain but a plant related to rhubarb. The rich, toasty flavors of kasha and nuts pair beautifully with the fresh, tart flavor of the orange. If you like this dish, you can experiment with different nut-fruit combinations (keeping to the same quantities as here, 1 ounce of nuts and about ¾ cup cut-up fruit). Try walnuts and red plums, pistachios and ruby grapefruit, peanuts and red grapes, or cashews and nectarines. Look for kasha in the aisle with bulgur and couscous.

Fat Releasers
Pecans, black pepper, orange, olive oil, garlic, whole-grain kasha

- ¼ cup (1 ounce) pecans
- 1 cup carrot juice
- 1 cup water
- ½ teaspoon ground coriander
- ½ teaspoon salt
- ¼ teaspoon ground black pepper
- 1 navel orange
- 2 teaspoons olive oil
- 3 cloves garlic, minced
- 1 cup whole-grain kasha

SAVE FOR A SNACK:
Have ½ cup leftover kasha topped with 1 tablespoon 0% Greek yogurt.

1. Toast the pecans in a toaster oven or small ungreased skillet until crisp and fragrant, 3 to 5 minutes. Set aside to cool.

2. In a small saucepan, combine the carrot juice, water, coriander, salt, and pepper. With a vegetable peeler, pull off 2 strips of orange zest and add them to the pan. Bring to a simmer while you start the kasha.

3. In a medium nonstick saucepan, heat the oil over medium-high heat. Add the garlic and cook until fragrant but not turning color, about 45 seconds. Stir in the kasha and cook until well coated and hot, about 2 minutes.

4. Add the simmering broth and bring to a boil. Reduce to a simmer, cover, and cook until the kasha is tender, 6 to 8 minutes.

5. Meanwhile, chop the cooled pecans and peel and cut the orange into dices.

6. When the kasha is done, discard the orange zest and stir in the pecans and orange.

Per ¾-cup serving: 171 calories • 4g protein • 6g fat (0.5g saturated) • 4g fiber
32mg calcium • 18mg vitamin C • 28g carbohydrate • 223mg sodium

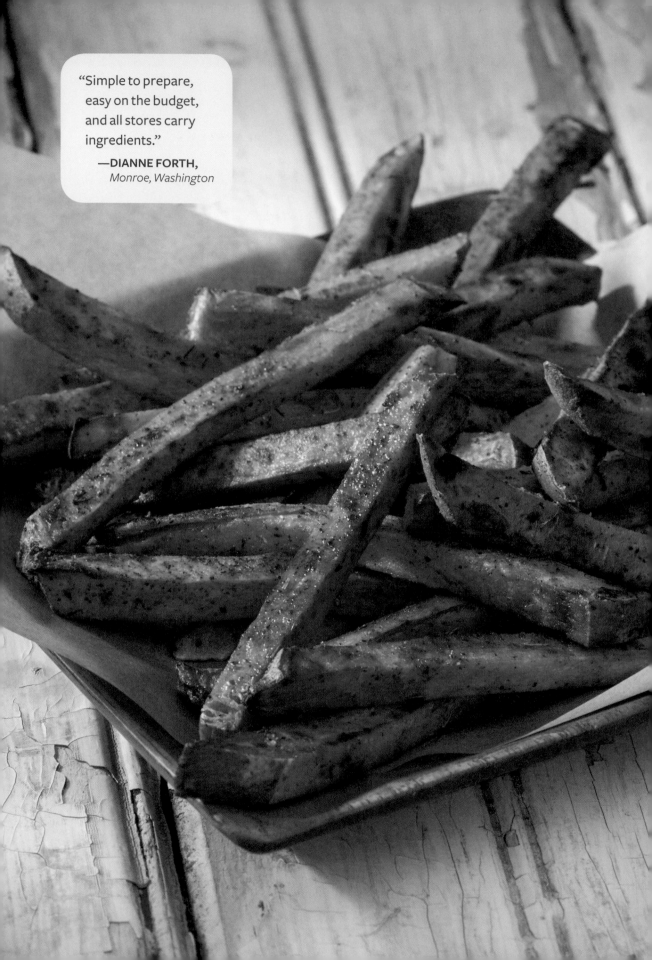

"Simple to prepare, easy on the budget, and all stores carry ingredients."
—DIANNE FORTH,
Monroe, Washington

Cajun Sweet Potato Fries

Hands-On Time: 10 minutes • **Total Time:** 50 minutes • **Makes:** 4 servings

Sweet potato skin is just as edible—and good for you—as the skin of regular potatoes; in this dish, it adds a sizable amount of fiber. Serve the potatoes with Confetti Meatloaf (page 123), Apple-Brined Roast Chicken (page 144), or Slow-Cooker Sunday Roast with Onion Gravy (page 114). If you prefer steak fries, cut the potatoes into 8 to 10 wedges and bake in a 425°F oven until firm-tender, about 30 to 40 minutes.

Fat Releasers
Sweet potatoes, olive oil, chili powder, thyme, black pepper, cayenne

4 small sweet potatoes (1½ pounds total), unpeeled and cut lengthwise into fries about ⅓ inch thick

1 tablespoon plus 1 teaspoon extra-virgin olive oil

2 teaspoons chili powder

½ teaspoon dried thyme

¼ teaspoon ground black pepper

⅛ teaspoon cayenne pepper

⅛ teaspoon salt

1. Preheat the oven to 475°F. Place a large wire cooling rack on a baking sheet.

2. In a large bowl, toss the sweet potatoes with the oil, making sure they all get coated. In a small bowl, stir together the chili powder, thyme, black pepper, cayenne, and salt. Sprinkle over the sweet potatoes and toss to coat.

3. Place the potatoes on the cooling rack and bake until firm-tender, 20 to 25 minutes.

Per serving: 134 calories • 2g protein • 4.5g fat (0.5g saturated) • 3.5g fiber 42mg calcium • 20mg vitamin C • 22g carbohydrate • 110mg sodium

Parmesan-Crumbed Roasted Root Vegetables

Hands-On Time: 20 minutes • **Total Time:** 50 minutes • **Makes:** 4 servings

Briefly cooking the hard root vegetables gives them a jump start to becoming tender before they bake. If you like, swap equal amounts of other root vegetables such as celeriac (celery root) or rutabaga for the turnips, carrots, and parsnips.

Fat Releasers
Sweet potatoes, whole-wheat bread, Parmesan cheese, marjoram, olive oil

- 2 **carrots, thinly sliced**
- 1 **white turnip (8 ounces), halved lengthwise and thinly sliced**
- 1 **parsnip (6 ounces), thinly sliced**
- 2 **sweet potatoes (8 ounces), peeled, halved lengthwise and thinly sliced**
- 1 **slice (1 ounce) whole-wheat bread, toasted**
- ⅓ **cup grated Parmesan cheese**
- ½ **teaspoon dried marjoram**
- ¼ **teaspoon salt**
- 1 **tablespoon extra-virgin olive oil**

1. Preheat the oven to 400°F.

2. In a large pot of boiling water, cook the carrots, turnip, and parsnip until they start to soften, about 5 minutes. Add the sweet potatoes and cook 2 minutes longer. Drain the vegetables and transfer them to a 9 x 9-inch baking dish.

3. Tear the toast into pieces and pulse in a food processor until finely ground. Add the Parmesan cheese, marjoram, and salt and pulse to combine. Add the oil and pulse until the crumbs are moistened.

4. Scatter the crumbs over the top of the vegetables and bake until the vegetables are tender, about 30 minutes.

Per serving: 170 calories • 5g protein • 6g fat (1.5g saturated) • 5g fiber 138mg calcium • 25mg vitamin C • 25g carbohydrate • 355mg sodium

Baked Stuffed Summer Squash

Hands-On Time: 20 minutes • **Total Time:** 55 minutes • **Makes:** 4 servings

You can make these squash several hours ahead and serve them at room temperature. Try the same general idea using zucchini. If you want to make this a Fade Away dish, leave out the cracker crumbs.

Fat Releasers
Squash, olive oil, garlic, tomatoes, black pepper, spinach, cheese, multigrain crackers

- 4 **yellow summer squash (½ pound each)**
- 3 **teaspoons extra-virgin olive oil**
- 2 **cloves garlic, minced**
- 6 **sun-dried tomato halves, finely chopped**
- 2 **teaspoons grated lemon zest**
- ¼ **teaspoon salt**
- ¼ **teaspoon ground black pepper**
- 2 **cups coarsely chopped baby spinach (about 2 ounces)**
- 6 **tablespoons shredded reduced-fat Cheddar cheese**
- 4 **multigrain crackers (½ ounce total), crushed into fine crumbs**

1. Preheat the oven to 350°F. Line a baking sheet with foil.

2. With a sharp knife, shave a thin slice off one side of the squash so they will sit flat. With the squash sitting horizontally, slice off the top third of the squash. With a small spoon or a melon baller, scoop out the flesh, leaving a ¼-inch wall all around. Finely chop the sliced-off portions and enough of the nonseedy scooped-out flesh to equal 1½ cups. (Discard the remainder or save for a soup.)

3. In a medium nonstick skillet, heat 2 teaspoons of the oil over medium-high heat. Add the garlic and cook until fragrant, about 45 seconds. Add the squash flesh, sun-dried tomatoes, lemon zest, salt, and pepper. Stir until the squash just begins to soften, 3 to 4 minutes.

4. Stir in the spinach and remove from the heat. Cover and let sit a minute or two to wilt the spinach.

5. In a small bowl, combine 3 tablespoons of the cheese, the cracker crumbs, and the remaining 1 teaspoon oil.

6. Arrange the squash shells on the baking sheet. Spoon the remaining 3 tablespoons cheese into the bottoms of the shells. Divide the stuffing mixture among the shells and top with the cracker crumb mixture.

7. Bake until the neck of the squash is tender, the filling is bubbling, and the topping is browned, 30 to 35 minutes. Serve hot or at room temp.

Per serving: 125 calories • 7g protein • 6g fat (2g saturated) • 4g fiber • 145mg calcium • 40mg vitamin C • 13g carbohydrate • 299mg sodium

Curried Lentils & Greens

Hands-On Time: 10 minutes • **Total Time:** 55 minutes • **Makes:** 6 servings

Lentils need no soaking before cooking, making them relatively quick-cooking in the land of dried beans and legumes. We've used brown lentils, the type that you'll typically find in bags alongside the dried beans in the supermarket. Mustard adds a nice bite to this dish, and mustard seeds add a nice crunch.

Fat Releasers
Olive oil, garlic, lentils, tomatoes, greens, yogurt

2 **teaspoons extra-virgin olive oil**

3 **cloves garlic, thinly sliced**

1 **teaspoon curry powder**

¾ **teaspoon mustard seeds or ¼ teaspoon dry mustard**

1 **cup lentils**

1 **can (14.5 ounces) no-salt-added diced tomatoes**

2 **cups water**

½ **teaspoon salt**

3 **cups torn greens, such as escarole, kale, spinach, or a combination (about 3 ounces)**

¼ **cup 0% Greek yogurt**

1. In a large nonstick saucepan or Dutch oven, heat the oil over medium-low heat. Add the garlic and cook, stirring frequently, until tender, about 2 minutes. Add the curry powder and mustard seeds (or dry mustard), and cook, stirring, for 1 minute.

2. Add the lentils, tomatoes, water, and salt and bring to a boil. Reduce to a simmer, cover, and cook until the lentils are tender, about 40 minutes.

3. Stir in the greens and cook until wilted, about 3 minutes. Serve topped with yogurt.

MAKE IT A MAIN: Serve a generous cup of lentils over ½ cup cooked brown rice per person. Add ½ cup reduced-fat feta cheese to the yogurt (mixing them together gives a tangy flavor) and use it to top the lentils for a one-dish meal.

Per ¾-cup serving: 148 calories • 10g protein • 2g fat (0.5g saturated) • 8g fiber
51mg calcium • 22mg vitamin C • 24g carbohydrate • 212mg sodium

Crispy Balsamic Potatoes

Hands-On Time: 5 minutes • **Total Time:** 1 hour • **Makes:** 4 servings

This is a fun way to get baked potatoes crispy without frying them. You cook the potatoes first and then, while they're still warm, you very gently squash them so the flesh breaks out of the skin a little bit. (Be careful not to press too hard or the potatoes will fall apart.) Next, you drizzle them with a little oil and balsamic mixture and bake until crispy.

Fat Releasers
Vinegar, olive oil, garlic, rosemary

Salt

24 small (1½-inch-diameter) red or Yukon Gold potatoes (about 1¼ pounds total)

2 tablespoons balsamic vinegar

1 tablespoon plus 1 teaspoon extra-virgin olive oil

1 small clove garlic, grated on a zester

½ teaspoon crumbled dried rosemary

SAVE FOR A SNACK: Like any baked potato, these make great leftovers. Have 3 of the potatoes for a midafternoon snack and top them with ¼ cup 0% Greek yogurt with some chopped grape tomatoes stirred in. Add a little black pepper, basil, or parsley, too.

1. Bring a large pot of lightly salted water to a boil. Add the potatoes and cook until firm-tender, about 20 minutes. Drain and set aside to cool slightly.

2. Meanwhile, whisk together the vinegar, oil, garlic, rosemary, and ¼ teaspoon salt.

3. When the potatoes are cool enough to handle (but still warm), gently but firmly press down on the potatoes with a water glass to squash them.

4. Lightly coat a baking sheet with cooking spray or line with parchment paper. Place the squashed potatoes on the baking sheet and drizzle the warm potatoes with the balsamic mixture. Let them sit while you preheat the oven to 350°F.

5. Bake the potatoes until crispy, about 30 minutes.

Per 6-potato serving: 148 calories • 3g protein • 4.5g fat (0.5g saturated) 2.5g fiber • 20mg calcium • 13mg vitamin C • 24g carbohydrate • 289mg sodium

Chapter
10

Desserts

Savor these sweet treats as a reward for your fat releasing efforts!

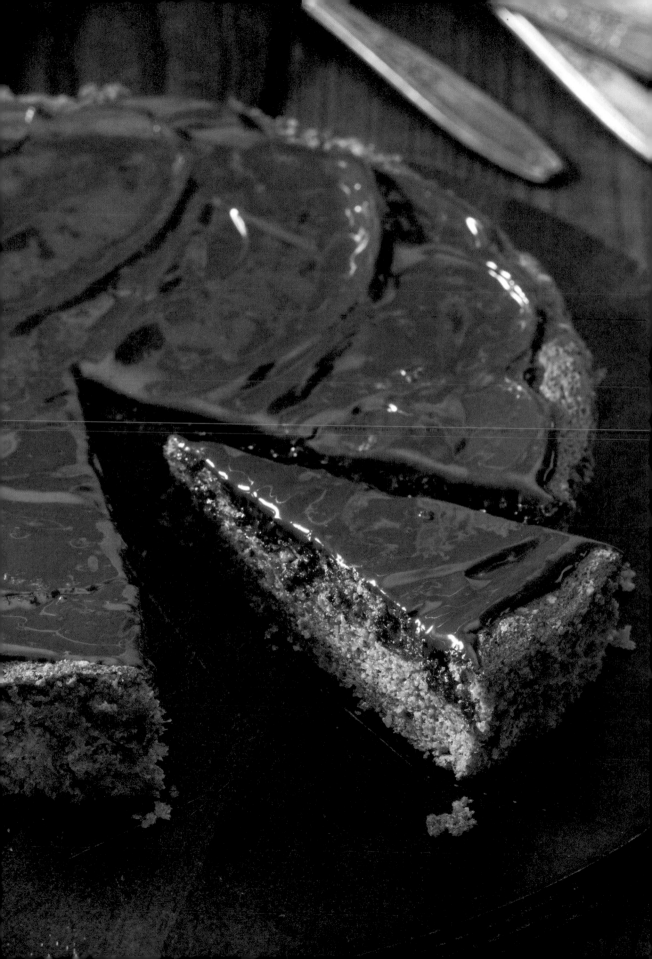

Pomegranate-Poached Pears

Hands-On Time: 15 minutes • **Total Time:** 1 hour + cooling time • **Makes:** 4 servings

By standing the pears up in their poaching liquid, only the bottom half gets colored by the pomegranate juice, providing a pretty contrast. You can make the pears well ahead of time; they will keep well in the fridge for a week.

Fat Releasers
Red wine, honey

1½ cups pomegranate juice
½ cup red wine
2 firm-ripe Bosc pears
2 teaspoons honey, preferably dark, such as buckwheat

1. Choose a small saucepan that is just big enough to fit the pears side by side (1½- to 2-quart). You also need to be able to cover the pan, so if your saucepan is too short, you can fashion a tall lid by using another upside-down saucepan. Add the pomegranate juice and wine to the saucepan.

2. Using an apple corer (or a melon baller), dig a small channel up through the blossom end (bottom) of the pear until you reach the seedy core. Scoop out the seeds. Peel the pears. Cut a slice off the bottom of the pears so they'll stand flat in the pan. As you work, place the pears in the wine mixture and ladle a little of the mixture over them to keep them from discoloring.

3. If the red wine mixture does not come up to where the pears start to narrow, add a little water. Cover and bring to a boil over medium-high heat. Reduce the heat to a gentle simmer and cook until the pears are firm-tender, 20 to 30 minutes (depending on the ripeness of the pears). You can slightly undercook them because they will continue to cook in the next step.

4. Remove from the heat, uncover the pan, and let the pears sit for 15 minutes in the hot liquid. Then carefully transfer the pears to a plate to cool completely.

5. Bring the poaching liquid to a full rolling boil and let boil for 12 minutes to reduce the liquid to ½ cup. Keep a close eye on the pan for the last 5 minutes because it will start to reduce very quickly and you don't want it to go too far. Stir the honey into the hot liquid. Let cool.

6. To serve, halve the pears lengthwise. Spoon 2 tablespoons of the pomegranate syrup onto a dessert plate and top with a pear half.

Per serving: 140 calories • 0g protein • 0g fat (0g saturated) • 3g fiber • 26mg calcium 4mg vitamin C • 31g carbohydrate • 14mg sodium

Warm Three-Berry Cream

Hands-On Time: 5 minutes • **Total Time:** 15 minutes • **Makes:** 4 servings

Bags of frozen mixed berries make this warm dessert easy to put together. Don't confuse evaporated milk with sweetened condensed milk, which is much higher in calories and very sweet. Any leftover evaporated milk should be transferred from the can to a freezer container and frozen for another use. The evaporated milk will keep in the freezer for up to 3 months. Thaw it in the refrigerator before using.

Fat Releasers
Milk, cream cheese, honey, berries

1 cup evaporated 2% milk

3 tablespoons ⅓-less-fat cream cheese

3 tablespoons honey

½ teaspoon vanilla extract

1 bag (12 ounces) frozen mixed berries, thawed

1. In a large skillet, combine the evaporated milk, cream cheese, honey, and vanilla and bring to a boil over medium-high heat. Boil until the bubbles are close together and the mixture is at a rolling boil, about 3 minutes.

2. Reduce the heat to medium-low. Add the thawed berries and any juices and cook until heated through, about 3 minutes. Spoon the fruit and sauce into bowls and serve.

Per ¾-cup serving: 193 calories • 5.5g protein • 3.5g fat (1.5g saturated) 3g fiber • 186mg calcium • 15mg vitamin C • 35g carbohydrate • 109mg sodium

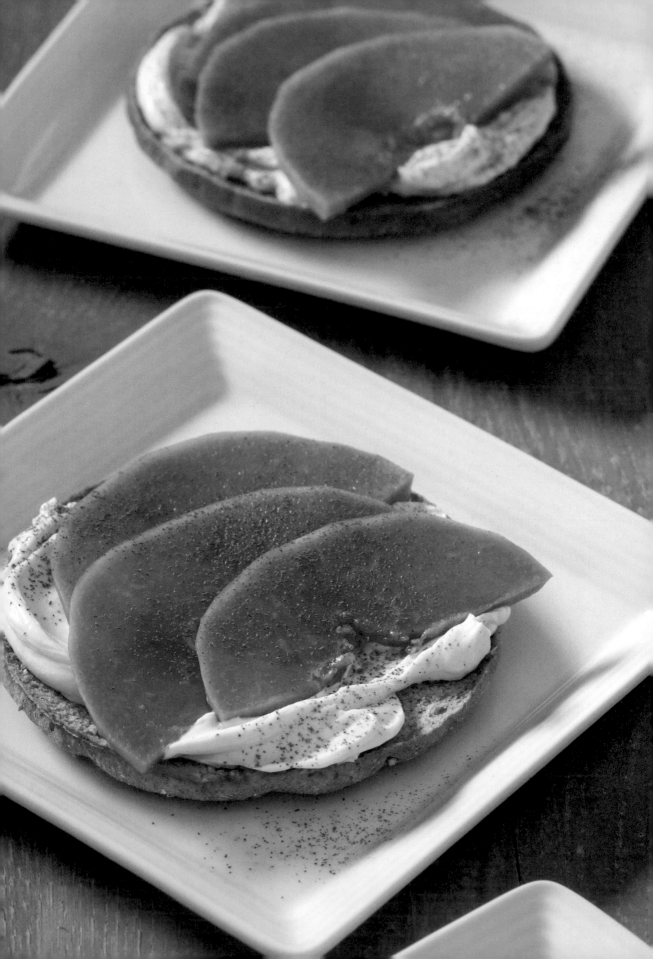

Papaya "Tarts"

Hands-On Time: 10 minutes • **Total Time:** 25 minutes • **Makes:** 4 tarts

Unless your market sells cut-up papaya, you will have leftover papaya. (A typical red papaya can weigh about 2 pounds.) Cut it up and save it for a snack, or freeze chunks of it and use them in your Fast Release or Fade Away Shakes. Try this simple "tart" idea with other fruits, too: nectarines, peaches, strawberries, or mangoes. You can find sandwich thins in the bread aisle at your supermarket.

Fat Releasers
Whole-wheat bread, coconut oil, honey, cream cheese, papaya, cinnamon

2 **whole-wheat or multigrain sandwich thins, split**

2 **teaspoons coconut oil**

1 **teaspoon honey, preferably dark**

6 **tablespoons (3 ounces) ⅓-less-fat cream cheese**

¼ **pound ripe papaya, seeded, peeled, and very thinly sliced crosswise**

Ground cinnamon, for dusting

1. Preheat the oven to 350°F.

2. Spread the cut sides of the sandwich thins with the coconut oil. Bake until golden and toasted, 10 to 12 minutes. Let cool.

3. Meanwhile, stir the honey into the cream cheese.

4. Spread the "tart shells" with the sweetened cream cheese. Arrange the papaya on top. Dust each tart with a small pinch of cinnamon.

Per tart: 137 calories • 5g protein • 7.5g fat (4.5g saturated) • 3g fiber 49mg calcium • 12mg vitamin C • 15g carbohydrate • 158mg sodium

Spicy Grilled Pineapple

Hands-On Time: 15 minutes • **Total Time:** 15 minutes • **Makes:** 4 servings

While you can certainly peel and core your own pineapple, today lots of supermarkets carry pineapple that's already been pared (and sometimes even sliced). Although perfect as a dessert, this can also be served as a side dish (if you're in Finish Strong) to accompany Roast Herb-Rubbed Turkey Breast (page 120), Jerk Steak (page 132), or Apple-Brined Roast Chicken (page 144).

Fat Releasers
Honey, limes, ancho chile powder, cayenne, olive oil, pineapple

---

2 tablespoons honey

1 tablespoon fresh lime juice

1 teaspoon ancho chile powder

Pinch of cayenne pepper

2 teaspoons extra-light olive oil, plus more for the grill

1¼ pounds peeled, cored pineapple, cut into eight 1-inch-thick half moons

¼ teaspoon salt

1. In a small bowl, whisk together the honey, lime juice, chile powder, and cayenne.

2. Preheat the grill or a grill pan to medium. Lightly oil the grates or the pan. In a shallow bowl, toss the pineapple with the 2 teaspoons oil and sprinkle with the salt. Grill the pineapple until heated through and softened slightly, about 3 minutes per side.

3. Transfer to a platter or serving plates and drizzle with the chile-lime mixture.

Per serving: 135 calories • 1g protein • 3.5g fat (0.5g saturated) • 2g fiber • 20mg calcium • 69mg vitamin C • 28g carbohydrate • 148mg sodium

Double Grape Gelatin

Hands-On Time: 15 minutes • **Total Time:** 45 minutes + chilling time

Makes: 4 servings

Wine for dessert? Yes! Combined with warm spices (much like mulled wine) and sweetened with orange juice and honey, red wine makes a great fat releaser dessert. And for a double dose of goodness, good-for-you red grapes are suspended in the wine gelatin.

Fat Releasers
Red wine, honey, cinnamon, oranges, grapes

1 envelope (¼ ounce) unflavored gelatin

1½ cups red wine

¼ cup plus 3 tablespoons honey

½ teaspoon ground cinnamon

⅛ teaspoon ground allspice

½ cup cold water

½ cup fresh orange juice, chilled

1 cup seedless red grapes, halved

1. In a small bowl, sprinkle the gelatin over ½ cup of the wine. Let stand until softened, about 5 minutes. Meanwhile, prepare an ice bath: Place several ice cubes in a large bowl and add enough cold water to cover.

2. In a medium saucepan, bring the remaining 1 cup wine, the honey, cinnamon, and allspice to a simmer over medium heat. Stir the softened gelatin into the simmering wine until the gelatin has dissolved, about 1 minute. Remove from the heat, transfer to a bowl that can sit in the ice bath without sinking in, and stir in the cold water and orange juice.

3. Let stand, stirring occasionally, until the gelatin starts to set up and thicken, about 30 minutes. Fold the grapes into the bowl, and then divide the mixture among 4 wineglasses. Refrigerate until set, at least 1 hour or overnight.

Per serving: 226 calories • 2g protein • 0g fat (0g saturated) • 0.5g fiber
21mg calcium • 15mg vitamin C • 47g carbohydrate • 11mg sodium

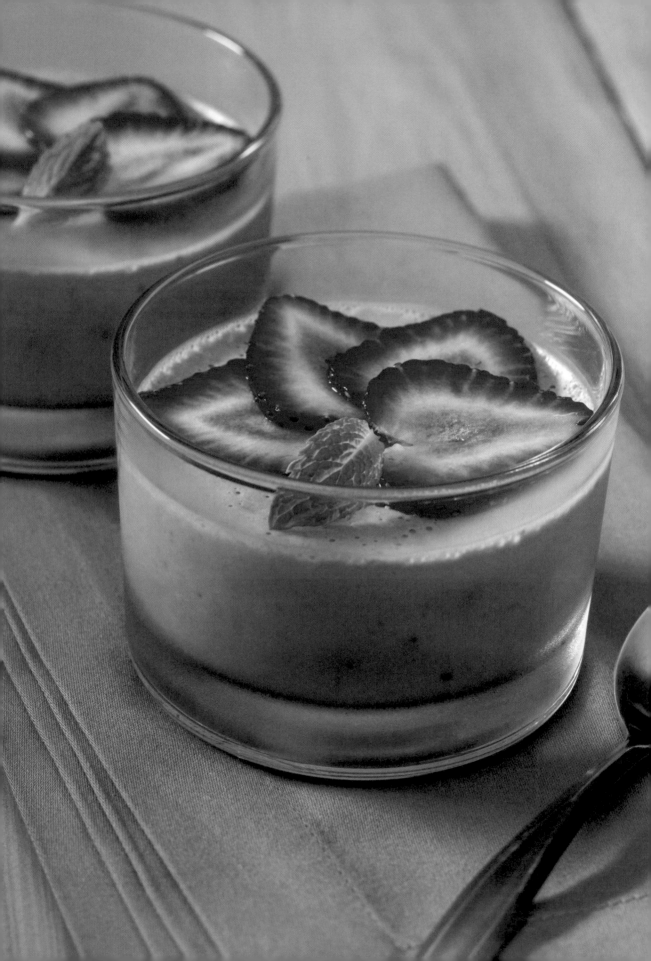

Strawberry Cheesecake Mousse

Hands-On Time: 20 minutes • **Total Time:** 20 minutes + chilling time

Makes: 4 servings

Gelatin is easy to work with, but there are a couple of tricks: Let the gelatin soften first in a little liquid before you melt it over heat. Then stir until you see no more granules; this tells you that the gelatin is completely dissolved. Look for packages of unflavored gelatin alongside boxes of pudding mix and Jell-O.

Fat Releasers
Strawberries, cream cheese, yogurt, honey, red wine

½ pound strawberries, thinly sliced (1½ cups), plus 4 for garnish

3 ounces ⅓-less-fat cream cheese

2 tablespoons 0% Greek yogurt

2 tablespoons honey

½ envelope (1⅛ teaspoons) unflavored gelatin

½ cup red wine or unsweetened cherry juice

Small mint leaves, for garnish (optional)

1. In a food processor, puree 1 cup of the sliced strawberries with the cream cheese, yogurt, and honey. Transfer to a bowl.

2. In a heatproof glass measuring cup, sprinkle the gelatin over the wine and let stand 5 minutes until softened. Place the measuring cup in a pan of simmering water and heat, stirring, until the gelatin has completely dissolved. Let cool to room temperature.

3. Slowly whisk the melted gelatin into the strawberry–cream cheese mixture until smooth and no streaks remain. Fold in the remaining ½ cup sliced strawberries. Spoon into 4 glasses or ramekins and chill until set, about 2 hours.

4. Slice the remaining 4 strawberries. Garnish the top of the mousse with the strawberry slices and a small mint leaf, if desired.

Per serving: 134 calories • 4g protein • 5g fat (2.5g saturated) • 1g fiber 41mg calcium • 31mg vitamin C • 15g carbohydrate • 77mg sodium

Slow-Cooker Fruit Compote

Hands-On Time: 30 minutes ● **Total Time:** 6 hours 30 minutes
Makes: 10 cups

This compote makes a lovely dessert, either chilled or warmed up a bit. Top it with a dollop of 0% Greek yogurt. Or use the compote as a waffle or pancake topping or in a breakfast parfait with Greek yogurt. You can even replace the fruit in one of your shakes with chunks of frozen compote: Freeze some compote in an ice cube tray and use about 6 compote cubes instead of the fruit.

Fat Releasers
Cinnamon, grapes

2 **teaspoons ground cinnamon**

¼ **teaspoon salt**

1 **bunch seedless red grapes (1¾ pounds), halved**

4 **pears, preferably red Bartlett, peeled, quartered, and sliced**

6 **tart-sweet apples (about 3 pounds), peeled, quartered, and sliced**

1. In a small bowl, blend the cinnamon and salt.

2. In a 6-quart slow cooker, layer the fruit in this order: grapes, pears, apples. Sprinkle each layer with some of the cinnamon-salt mixture. Cover and cook on high for 1 hour, then cook on low for 5 hours.

3. Lightly mash the fruit, but leave it pretty chunky. Let cool to room temperature (it will thicken as it cools). Then ladle into 1-cup containers and freeze what you won't use in a week.

Per cup: 152 calories ● 1g protein ● 0.5g fat (0g saturated) ● 5g fiber ● 25mg calcium ● 10mg vitamin C ● 40g carbohydrate ● 60mg sodium

Individual Blueberry-Apple Crisps

Hands-On Time: 15 minutes • **Total Time:** 30 minutes • **Makes:** 4 servings

This super-simple dessert can be easily varied. Use pear, peach, or nectarine for the apple. Use raspberries, chopped mango, or diced strawberries for the blueberries. Just be sure to use only the quantities listed. (This is where a kitchen scale will come in handy.)

Fat Releasers
Cinnamon, honey, oats, coconut oil

1 apple, peeled and diced (size of blueberries)

½ teaspoon ground cinnamon

1 container (6 ounces) blueberries

4 teaspoons honey

¼ cup quick-cooking oats

2 teaspoons turbinado sugar

⅛ teaspoon salt

1½ teaspoons coconut oil

1. Preheat the oven to 375°F.

2. Divide the apple among four 6-ounce ramekins. Sprinkle with ¼ teaspoon of the cinnamon (about a pinch each). Top with the blueberries. Drizzle 1 teaspoon of honey over each ramekin.

3. In a small bowl, stir together the oats, turbinado sugar, salt, and remaining ¼ teaspoon cinnamon. Work the coconut oil in with your fingers. Spread 1 tablespoon of the mixture over each ramekin.

4. Place the ramekins on a baking sheet and bake until the fruit is bubbling, about 15 minutes.

Per serving: 109 calories • 1g protein • 2.5g fat (1.5g saturated) • 2.5g fiber 2mg calcium • 6mg vitamin C • 23g carbohydrate • 73mg sodium

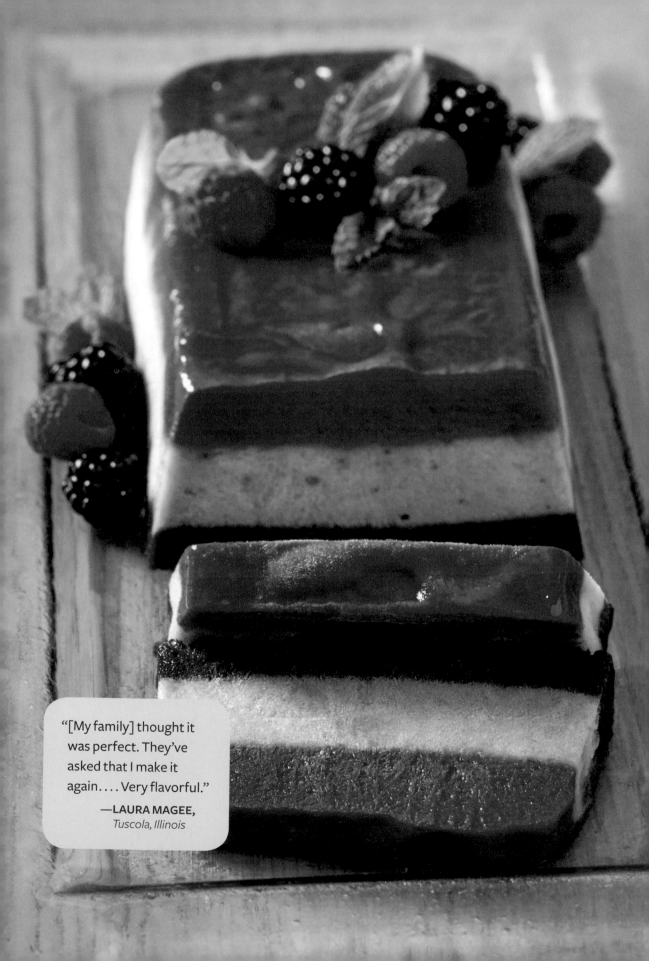

"[My family] thought it was perfect. They've asked that I make it again. . . . Very flavorful."

—LAURA MAGEE,
Tuscola, Illinois

Frozen Berry Terrine

Hands-On Time: 30 minutes

Total Time: 30 minutes + freezing time • **Makes:** 8 servings

Fat Releasers
Raspberries, honey, yogurt, blackberries, lemons

While this takes a bit of time to set up, it looks beautiful on the plate and tastes even better. You can swap strawberries for the raspberries or blueberries for the blackberries. The banana, silky smooth when pureed and frozen, provides a nice contrast in color, flavor, and texture.

1 package (12 ounces) frozen unsweetened raspberries, thawed

8 tablespoons honey

5 tablespoons 0% Greek yogurt

1 package (10 ounces) frozen unsweetened blackberries, thawed

¼ teaspoon vanilla extract

2 bananas (¾ pound total), cut up

2 teaspoons fresh lemon juice

Fresh raspberries and blackberries, for garnish (optional)

Fresh mint leaves, for garnish (optional)

1. Line a 9 x 5-inch loaf pan with plastic wrap, leaving an overhang on all sides.

2. In a food processor, combine the raspberries, 3 tablespoons of the honey, and 4 tablespoons of the yogurt and puree. Transfer the mixture to a fine-meshed sieve and strain, pressing to leave the seeds behind. Discard the seeds. Transfer the puree to the loaf pan; spread to make an even layer; freeze.

3. In the same processor bowl (no need to clean), puree the blackberries, 3 tablespoons of the honey, the remaining 1 tablespoon yogurt, and the vanilla. Strain through a fine-mesh sieve to leave the seeds behind. Refrigerate the blackberry mixture while you make the banana layer.

4. Clean the processor bowl and puree the bananas with the lemon juice and the remaining 2 tablespoons of honey. Spoon the banana mixture over the raspberry mixture in the pan and spread it to the edges. Freeze until beginning to set, about 1 hour.

5. Spread the blackberry mixture over the banana mixture. Fold the plastic wrap over the top. Freeze until firm, at least 8 hours.

6. To serve, invert the terrine onto a serving platter. Remove the plastic wrap and cut the terrine into 8 slices. If desired, garnish with fresh raspberries, blackberries, and mint leaves.

Per serving: 132 calories • 2g protein • 0g fat (0g saturated) • 4.5g fiber • 25mg calcium 10mg vitamin C • 35g carbohydrate • 5mg sodium

Mango Melba

Hands-On Time: 10 minutes • **Total Time:** 10 minutes • **Makes:** 4 servings

There are so many varieties of mango out there that if one isn't in season you'll be able to find another. But, if you do see them, choose the smaller, thinner Ataulfo variety (also called Champagne mangoes), as they are silky smooth and very sweet. This preparation would also work with peaches or nectarines in place of the mangoes.

Fat Releasers
Yogurt, honey, raspberries, limes, mangoes

½ cup 0% Greek yogurt

3 tablespoons honey

2 teaspoons grated lime zest

2 cups frozen unsweetened raspberries, thawed

1½ teaspoons fresh lime juice

2 mangoes (about 10 ounces each), peeled and cut into ½-inch wedges

1. In a medium bowl, mix together the yogurt, 2 tablespoons of the honey, and the lime zest.

2. In a food processor, puree the raspberries, the remaining 1 tablespoon honey, and the lime juice. Transfer to a fine-mesh sieve and push on the fruit, leaving the seeds behind.

3. Arrange the mango slices on 4 dessert plates, and spoon the raspberry sauce over the top. Top each serving with 2½ tablespoons of the yogurt mixture.

Per serving: 148 calories • 4g protein • 0.5g fat (0g saturated) • 4g fiber 39mg calcium • 46mg vitamin C • 36g carbohydrate • 12mg sodium

Honey-Walnut Fudge Bites

Hands-On Time: 10 minutes • **Total Time:** 30 minutes • **Makes:** 20 cookies

Honey keeps baked goods exceptionally moist, and these little chocolate and walnut cookies will stay moist and chewy for at least 3 weeks. Freeze or store at room temperature in an airtight container.

Fat Releasers
Almond flour, cocoa powder, walnuts, honey, eggs

- 1 cup almond flour
- 2 tablespoons unsweetened cocoa powder
- ¼ cup coarsely chopped walnuts
- Pinch of salt
- ¼ cup honey
- 1 large egg white
- ¼ teaspoon almond extract

1. Preheat the oven to 325°F. Line a baking sheet with parchment paper or a nonstick liner.

2. In a medium bowl, stir together the almond flour, cocoa powder, walnuts, and salt. Stir in the honey, egg white, and almond extract.

3. Drop the dough in small, walnut-sized mounds onto the baking sheet about 2 inches apart. Bake until firm and set, 17 to 19 minutes. (If you use the shorter time, you'll get a fudgier cookie.) Let cool on the baking sheet.

Per cookie: 57 calories • 2g protein • 4g fat (0.5g saturated) • 1g fiber
14mg calcium • 0mg vitamin C • 5g carbohydrate • 12mg sodium

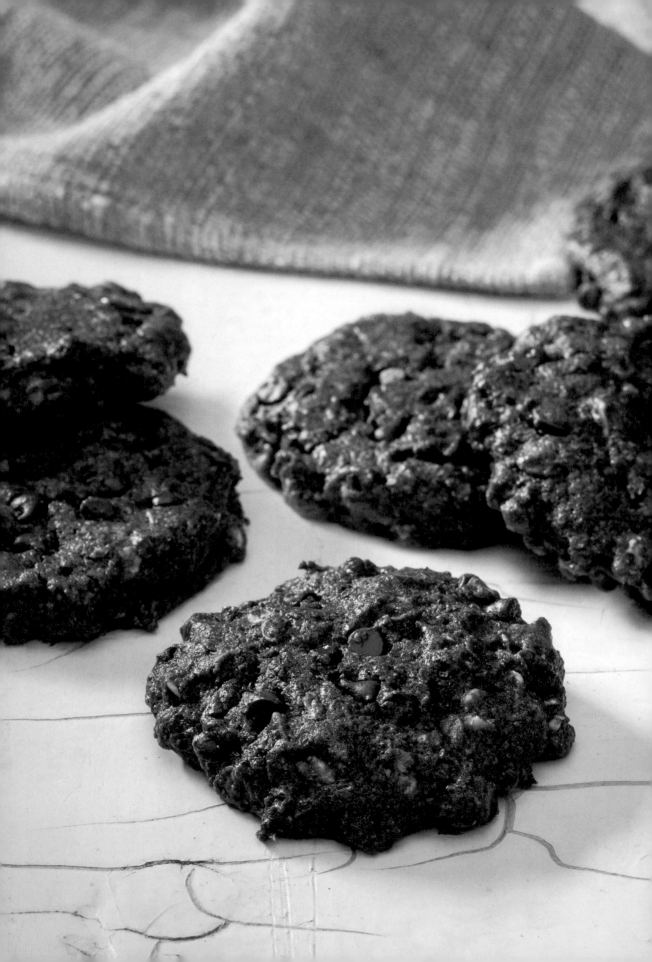

Chocolate Chocolate-Chip Cookies

Hands-On Time: 30 minutes • **Total Time:** 50 minutes • **Makes:** 30 cookies

Toasted oats mimic the flavor and crunch of nuts in these cookies while making them good for you, too. Unsweetened cocoa powder and chocolate chips pair up to make the cookies especially chocolaty.

Fat Releasers
Oats, whole-wheat flour, cocoa, olive oil, flaxseed meal, eggs, chocolate

½ cup old-fashioned rolled oats

1 cup whole-wheat pastry flour, spooned into the cup and then leveled

2 tablespoons unsweetened cocoa powder

½ teaspoon baking soda

½ teaspoon salt

¼ cup extra-light olive oil

⅓ cup flaxseed meal

⅓ cup maple syrup

2 tablespoons turbinado sugar

2 large egg whites

1½ teaspoons vanilla extract

2 tablespoons water

1 cup (6 ounces) mini chocolate chips

1. Preheat the oven to 350°F. On a rimmed baking sheet, toast the oats until golden brown and crisp, about 15 minutes.

2. Meanwhile, in a medium bowl, combine the flour, cocoa powder, baking soda, and salt.

3. In a large bowl, stir together the oil, flaxseed meal, maple syrup, turbinado sugar, egg whites, vanilla, and water until well combined. Fold in the flour mixture, oats, and chocolate chips.

4. Line 2 baking sheets with parchment paper. Drop the dough by rounded teaspoonsful 2 inches apart onto the baking sheets and flatten slightly with dampened hands. Bake until the cookies are set, 10 to 12 minutes, rotating the sheets from top to bottom halfway through. Remove from the baking sheets to cool on racks.

SAVE FOR A SNACK: These cookies freeze well. Serve what you want, then freeze the remainder. They're good straight from the freezer, or thaw at room temperature before eating.

Per cookie: 81 calories • 2g protein • 4g fat (1g saturated) • 1g fiber • 8mg calcium 0mg vitamin C • 11g carbohydrate • 64mg sodium

Flourless Chocolate–Peanut Butter Cakelets

Hands-On Time: 15 minutes • **Total Time:** 30 minutes • **Makes:** 12 cakelets

Nuts and chocolate, in addition to being delicious, have the ability to help baked goods rise. So these little cakes, which have no flour in them at all, are leavened by eggs, peanut butter, and cocoa. The cakes store well in the fridge or freezer. If freezing, spread them out on a tray to freeze solid, then store them in a plastic resealable bag. When you're ready to have one for dessert, just leave it at room temperature for 10 minutes or so.

Fat Releasers
Honey, chocolate, peanut butter, cocoa, eggs

- ½ cup honey
- ⅓ cup (about 2 ounces) mini semisweet chocolate chips
- ¼ cup creamy natural peanut butter
- 5 tablespoons unsweetened cocoa powder
- 2 large eggs, separated
- 2 teaspoons vanilla extract
- ¼ teaspoon salt
- 2 egg whites
- ¼ teaspoon cream of tartar

1. Preheat the oven to 375°F. Line 12 cups of a muffin tin with paper liners.

2. In a small saucepan, combine the honey, chocolate chips, peanut butter, and cocoa and stir over low heat until smooth.

3. In a large bowl, beat the egg yolks with the vanilla and salt. Whisk about ¼ cup of the chocolate mixture into the egg yolks to warm them. Scrape the remaining chocolate mixture into the egg yolks and stir to combine.

4. In a large bowl, with an electric mixer, beat the 4 egg whites until foamy. Add the cream of tartar and beat until stiff peaks form.

5. Stir one-third of the egg whites into the chocolate mixture to lighten it, then gently but thoroughly fold in the remaining egg whites.

6. Divide the batter among the muffin cups and bake until a wooden pick inserted in the center comes out with a few moist crumbs clinging to it, 12 to 14 minutes. Let cool completely in the pan on a rack. The cakes will fall a little as they cool.

Per cakelet: 124 calories • 4g protein • 5g fat (1.5g saturated) • 1g fiber • 7mg calcium • 0mg vitamin C • 17g carbohydrate • 71mg sodium

Chocolate Zucchini Squares

Hands-On Time: 15 minutes

Total Time: 45 minutes + cooling time • **Makes:** 16 squares

Fat Releasers
Coconut oil, zucchini, honey, almond oil, eggs, cocoa powder, cinnamon, chocolate

Super moist because of the zucchini (and the coconut oil), this cake takes really well to being frozen. After cooling the cake, cut it into squares and spread them out on a tray. Place in the freezer until frozen solid, then pop into storage bags. They will keep for quite a long time in the freezer, but chances are you'll never find out how long they can go. You can eat them straight from the freezer or thaw at room temperature for a few minutes.

5 tablespoons coconut oil, plus extra for the pan

1 medium zucchini (12 ounces)

½ cup honey

¼ cup turbinado sugar

2 tablespoons almond oil or extra-light olive oil

1 large egg

1 large egg white

½ teaspoon vanilla extract

2 tablespoons water

¾ cup white whole-wheat flour, spooned into the cup and then leveled

½ cup all-purpose flour, spooned into the cup and then leveled

2 tablespoons unsweetened cocoa powder

1 teaspoon baking soda

½ teaspoon ground cinnamon

¼ teaspoon salt

⅓ cup mini chocolate chips

1. Preheat the oven to 325°F. Coat a 9-inch square baking pan with some coconut oil.

2. Place a clean kitchen towel on a work surface. Grate the zucchini on the large holes of a box grater onto the towel (you'll have about 2 cups). Wrap the zucchini up in the towel and twist to squeeze out excess water.

3. In a large bowl, beat together the honey, sugar, 5 tablespoons coconut oil, and the almond oil. Beat in the whole egg, egg white, vanilla, and water.

4. In a small bowl, whisk together the flours, cocoa powder, baking soda, cinnamon, and salt.

5. Stir the flour mixture into the honey mixture. Fold in the zucchini. Scrape the batter into the baking pan and spread out. Sprinkle with the chocolate chips.

6. Bake until a wooden pick inserted into the cake comes out clean (or with some moist crumbs clinging if you like a denser cake), 25 to 30 minutes.

7. Let cool in the pan on a rack, then cut into 16 squares.

Per square: 165 calories • 3g protein • 8g fat (5g saturated) • 1.5g fiber • 11mg calcium 4mg vitamin C • 23g carbohydrate • 129mg sodium

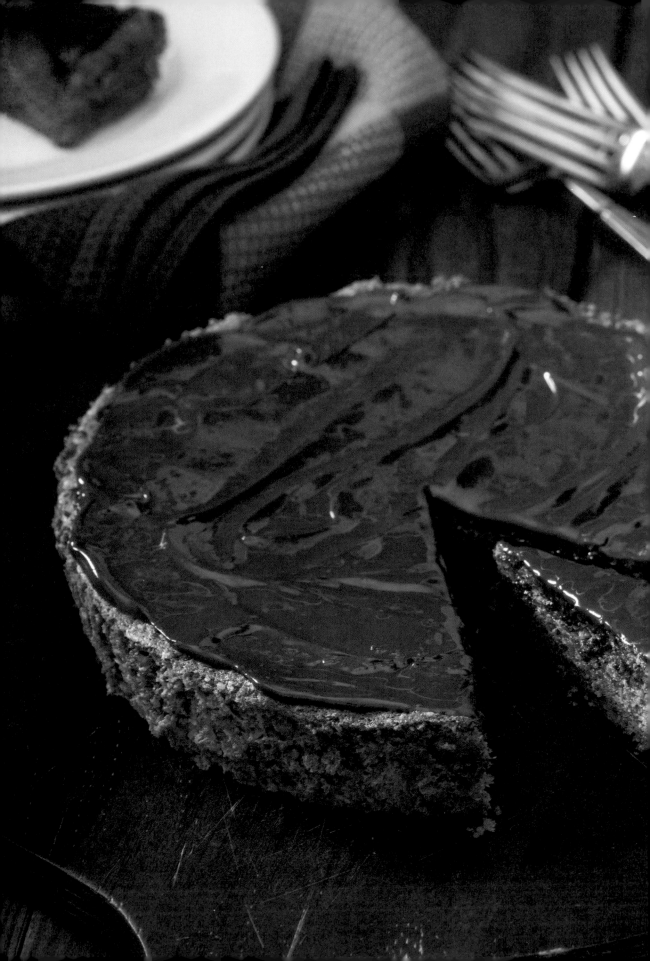

Chocolate-Glazed Espresso Nut Torte

Hands-On Time: 35 minutes

Total Time: 1 hour 10 minutes + cooling time • **Makes:** 12 servings

This dense, nut-based cake will stay moist for at least a week. Refrigerate the unglazed cake right in the pan. When you're ready to serve, unmold it from the springform and glaze the cake.

Fat Releasers
Honey, almond oil, walnuts, almonds, multigrain bread, eggs, chocolate

TORTE

- ½ **cup turbinado sugar**
- ⅓ **cup honey**
- 5 **teaspoons almond oil or extra-light olive oil**
- 2 **teaspoons vanilla extract**
- ½ **cup finely ground walnuts (2 ounces)**
- ½ **cup finely ground raw almonds (2 ounces)**
- 2 **slices (1 ounce each) multigrain bread, toasted and finely ground**
- ½ **teaspoon salt**
- 8 **large egg whites**
- ¼ **teaspoon cream of tartar**
- 2 **teaspoons espresso powder**

GLAZE

- ⅓ **cup semisweet mini chocolate chips**
- 1 **teaspoon almond oil**

1. *To make the torte:* Preheat the oven to 350°F. Generously coat the bottom (not the sides) of an 8½-inch springform pan with cooking spray. Line the bottom with waxed or parchment paper and coat the paper.

2. In a large bowl, stir together the sugar, honey, oil, and vanilla. Stir in the walnuts, almonds, bread crumbs, and salt.

3. In a separate bowl, beat the egg whites and cream of tartar until soft peaks form. Sprinkle with the espresso powder and beat on high speed until stiff (but not dry) peaks form.

4. Stir one-third of the beaten egg whites into the nut mixture to lighten it. Then, gently fold in the remaining beaten whites. Scrape the batter into the springform pan.

5. Bake until a wooden pick inserted in the center comes out clean, 30 to 35 minutes. Let cool completely in the pan on a rack. The cake will fall, especially the center. With a knife, loosen the edges of the torte from the pan and gently press down around the edges to make the top of the torte even.

6. To unmold, release the sides of the springform. Carefully invert the torte and remove the springform bottom and paper, then reinvert onto a serving plate.

7. *To make the glaze:* In a small saucepan, melt the chocolate chips and almond oil over very low heat, stirring until smooth. Spread the chocolate glaze over the top of the cooled torte.

Per serving: 194 calories • 5g protein • 10g fat (2g saturated) • 1.5g fiber • 0mg calcium 0mg vitamin C • 24g carbohydrate • 151mg sodium

Chocolate-Coconut Pudding

Hands-On Time: 15 minutes

Total Time: 15 minutes + chilling time • **Makes:** 4 servings

For an extra indulgence, dollop the top of the puddings with a spoonful of 0% Greek yogurt sweetened with a whisper of honey. Sprinkle the yogurt with a little cinnamon.

Fat Releasers
Coconut milk, cocoa powder

---

1 can (14 ounces) light coconut milk

3 tablespoons unsweetened cocoa powder

¼ teaspoon salt

¼ cup agave syrup or honey

1 envelope (¼ ounce) unflavored gelatin

¼ cup water

½ teaspoon vanilla extract

1. In a saucepan, whisk the coconut milk into the cocoa powder and salt. Whisk in the agave syrup. Bring to a low simmer over medium-low heat.

2. Meanwhile, sprinkle the gelatin over the water to soften.

3. Add the softened gelatin to the coconut milk and stir 1 minute over low heat to dissolve the gelatin. Stir in the vanilla.

4. Divide the mixture among four 6-ounce dessert bowls, ramekins, or custard cups. Let cool to room temperature, then cover and refrigerate until set, about 6 hours.

Per serving: 144 calories • 3g protein • 6g fat (5g saturated) • 0.5g fiber 1mg calcium • 0mg vitamin C • 20g carbohydrate • 167mg sodium

Spiced Carrot-Almond Cake

Hands-On Time: 20 minutes • **Total Time:** 55 minutes • **Makes:** 12 servings

Pastry flour, which is made from a softer wheat (meaning it's lower in gluten), makes for a tender cake, as does the addition of yogurt. When shopping for carrots, don't bother with those that still have their green tops attached; they may look fresher, but a good portion of the nutrients go into the greens, which are then tossed out. Grate the carrots on the large holes of a box grater. Leftover cake can be stored, either iced or not, in the fridge for 3 days or in the freezer for up to 3 weeks.

Fat Releasers
Whole-wheat flour, almonds, ginger, cinnamon, eggs, yogurt, olive oil, cream cheese

- ¾ cup plus 2 tablespoons whole-wheat pastry flour
- ½ cup raw almonds
- 1 teaspoon baking soda
- 1 teaspoon ground ginger
- 1 teaspoon ground cinnamon
- ¼ teaspoon salt
- ⅛ teaspoon ground allspice
- 1 large egg
- 2 large egg whites
- ½ cup plus 1 tablespoon maple syrup
- ¼ cup plus 1 tablespoon 0% Greek yogurt
- 3 tablespoons extra-light olive oil
- 1½ cups shredded carrots (5 ounces)
- 3 ounces ⅓-less-fat cream cheese

1. Preheat the oven to 350°F. Coat an 8 x 8-inch baking pan with cooking spray. Line the bottom of the pan with parchment paper.

2. In a food processor, pulse the flour and almonds together until finely ground, about 2 minutes. Transfer to a large bowl and whisk in the baking soda, ginger, cinnamon, salt, and allspice.

3. In a separate bowl, whisk together the whole egg, egg whites, ½ cup of the maple syrup, ¼ cup of the yogurt, and the oil. Fold the wet ingredients into the flour mixture, and then fold in the carrots.

4. Scrape the batter into the prepared pan and bake until the cake is set and a wooden pick inserted in the center comes out clean, 30 to 35 minutes. Cool 15 minutes in the pan on a rack, then invert the cake onto the rack to cool completely.

5. In a small bowl, with an electric mixer, beat the cream cheese and the remaining 1 tablespoon yogurt together until smooth. Beat in the remaining 1 tablespoon maple syrup. Spread the frosting over the top of the cake. Cut the cake into 12 pieces (roughly 2 inches square).

Per serving: 172 calories • 5g protein • 8.5g fat (1.5g saturated) • 2.5g fiber 59mg calcium • 1mg vitamin C • 20g carbohydrate • 206mg sodium

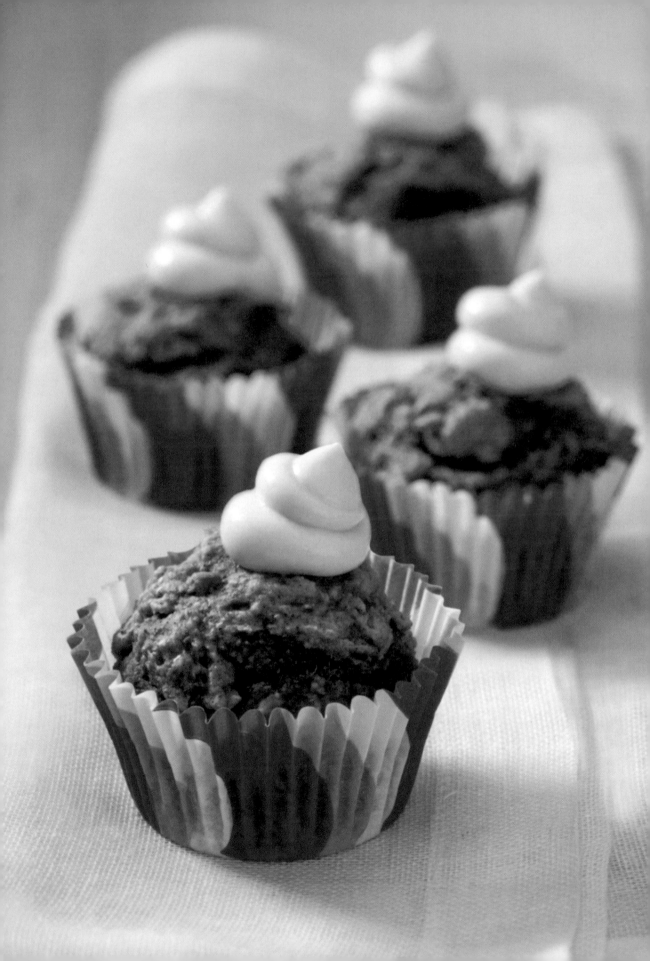

Spice Cupcakes with Honey-Cream Frosting

Hands-On Time: 25 minutes • **Total Time:** 45 minutes • **Makes:** 12 cupcakes

Measure out the olive oil first, then use the same measuring cup for the honey. The thin coating of oil will make the honey slide right out. Use a kitchen scale to make sure you get exactly 10 ounces of sweet potatoes, most likely from just one. (Toss any leftover sweet potato into a soup.) These cupcakes freeze quite well even after frosting. (Tightly covered, they should keep for a month.) Make the whole batch, place the frosted cupcakes on a tray and freeze solid. Transfer them to an airtight freezer container.

Fat Releasers
Sweet potatoes, whole-wheat flour, cinnamon, ginger, olive oil, honey, eggs, cream cheese

CUPCAKES

- 10 **ounces sweet potatoes, peeled and thinly sliced**
- 2 **cups white whole-wheat flour**
- 1 **teaspoon ground cinnamon**
- ¾ **teaspoon ground ginger**
- ¾ **teaspoon baking powder**
- ½ **teaspoon baking soda**
- ¼ **teaspoon salt**
- ⅛ **teaspoon ground allspice**
- ¼ **cup extra-light olive oil**
- ⅓ **cup honey**
- 1 **large egg**
- 2 **large egg whites**
- ¼ **cup water**

FROSTING

- 6 **ounces ⅓-less-fat cream cheese, at room temperature**
- 2 **tablespoons honey**
- 1 **teaspoon vanilla extract**

1. *To make the cake:* Preheat the oven to 350°F. Line 12 muffin cups with paper liners.

2. In a small pot of boiling water, cook the sweet potatoes until tender, about 5 minutes. Drain well, return to the pot, and mash. Set aside to cool slightly.

3. In a medium bowl, whisk the flour, cinnamon, ginger, baking powder, baking soda, salt, and allspice.

4. In a large bowl, with an electric mixer, beat the oil and honey until well blended. Add the whole egg and egg whites, one at a time, beating well after each addition. Beat in the sweet potatoes and water. Fold in the flour mixture.

5. Divide the batter among the muffin cups and bake until a wooden pick inserted in the center comes out clean, 15 to 17 minutes. Cool for 10 minutes in the pan on a rack, and then transfer to the rack to cool completely.

6. *To make the frosting:* In a medium bowl, with an electric mixer, beat the cream cheese with the honey and vanilla. Spread the cooled cupcakes with the frosting.

Per cupcake: 206 calories • 5g protein • 8.5g fat (2.5g saturated) • 3.5g fiber • 47mg calcium 2mg vitamin C • 29g carbohydrate • 217mg sodium

I've tried my best to make the Digest Diet as accessible and delicious for as many kinds of eaters as possible. Some of you, however, simply can't stick to the diet exactly as written. And that's okay! The Digest Diet is about making healthy and sustainable lifestyle changes using wholesome, nutrient-packed foods that you can incorporate into your diet for life. And, as I hope you've learned by now, accepting "not perfect" and striving for the "middle ground" is key to your success on the Digest Diet. So, we've also identified common dieting hurdles many of you face: Quick-Fix, Vegetarian, Dairy-Free, Cooking for One, and On a Budget.

For each dieting challenge, we've included 2 days' worth of menus for Phase 2 and Phase 3. Please note that these are intended only as examples. You should feel free to swap out recipes or meals (just keep them within the same phase) and substitute ingredients (check out our list of suitable swaps on page 52) as you like. Also, in the recipe index that follows, you'll see that we've flagged the recipes that are best suited for each dieting challenge.

Men, note that these menus are designed to meet the ladies' calorie requirements. If you find the menus satisfying as written, that's fine; but if you find that you're hungry, try adding another 150 to 200 calories per day (either in the form of an extra snack or a slightly bigger portion of your meals). Also, if you choose to have red wine for dinner, you can opt for a 6-ounce glass.

Here are some other things to keep in mind when designing your own menus:

● QUICK FIX

In addition to choosing recipes that take a short amount of time to prepare, here are some tips for saving time in the kitchen.

▶ Choose recipes that can be prepared ahead or in stages. Put them together on the weekend, or whenever you have spare time. Then, at mealtime, you'll have little to no prep to get dinner on the table.

▶ Buy vegetables or meat that has already been trimmed and cut up.

▶ You can use frozen vegetables to save time, but avoid canned unless the vegetables are "no-salt-added."

▶ Grilling and broiling are fast cooking methods with minimal cleanup. Microwaving or steaming vegetables is another timesaver.

● VEGETARIAN

Protein is a key nutrient for successful weight loss. So in planning your vegetarian menus for the Digest Diet, choose foods that provide significant amounts of protein, such as eggs and dairy (extremely important for calcium, too). For plant sources of protein, concentrate on soy products and quinoa because both have what is called "complete protein" (significant amounts of all the essential amino acids). Legumes (such as beans, lentils, or chickpeas) are also good plant sources of protein.

● DAIRY-FREE

Calcium is a cornerstone of the Digest Diet (you should strive to get at least 1,000 milligrams daily), and dairy is one of the best sources of calcium, so we do encourage you to try to consume some dairy if you can. Some people find that they can tolerate ice cream or hard cheese but not milk or yogurt. If you truly can't eat dairy products, there are plenty of substitutions you can make. And take special care to consume other foods that are either naturally rich in calcium, such as dark leafy greens, or that have been fortified with calcium. See the list on page 55.

● COOKING FOR ONE

Most of the recipes in this book are designed to serve 4 so that you can make them for your whole family. But if you're on your own and don't want to be stuck with lots of leftovers (or your family just doesn't want to eat your "diet" food—though they may change their minds once they taste it!), look for recipes that have "Cooking for One" instructions to help you scale down the quantities. In addition:

▶ Choose recipes that will keep well so you can refrigerate or freeze the remainder for future meals.

▶ When shopping for meat and poultry that come prepackaged, remove what you don't need right away, divide it into single servings (about 4 ounces each), spread it out on a parchment-lined tray, and freeze it. Once the meat or poultry is frozen, place it in plastic food storage bags labeled with the date.

▶ If buying fresh vegetables in quantities larger than you can consume in the space of 2 or 3 days, briefly cook them in a vegetable steamer or a pot of boiling water; they should still be slightly on the raw side, since you will be cooking them more later. This will help them last longer in the fridge.

BONUS!

ENJOY A FULL YEAR
FREE
$47.88 VALUE

Thanks for adding our book to your family library! We hope you've discovered smart ideas and advice to help you jumpstart your weight loss, direct from the editors of America's favorite magazine, Reader's Digest. And now you can keep the best info and tips from sources you trust coming to your home all year long—FREE! Here's how.

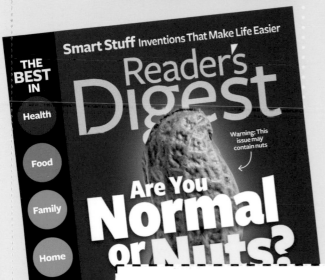

FREE SUBSCRIPTION

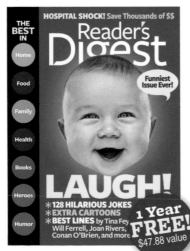

Return this card today to claim your Free Subscription (a $47.88 value) to Reader's Digest magazine. You'll enjoy a full-year of the only true family magazine delivered to your home, along with instant access to our exclusive website, rd.com.

YES! PLEASE START MY **FREE 1-YEAR SUBSCRIPTION** TO READER'S DIGEST MAGAZINE!

NAME _____
(please print)

ADDRESS _____

CITY _____

STATE _____ ZIP _____

E-MAIL _____

MAIL THIS CARD TODAY!

Get the Best News & Advice, from a source you trust.
FREE YEAR of Reader's Digest!

As a Reader's Digest subscriber, you'll look forward to:

▶ **Everything You Need, In One Easy Read**...Your #1 trusted source for the latest news on the topics that matter most to you, selected and condensed for quick reading

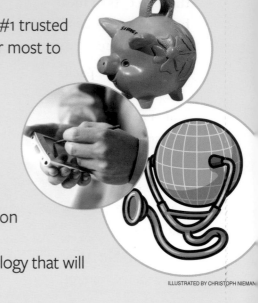

▶ **Feel-Good Humor and Stories**...Laugh out loud with over 400 family-friendly jokes, cartoons and heart-warming stories about hometown heroes

▶ **Thousands of Tips for Living a Richer, More Satisfying Life**...Discover the best in health, nutrition and prevention, plus surprising ideas in food, money and technology that will simplify your life

ILLUSTRATED BY CHRISTOPH NIEMAN

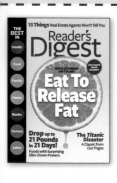

▶ **Exclusive Best of America Issue**...enjoy our bigger-than-ever special issue featuring the Top 100 Things We Love About America

---

● ON A BUDGET

Dieting can sometimes be a pretty expensive proposition. Luckily, the lean cuts of meat that are called for in this diet also happen to be the most modestly priced. Here are some tips for saving money on other ingredients:

▶ Buy family packs of skinless, boneless chicken breast halves, remove them from the packaging, spread them out on a parchment-lined tray, and freeze them. Pop them into a large plastic food storage bag and label it with the date.

▶ Although fish is a good, low-calorie source of protein, it can be quite costly. Choose fish on special at your market, since most white-fleshed fish are interchangeable in recipes.

▶ Buy frozen, farmed shrimp; they are considerably less expensive than other shrimp.

▶ Buy one type of nut in bulk and sub it in for other nuts. Just be sure to get unsalted nuts (whether roasted or raw).

▶ Buy large bags of your favorite nonstarchy frozen vegetables (for example, cauliflower, mixed stir-fry vegetables, spinach) and use them as regular side dishes.

▶ Fresh herbs can certainly make a difference to a dish, but in most cases you can sub in dried. As a general rule, use one-third the quantity of the fresh.

Menu 1

Breakfast

Salsa Omelet: Whisk together 1 egg, 2 egg whites, 1 tablespoon fat-free milk, ¼ teaspoon ground cumin, and a pinch each of salt and ground black pepper. Coat a medium nonstick skillet with cooking spray and cook the egg mixture, without stirring, over medium heat until set around the edges but a little wet in the center (1 to 2 minutes). Sprinkle the omelet with 1 tablespoon Parmesan, cover, and cook until the top is set, about 1 minute. Spread the finished omelet with 1 tablespoon salsa and fold in half to serve. Serve with 2 ounces deli-sliced roast turkey and 1 cup fat-free milk.

Snack 1

1 mini cheese (page 35), 10 raw almonds, ½ bell pepper (any color)

Lunch

Fade Away Shake (page 69)

Snack 2

2 teaspoons natural peanut butter spread on 1 high-fiber cracker (page 27). Serve with ½ cup fat-free milk.

Dinner

Chicken Piccata with Capers & Olives (page 125) and 2 cups steamed broccoli. Have a 4-ounce glass of red wine with dinner or a handful of red grapes for dessert.

QUICK-FIX | Fade Away

Menu 2

Breakfast

Fade Away Shake (page 69)

Snack 1

10 baby carrots, 20 pistachio nuts, ½ cup fat-free milk

Lunch

Golden Gazpacho (page 99) and **Turkey-Swiss Sticks:** Halve 2 thin stalks of celery crosswise and then halve again to make 4 sticks. Spread ¼ teaspoon Dijon mustard on to each of the celery sticks. Top each of 4 slices (2 ounces total) of reduced-sodium deli-sliced turkey with ½ slice reduced-fat Swiss cheese (2 ounces total) and roll a turkey-cheese stack around each celery stick.

Snack 2

1 tablespoon sunflower seeds and a pinch of Fat Releaser Seasoning (page 31; optional) stirred into ½ cup nonfat yogurt. Serve with 1 plum tomato cut into wedges.

Dinner

Indian-Spiced Shrimp (page 129), 2 cups steamed Chinese stir-fry vegetables (from the frozen foods aisle), and 2 cups salad greens tossed with 1 tablespoon **Digest Diet Vinaigrette** (page 50). Have a 4-ounce glass of red wine with dinner or a handful of red grapes for dessert.

QUICK-FIX | Finish Strong

Menu 1

Breakfast
Homemade Instant Oatmeal (page 79) with ½ cup chopped fresh fruit (whatever you have on hand). Have with ½ cup fat-free milk.

Snack 1
2 clementines, 1 mini cheese (page 35), 1 high-fiber cracker (page 27)

Lunch
Tuna Melts: Mix together 1 pouch (2.5 ounces) water-packed white tuna, 1 tablespoon store-bought ranch dressing, 1 teaspoon pickle relish (or chopped capers or chopped pickled jalapeños), and 1 chopped scallion. Split a multigrain sandwich thin and lightly toast. Top with the tuna mixture and 2 thin slices (1 ounce total) reduced-fat deli-sliced cheese (whatever you have on hand). Heat under the broiler or in a toaster oven for 1 or 2 minutes, or long enough to just melt the cheese.

Snack 2
Stir ½ cup blueberries, 1 teaspoon slivered almonds, 1 teaspoon honey, and a pinch of cinnamon into ½ cup nonfat yogurt.

Dinner
Turkey Milanese (page 211) and 2 slices (1 ounce each) whole wheat baguette. Have a 4-ounce glass of red wine with dinner or a handful of red grapes for dessert.

Menu 2

Breakfast

Tropical Fruit & Berry Salad with Yogurt Dressing (page 87). Serve with 1 light multigrain English muffin, toasted and spread with 2 teaspoons natural almond or peanut butter.

Snack 1

¼ cup fat-free ricotta cheese mixed with 1 tablespoon raisins and 1 tablespoon sunflower seeds

Lunch

Single portion of soup; choose a soup with a serving size that comes close to 250 calories, such as **Spicy Garlic-Tomato Soup with Chicken** (page 90) or **Winter Vegetable Soup with Smoked Pork** (page 103). Make it ahead so you can just grab your lunch portion from the fridge and reheat it. (You'll have enough soup for leftovers for several days.) Serve with 1 multigrain sandwich thin, toasted and spread with 1 wedge Laughing Cow Light (any flavor).

Snack 2

1 tangerine, 20 pistachios

Dinner

Flank Steak with Scallion Chimichurri (page 113), 2 cups steamed green beans, and 2 cups field greens tossed with 1 tablespoon **Digest Diet Vinaigrette** (page 50). Have **Spicy Grilled Pineapple** (page 258) with ¼ cup 0% frozen Greek yogurt for dessert.

VEGETARIAN | Fade Away

Menu 1

Breakfast

Sesame-Walnut Tofu Scramble: Use the mixture for the **Sesame-Walnut Tofu Burgers** (page 130), but do not form it into burgers; instead, cook it in a nonstick skillet with 4 teaspoons olive oil, the way you would scramble eggs. If you're not making breakfast for 4 people, just divide the uncooked mixture into 4 portions and use one-fourth for the scramble, cooking it in a small skillet with 1 teaspoon oil. Freeze or refrigerate the remaining portions for future breakfasts; or form it into burgers for a future dinner. Have with 1 cup fat-free milk.

Snack 1

1 bell pepper (any color) with ¼ cup hummus for dipping

Lunch

Fade Away Shake (page 69)

Snack 2

4 teaspoons almond butter or natural peanut butter spread on 4 small stalks celery

Dinner

Meatless Sloppy Joes (page 131; use vegetarian Worcestershire sauce) and 2 cups steamed asparagus. Have a 4-ounce glass of red wine with dinner or a handful of red grapes for dessert.

Menu 2

Breakfast
Fade Away Shake (page 69)

Snack 1
10 baby carrots, 1 tablespoon hulled sunflower seeds, ¼ cup fat-free ricotta cheese (stir in a Fat Releaser Seasoning, page 31, if you'd like)

Lunch
Quinoa Salad: ¾ cup cooked and cooled quinoa (white or red) tossed with 1 tablespoon toasted hulled pumpkin seeds, 1 cup baby spinach (chopped), ¼ cup crumbled reduced-fat feta cheese, and a dressing made with 1 tablespoon 0% Greek yogurt, 2 to 3 teaspoons (to taste) balsamic vinegar, 1½ teaspoons extra-virgin olive oil, and ground black pepper to taste.

Snack 2
1 cup grape tomatoes, 1 mini cheese (page 35), 1 high-fiber cracker (page 27)

Dinner
Moroccan Chickpea Stew (page 163) and 2 cups shredded romaine tossed with 1 tablespoon **Digest Diet Vinaigrette** (page 50). Have a 4-ounce glass of red wine with dinner or a handful of red grapes for dessert.

VEGETARIAN Finish Strong

Menu 1

Breakfast

Quinoa & Walnut Muffins (page 82) spread with 2 tablespoons unsweetened applesauce and 1 tablespoon natural peanut butter. Serve with ½ cup fat-free milk.

Snack 1

20 pistachios, 1 cup high-fiber mixed vegetable juice

Lunch

Sweet Potato & Tomato Soup (page 108) and 1 light multigrain English muffin, split, toasted, and topped with 2 ounces reduced-fat cheese (your favorite). Heat in the broiler or toaster oven just long enough to melt the cheese.

Snack 2

¼ cup blueberries, 1 teaspoon honey, and a pinch of cinnamon stirred into ½ cup nonfat yogurt

Dinner

Breaded Tofu Steaks (page 149), **Double-Sesame Bok Choy** (page 225), and ½ cup cooked brown basmati rice. Have a 4-ounce glass of red wine with dinner or a handful of red grapes for dessert.

Menu 2

Breakfast

California Breakfast Wrap (page 85). Have with ½ cup fat-free milk.

Snack 1

2 dates, pitted and stuffed with 2 teaspoons natural peanut butter

Lunch

Black Bean Salad: Toss ¾ cup canned no-salt-added black beans with ¼ cup shredded part-skim mozzarella, ½ cup chopped grape tomatoes, 4 teaspoons chopped toasted walnuts, and 4 teaspoons **Digest Diet Vinaigrette** (page 50).

Snack 2

1 orange, 1 mini cheese (page 35), 1 high-fiber cracker (page 27)

Dinner

Eggplant "Meatballs" with Pasta (page 183). For dessert, have ½ cup **Slow-Cooker Fruit Compote** (page 262) topped with 1 tablespoon fat-free vanilla yogurt.

Menu 1

Breakfast

Homemade Breakfast Sausage (page 75) and 1 egg scrambled in 1 teaspoon olive oil. Have with 1 cup calcium-enhanced mixed vegetable juice.

Snack 1

1 tablespoon almond butter and 1 bell pepper (any color)

Lunch

Fade Away Shake (page 69) made with unflavored soy protein powder instead of powdered milk and soy yogurt instead of regular yogurt

Snack 2

2 tablespoons chopped tomatoes mixed with 2 tablespoons hummus, spread on 2 high-fiber crackers (page 27). Serve with ½ cup unflavored almond milk.

Dinner

Baked Pistachio-Lime Chicken Pockets (page 126) and 2 cups steamed greens (spinach, collard greens, or turnip greens). Have a 4-ounce glass of red wine with dinner or a handful of red grapes for dessert.

Menu 2

Breakfast

Fade Away Shake (page 69) made with unflavored soy protein powder instead of powdered milk and soy yogurt instead of regular yogurt

Snack 1

2 cups cooked broccoli and ½ cup tomato salsa for dipping

Lunch

Sardine Salad: 1 can (3.75 ounces) water-packed sardines (drained and flaked), 1 tablespoon light mayonnaise, 1 teaspoon grated lemon zest (optional), 2 teaspoons lemon juice, 1 celery stalk (diced), ¼ cup chopped grape tomatoes, 1 tablespoon toasted slivered almonds, and black pepper to taste. If you're making the salad to take to work, pack inside a hollowed-out large red bell pepper (and then eat the pepper with the salad). If you're having the salad at home, just cut the bell pepper into wedges and top with the salad.

Snack 2

2 teaspoons almond butter spread on 1 high-fiber cracker (page 27). Have with ½ cup unflavored soy milk (with added calcium).

Dinner

Grill or broil boneless loin pork chops (4 ounces each) and serve with **Roasted Winter Vegetable Salad** (page 201) and 1 cup field greens tossed with 1½ teaspoons **Digest Diet Vinaigrette** (page 50). Have a 4-ounce glass of red wine with dinner or a handful of red grapes for dessert.

Menu 1

Breakfast

Bean & Egg Roll-Up: Whisk together 1 egg, 2 egg whites, 1 tablespoon water, and a pinch each of salt, black pepper, and chili powder. Coat a medium nonstick skillet with cooking spray and cook the egg mixture, without stirring, over medium heat until set around the edges but a little wet in the center (1 to 2 minutes). Cover and cook until the top is set, about 1 minute. In a small bowl, mash together 3 tablespoons canned no-salt-added white beans with a pinch of salt, a generous pinch of smoked paprika, 1 teaspoon cider vinegar, and ½ teaspoon honey. Spread the mixture over a high-fiber wrap, top with the omelet, and roll up. Have with ½ cup unflavored almond milk.

Snack 1

½ cup calcium-fortified orange juice, 10 raw almonds

Lunch

Make the whole recipe of **Bulgur Salad with Tomatoes & Olives** (page 215). Have 1 serving for lunch and save the rest for lunches for the rest of the week.

Snack 2

1 cup calcium-enhanced mixed vegetable juice, 1 high-fiber cracker (page 27), 1 ounce soy Cheddar

Dinner

Dilled Salmon Cakes: Make 4 patties with a mixture of canned salmon (14.75 ounces), ¾ cup fresh whole-grain bread crumbs (from 1½ slices bread), ¼ cup each minced dill and scallions, 2 egg whites, and a generous pinch of black pepper. Cook in a nonstick skillet in 4 teaspoons olive oil. Serve 1 patty per person with 2 cups steamed broccoli and 1 cup coleslaw mix tossed with 1½ teaspoons **Digest Diet Vinaigrette** (page 50) and 2 teaspoons toasted slivered almonds. Have a 4-ounce glass of red wine with dinner or a handful of red grapes for dessert.

Menu 2

Breakfast

One slice **Butternut Breakfast Bread** (page 81) spread with
2 tablespoons soy cream cheese. Have with 1 cup calcium-
fortified orange juice.

Snack 1

½ cup coconut milk yogurt, 1 kiwifruit

Lunch

Two-cup serving of **Creamy Double-Mushroom Barley Soup**
(page 109) and 2 high-fiber crackers (page 27) topped with 1 plum
tomato (sliced and sprinkled with a Fat Releaser Seasoning,
page 31, if desired)

Snack 2

White Bean–Spinach Spread: This makes enough for 2 snacks
(½ cup each). Save half for the next day. Cook 1 clove garlic
(grated) in 1 teaspoon olive oil until fragrant. Add 1 cup canned
no-salt-added white beans and ⅓ cup calcium-enhanced mixed
vegetable juice. Stir in 1 cup chopped baby spinach, cover, and
cook to wilt the spinach. Mash with 1 teaspoon grated lemon
zest (optional) and ⅛ teaspoon salt. Serve warm or chilled, with
½ bell pepper (any color).

Dinner

Grill or broil a ¾-pound flank steak (3 ounces per serving) and
serve with steamed green beans (2 cups per person) and **Lemony
Quinoa & Butternut Pilaf** (page 239). Have **Chocolate-Coconut
Pudding** (page 274) for dessert.

Menu 1

Breakfast

Spicy Tomato Omelet: Whisk together 1 egg, 2 egg whites, 1 tablespoon fat-free milk, 1 large pinch oregano, and a pinch each of salt and cayenne pepper. Coat a medium nonstick skillet with cooking spray and cook the egg mixture, without stirring, over medium heat until set around the edges but a little wet in the center (1 to 2 minutes). Top the finished omelet with 2 tablespoons diced grape or cherry tomatoes. Fold the omelet in half to serve. Serve with 2 slices turkey bacon cooked in 1 teaspoon olive oil in a nonstick skillet. Have with ½ cup fat-free milk.

Snack 1

10 baby carrots, 1 mini cheese (page 35), 1 high-fiber cracker (page 27)

Lunch

Fade Away Shake (page 69)

Snack 2

½ bell pepper (any color) spread with 3 tablespoons hummus. Serve with ½ cup fat-free milk.

Dinner

Herb-Crusted Salmon (page 127; follow the directions for Cooking for One), 2 cups steamed green beans or asparagus, and 1 tomato (sliced) drizzled with 1 teaspoon balsamic vinegar. Have a 4-ounce glass of red wine with dinner or a handful of red grapes for dessert.

Menu 2

Breakfast

Fade Away Shake (page 69)

Snack 1

½ cup chopped grape tomatoes, ¼ teaspoon dried oregano, and a pinch of black pepper stirred into ½ cup nonfat yogurt. Serve with 2 high-fiber crackers (page 27).

Lunch

Smoked Ham Roll-Ups: Top 2 large romaine lettuce leaves with 2 ounces each reduced-sodium deli-sliced smoked ham. Spread each with 1 tablespoon hummus. Top each with 1 slice (¾ ounce) reduced-fat Swiss cheese, 1 teaspoon minced pickled jalapeño or hamburger relish, and very thinly sliced sweet onion (optional) and then roll it up.

Snack 2

10 pistachios, 1 mini cheese (page 35), 1 cup high-fiber mixed vegetable juice

Dinner

Parmesan-Pecan Pork (page 117); follow the directions for Cooking for One), 2 cups steamed cauliflower florets, 2 cups field greens tossed with 1 tablespoon **Digest Diet Vinaigrette** (page 50). Have a 4-ounce glass of red wine with dinner or a handful of red grapes for dessert.

Menu 1

Breakfast

California Breakfast Wrap (page 85) and 1 cup fat-free milk

Snack 1

1 orange, 10 raw almonds

Lunch

Turkey & Carrot Couscous: Cook ¼ cup whole-wheat couscous in a small saucepan according to package directions. Fluff with a fork and let cool slightly, then stir in 1 small grated carrot (about ¾ cup), 2 ounces slivered deli-sliced reduced-sodium smoked turkey, 1 tablespoon Parmesan, 2 teaspoons chopped nuts (pecans, if you have them), and 2 teaspoons **Digest Diet Vinaigrette** (page 50).

Snack 2

1 sliced pear, 1 mini cheese (page 35)

Dinner

Grill or pan-grill a small (4-ounce) sirloin steak and serve with **Honey-Mustard Cabbage Slaw** (page 216) and 5 boiled small red potatoes (3 ounces total). Have a 4-ounce glass of red wine with dinner or a handful of red grapes for dessert.

Menu 2

Breakfast

Homemade Instant Oatmeal (page 79) with ½ cup blueberries. Have with ½ cup fat-free milk.

Snack 1

2 teaspoons sunflower seeds and 2 dates (chopped) stirred into ½ cup nonfat yogurt

Lunch

One-cup serving of soup that comes close to 150 calories, such as **Hearty Minestrone with Quinoa** (page 95) or **Spicy Garlic-Tomato Soup with Chicken** (page 90). (You'll have enough soup for leftovers for several days.) Serve with **PB & K Roll-Ups:** Spread 1 high-fiber wrap with 1 tablespoon natural peanut butter. Peel 1 kiwifruit and coarsely chop. Sprinkle over the peanut butter and roll up. Serve with ½ cup fat-free milk.

Snack 2

10 baby carrots, 1 mini cheese (page 35), 1 high-fiber cracker (page 27)

Dinner

One **Chicken Burger** (page 143; without the bun), slabs of grilled zucchini (1 large) with a squeeze of lemon, 2 cups field greens tossed with 1 tablespoon **Digest Diet Vinaigrette** (page 50). Have a **Flourless Chocolate–Peanut Butter Cakelet** (page 270) for dessert.

Menu 1

Breakfast

Cheese Omelet: Whisk together 1 egg, 2 egg whites, 1 tablespoon fat-free milk or water, and a pinch each of salt and black pepper. Coat a medium nonstick skillet with cooking spray and cook the egg mixture, without stirring, over medium heat until set around the edges but a little wet in the center (1 to 2 minutes). Top with 2 tablespoons shredded reduced-fat cheese (whatever you have on hand). Fold the omelet in half to serve. Serve with 1 cup fat-free milk and 2 high-fiber crackers (page 27) spread with 2 tablespoons hummus.

Snack 1

1 mini cheese (page 35), 1 cup high-fiber mixed vegetable juice

Lunch

Fade Away Shake (page 69)

Snack 2

½ ounce dry-roasted, unsalted nuts (10 almonds, 13 peanuts, or 25 pistachios), ½ bell pepper (any color), ½ cup fat-free milk

Dinner

Mexican Slow-Cooked Turkey Breast (page 138; save leftovers for lunches), 1 cup steamed broccolini or broccoli florets, and **Tomato-Scallion Salad** (2 diced plum tomatoes tossed with 2 sliced scallions, 1 teaspoon balsamic vinegar, black pepper to taste, and a pinch of Fat Releaser Seasoning, page 31, if you'd like). Have a 4-ounce glass of red wine with dinner or a handful of red grapes for dessert.

Menu 2

Breakfast
Fade Away Shake (page 69)

Snack 1
1 cup grape tomatoes, 1 mini cheese (page 35), 1 high-fiber cracker (page 27)

Lunch
Mini Chef's Salad: 2 cups chopped lettuce (iceberg or romaine), 1 cup (about 3.5 ounces) shredded cooked turkey (left over from previous night's dinner), 1 ounce reduced-fat cheese (shredded or slivered deli-sliced), ½ cup chopped tomatoes (whatever type you have available), 1 tablespoon chopped nuts (your favorite). Toss everything with 2 tablespoons **Digest Diet Vinaigrette** (page 50). Serve with 2 high-fiber crackers (page 27).

Snack 2
½ ounce dry-roasted, unsalted nuts (10 almonds, 13 peanuts, or 25 pistachios), 10 baby carrots, ½ cup fat-free milk

Dinner
Confetti Meatloaf (page 123; save leftovers for lunches) and 2 cups coleslaw mix tossed with 1 tablespoon **Digest Diet Vinaigrette** (page 50). Have a 4-ounce glass of red wine with dinner or a handful of red grapes for dessert.

Menu 1

Breakfast

Breakfast Egg Salad (page 70; make the full amount and save half for the next day) and 1 multigrain sandwich thin, split and toasted. Enjoy with 1 cup fat-free milk.

Snack 1

1 small apple (diced), 1 teaspoon honey, and a pinch of cinnamon mixed with ¼ cup nonfat yogurt

Lunch

Sub-Style Roll-Up: Make a dressing with 1 tablespoon light mayonnaise, ½ teaspoon balsamic vinegar, and a generous pinch each of dried oregano and ground black pepper. Spread the dressing over a high-fiber wrap. Layer the bread generously with lettuce leaves (or whatever greens you have on hand), 4 ounces reduced-sodium deli-sliced meat (your favorite), very thinly sliced red onion, and/or 2 teaspoons chopped dill pickle. Have with ½ cup fat-free milk.

Snack 2

2 clementines, ½ ounce dry-roasted, unsalted nuts (10 almonds, 13 peanuts, or 25 pistachios)

Dinner

Eggplant "Meatballs" with Pasta (page 183). Have a 4-ounce glass of red wine with dinner or a handful of red grapes for dessert.

Menu 2

Breakfast

Homemade Instant Oatmeal (page 79) with 2 tablespoons raisins and 1 tablespoon chopped nuts (your favorite) stirred in

Snack 1

½ cup grapes, ½ cup nonfat yogurt with 1 teaspoon honey stirred in

Lunch

A serving of soup that comes close to 250 calories, such as 1 cup **Turkey, Black Bean & Winter Squash Soup** (page 96) or 2 cups **Russian Cabbage & Beef Soup** (page 102). (You'll have enough soup for leftovers for several days.) Serve with 1 light multigrain English muffin, toasted and spread with 2 wedges Laughing Cow Light (any flavor).

Snack 2

2 teaspoons natural peanut butter, 1 high-fiber cracker (page 27), ½ cup fat-free milk

Dinner

Southwestern Turkey Tacos (page 179). For dessert, enjoy 2 **Chocolate Chocolate-Chip Cookies** (page 269).

Recipe Index

⏱=Quick-Fix   🌱=Vegetarian   🚫=Dairy-Free   🍽①=Cooking for One $=On a Budget

Jamaican Grilled Tuna with Avocado-Mango Relish, 147 ⏱⊘‖①‖

Pan-Fried Scallops with Citrus Dressing, 148 ⏱⊘

Breaded Tofu Steaks, 149 ⊛⊘⑤

ONE-DISH MAINS

Beef & Portobello Saute, 169 ⏱⊘

Beef & Tomatillo Chili, 170 ⊘

Chipotle Pork Stew, 171 ⏱⊘‖①‖⑤

Pasta with Pork & Caramelized Onions, 172 ⑤

Garlicky Chicken Stew with Artichokes, 173 ⊘‖①‖

Pasta with Chicken, Broccoli Rabe & Sun-Dried Tomatoes, 175 ⊘

Country Captain, 176-177 ⊘⑤

Penne & Turkey with Creamy Broccoli Pesto, 178 ⑤

Southwestern Turkey Tacos, 179 ⏱⑤

Tangy Shrimp and Vegetables with Linguine, 180 ⊘

Asparagus & Tuna Bake, 181 ⑤

Eggplant "Meatballs" with Pasta, 183 ⊛⑤

Vegetarian Posole, 184 ⊛

Orzo Primavera, 185 ⊛

Chickpea & Arugula Pizza, 187 ⏱⊛

SALADS AND SALAD DRESSINGS

Grilled Pork & Pear Salad with Walnuts, 205 ⏱⊘‖①‖

Grilled Lamb & Asparagus Salad, 207-208 ⊘‖①‖

Marinated Grilled Chicken Salad, 209 ⊘⑤

Turkey Milanese, 211 ⏱

Salmon Nicoise, 213 ⏱⊘

Italian Tuna & Fennel Salad, 214 ⏱⊘

Bulgur Salad with Tomatoes & Olives, 215 ⊛⊘‖①‖

Honey-Mustard Cabbage Slaw, 216 ⊛‖①‖⑤

Lentil Salad with Feta, 217 ⊛‖①‖⑤

Creamy Potato Salad, 218 ‖①‖⑤

Caesar Salad with Roasted Cauliflower & Pasta, 219 ⑤

Chickpea Salad with Carrot Dressing, 220 ⊛‖①‖⑤

Belgian Endive & Grapes, 221 ⏱⊘

SIDE DISHES

Sweet & Sour Greens with Bacon, 237 ⊘⑤

Lemony Quinoa & Butternut Pilaf, 239 ⊛⊘

Hoppin' John, 240 ⊘‖①‖

Barley Risotto with Collards, 241 ⊛

Honey-Roasted Acorn Squash, 243 ⊘‖①‖

Brown Basmati Risi e Bisi, 244 ⑤

Kasha & Orange Pilaf with Pecans, 245 ⊛⊘‖①‖

Cajun Sweet Potato Fries, 247 ⊛⊘⑤

Parmesan-Crumbed Roasted Root Vegetables, 248 ‖①‖⑤

Baked Stuffed Summer Squash, 249 ‖①‖

Curried Lentils and Greens, 250 ‖①‖⑤

Crispy Balsamic Potatoes, 251 ⊛⊘‖①‖⑤

DESSERTS

Pomegranate-Poached Pears, 254 ⊘

Warm Three Berry Cream, 255 ⊛

Papaya "Tarts", 257

Spicy Grilled Pineapple, 258 ⏱⊘‖①‖

Double Grape Gelatin, 259 ⊘‖①‖

Strawberry Cheesecake Mousse, 261 ‖①‖

Slow-Cooker Fruit Compote, 262 ⊘⑤

Individual Blueberry-Apple Crisps, 263 ⊘

Frozen Berry Terrine, 265

Mango Melba, 266 ⏱

Honey-Walnut Fudge Bites, 267 ⊘‖①‖

Chocolate Chocolate Chip Cookies, 269 ⊘‖①‖

Flourless Chocolate-Peanut Butter Cakelets, 270 ⊘‖①‖⑤

Chocolate Zucchini Squares, 271 ⊘‖①‖

Chocolate-Glazed Espresso Nut Torte, 273 ⊘

Chocolate-Coconut Pudding, 274 ⊘⑤

Spiced Carrot-Almond Cake, 275 ‖①‖⑤

Spice Cupcakes with Honey-Cream Frosting, 277 ‖①‖⑤

Index

swaps (substitutions), 52
sweeteners, 32, 42, 54, 61
sweet potatoes
    in recipes, 108, 247, 248, 277
    as vitamin C source, 12
Sweet & Sour Greens with Bacon, 237
Swiss cheese
    buying and storing, 34
    as calcium source, 13
    in recipe, 86

T

tacos, 179
Tangy Shrimp and Vegetables with Linguine, 180
Thai Beef Salad, 190
tofu, in recipes, 93, 109, 130, 149, 167, 215
tomatillos, 170
tomatoes and tomato products
    in breakfast recipes, 70, 74, 85
    canned, 27
    as fiber source, 16
    in main dish recipes, 135–136
    in one-dish main recipes, 165, 166, 175
    in salad recipes, 193, 211, 213, 215
    in side dish recipes, 227, 236
    in soup recipes, 90, 92, 97, 99, 108
    as vitamin C source, 12
tortillas, 14, 101
toxins, 5
trans fats, 15, 42
Tropical Fruit & Berry Salad with Yogurt Dressing, 87
tuna
    buying and storing, 27
    as protein source, 14
    in recipes, 147, 181, 214
turbinado sugar, 32
turkey
    in breakfast recipe, 86
    in main dish recipes, 120, 123, 138
    in one-dish main recipes, 162, 178, 179
    as protein source, 14
    in salad recipe, 211
    in soup recipes, 91, 92, 96
turkey bacon, in recipes, 193, 197, 237

turnip greens
    as calcium source, 13
    as fiber source, 16
    in recipe, 237
    as vitamin C source, 12
turnips, in recipes, 103, 201, 248
21-day plan. *See also specific phases*
    food choices in, 11–12, 42–43
    individualizing, 53–58
    phases in, 46–53, 56–57
    problems following, 61
    rules and guidelines, 41–42

U

"use by" dates, 33, 34

V

veal, 14
vegetable peelers, 24
vegetables. *See also specific types*
    buying and storing, 34
    as calcium source, 13
    cooking methods for, 36
    as fiber source, 16
    frozen, 27, 281
    leftover, 235
    in one-dish main recipes, 153, 161, 180
    in salad recipe, 201
    in side dish recipe, 234–235, 248
    in soup recipes, 103
    as vitamin C source, 12
Vegetarian Double-Pea Soup, 100
vegetarians
    diet suitability for, 62
    menus for, 286–289
    protein sources for, 14, 279
    Vegetarian Posole, 184
Vietnamese Pho with Chicken & Spaghetti Squash, 158
vinegar
    buying and storing, 30
    as fat releaser, 16–17
    in recipes, 50, 70, 202, 251
    types of, 17
vitamin C
    deficiencies in, 4
    as fat releaser, 12
    food sources, 12, 45
    intake guidelines, 46
vitamin E, 4
vitamin supplements, 63

W

walnuts, in recipes, 82, 130, 205, 231, 267, 273
Warm Broccolini Salad with Cashew Pesto, 203
Warm Goat Cheese on a Bed of Greens, 198
Warm Three-Berry Cream, 255
water, drinking. *See* hydration
watercress, 13, 198
watermelon, 63
watermelon seeds, 14
weight loss, 60, 61
wheat berries, 29
white beans
    as protein source, 14
    in recipe, 95
    substitutions for, 52
whole foods, 3, 41
wine
    buying and storing, 30
    fade away phase, 49–50, 51
    finish strong phase, 51
    in recipes, 116, 159, 259
    as resveratrol source, 15–16
Wine-Braised Chicken & Leeks, 159
Winter Vegetable Soup with Smoked Pork, 103
wraps, 28, 85

Y

yellow squash, in recipes, 95, 99, 157, 185, 249
yogurt. *See also* dairy products
    in breakfast recipes, 67, 69, 70, 77, 87
    buying and storing, 33, 34
    as calcium source, 13
    Greek vs. regular, 62
    in main dish recipes, 121
    in salad recipe, 193
    substitutes for, 52

Z

zinc, 4
zucchini
    in dessert recipe, 271
    in one-dish main recipes, 161, 163, 165, 185
    in salad recipe, 190
    in side dish recipe, 236
    substitutes for, 52

Conversion Charts

ABBREVIATIONS

C	Celsius
cm	centimeter
F	Fahrenheit
fl oz	fluid ounce
ft	foot
g	gram
gal	gallon
in.	inch
kg	kilogram
L	liter
lb	pound
m	meter
mL	milliliter
mm	millimeter
oz	ounce
qt	quart
tbsp	tablespoon
tsp	teaspoon

TEASPOONS

⅛ tsp	0.5 mL
¼ tsp	1 mL
½ tsp	2 mL
¾ tsp	4 mL
1 tsp	5 mL
1½ tsp	7 mL
2 tsp	10 mL

TABLESPOONS

1 tbsp	15 mL
1½ tbsp	20 mL
2 tbsp	30 mL
3 tbsp	45 mL
4 tbsp	60 mL
5 tbsp	75 mL
6 tbsp	90 mL
8 tbsp	125 mL

WEIGHTS

1 oz	30 g
2 oz	60 g
3 oz	90 g
4 oz	125 g
5 oz	150 g
6 oz	175 g
8 oz	250 g
10 oz	300 g
12 oz	375 g
16 oz	500 g
32 oz	1 kg
¼ lb	125 g
½ lb	250 g
⅔ lb	300 g
¾ lb	375 g
1 lb	500 g
2 lb	1 kg
3 lb	1.5 kg

LENGTHS

¼ in.	5 mm
½ in.	1 cm
1 in.	2.5 cm
2 in.	5 cm
6 in.	15 cm
1 ft	30 cm

VOLUME

1 fl oz	30 mL
2 fl oz	50 mL
5 fl oz	150 mL
10 fl oz	300 mL
1 pint	500 mL
1 qt	1 L
1 gal	4 L
¼ cup	60 mL
⅓ cup	75 mL
½ cup	125 mL
⅔ cup	150 mL
¾ cup	175 mL
1 cup	250 mL
1¼ cups	300 mL
1½ cups	375 mL
2 cups	500 mL
4 cups	1 L
6 cups	1.5 L

OVEN TEMPERATURES

°F	°C
175°F	80°C
200°F	95°C
225°F	110°C
250°F	120°C
275°F	140°C
300°F	150°C
325°F	160°C
350°F	180°C
375°F	190°C
400°F	200°C
425°F	220°C
450°F	230°C
475°F	240°C
500°F	260°C

BAKING PANS

8 x 8 in.	20 x 20 cm
9 x 9 in.	22 x 22 cm
9 x 13 in.	22 x 33 cm
10 x 15 in.	25 x 38 cm
11 x 17 in.	28 x 43 cm
8 x 2 in. (round)	20 x 5 cm
9 x 2 in. (round)	22 x 5 cm
10 x 4½ in. (tube)	25 x 11 cm
8 x 4 x 3 in. (loaf)	20 x 10 x 7.5 cm
9 x 5 x 3 in. (loaf)	22 x 12.5 x 7.5 cm

CASSEROLE DISHES

Recipe calls for	Substitute
1 qt (4 cups)	900 mL
1½ qt (6 cups)	1.35 L
2–2½ qt (8–10 cups)	2.25 L
3 qt (12 cups)	2.7 L
4–5 qt (16–20 cups)	4.5 L

The Digest Diet.

Get everything you need to stay
slim for life!

Visit our online store and find unique ingredients, the best kitchen accessories, every book in the Digest Diet series, and so much more!

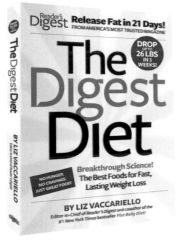

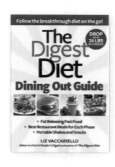

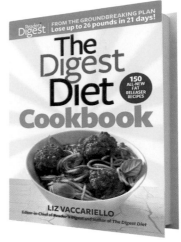

The Digest Diet
Jump-start weight loss and get your body into "fat release" mode.

The Digest Diet Dining Out Guide
Eat well anytime, anywhere with this handy pocket guide.

The Digest Diet Cookbook
Enjoy 150 NEW recipes to maintain weight loss and still enjoy every bite.

One-Click Shopping
All the essentials, shipped right to you! Shop for ingredients by each phase of the diet, plus handy travel containers, kitchen tools, accessories, and more.

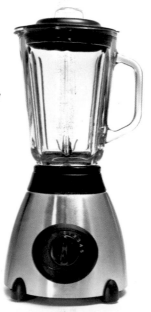

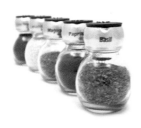

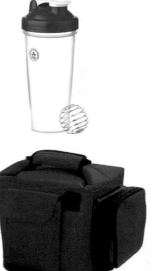

Get it all at **DigestDietShop.com**
Books can be purchased through retail and online bookstores